Dr. Newbold's
NUTRITION FOR
YOUR NERVES

Dr. Newbold's
NUTRITION FOR
YOUR NERVES

H. L. Newbold, M.D.

KEATS PUBLISHING, INC. New Canaan, Connecticut

Dr. Newbold's Nutrition for Your Nerves is not intended as medical advice. Its intent is solely informational and educational. Please consult a health professional should the need for one be indicated.

DR. NEWBOLD'S NUTRITION FOR YOUR NERVES

Library of Congress Cataloging-in-Publication Data

Newbold, H. L. (Herbert Leon)
   (Nutrition for your nerves)
   Dr. Newbold's nutrition for your nerves / H.L. Newbold.
     p.   cm.
   Includes bibliographical references and index.
   ISBN 0-87983-606-7 : $14.95
   1. Mental illness—Nutritional aspects 2. Food allergy—
Psychological aspects. 3. Mental illness—Diet therapy.
I. Title. II. Title: Doctor Newbold's nutrition for your nerves.
III. Title: Nutrition for your nerves.
RC455.4.N8N48   1993
616.89'071—dc20   93-3318
                                                              CIP

Printed in the United States of America

Published by Keats Publishing, Inc.
27 Pine Street (Box 876)
New Canaan, Connecticut 06840-0876

Dedicated to
Susan Deena Hecht Newbold

"All our provisional ideas in psychology will someday be based on organic structure. This makes it probable that special substances and special chemicals control the operation."
—SIGMUND FREUD

"Each patient carries his own doctor inside him. We are at our best when we give the doctor who resides within a chance to work."
—ALBERT SCHWEITZER
Nobel Prize, medicine

"The laws of Nature are so simple, we have to rise above the complexity of scientific thought to see them."
—RICHARD FEYNMAN
Nobel Prize, physics

CONTENTS

AUTHOR'S NOTE

When writing a book on a medical subject, I must give advice that applies generally. I cannot directly give any one person medical advice without first taking a medical history, doing a physical examination, and ordering laboratory tests.

Since it is not possible for me to carry out those procedures before allowing you to read this book, you must check with your physician before taking any of the advice given in this or in any other book.

Your physician, the doctor who examines you, must take the responsibility for your health and anything that you do to improve it.

To preserve their privacy, except where stated, the names and identifying facts about patients mentioned in this book have been changed.

Those of you who read the complete book—and I hope all of you will—might notice that a few points are repeated several times. I have purposely made the repetitions because they deal with crucial points that a pick-and-chose reader might miss.

H. L. NEWBOLD, M.D.
New York, New York

Dr. Newbold's
NUTRITION FOR
YOUR NERVES

CHAPTER ONE

WHAT CAUSES EMOTIONAL PAIN?

In every age there are certain articles of faith which society accepts unquestioningly, with or without evidence; often, indeed, in the face of inconvenient facts.

WILLIAM MANCHESTER

Mrs. Keenan recently brought her son James to my office for a consultation. James, age 27, was from Connecticut but had been working for an architectural firm in Dallas for three years. Six weeks earlier he had broken with his girl friend and moved out of the apartment they shared. He became increasingly tense, depressed, and unable to focus on his work. His supervisor asked him to take a leave of absence.

When I spoke with James alone, he wept as he told me how deeply he loved his girl friend. Life had lost all meaning. He could think of nothing except Pauline. He had no appetite and could eat only "light foods" such as ice cream and cookies. He drank a pint of bourbon to fall asleep. Even then, he slept for only a few restless hours.

At this point I knew what caused his distress. I knew how to cure him.

Causes

The human mind has a need to explain what happens: why the sun rises, why people fall sick, why people develop emotional pain. To satisfy, the explanation need not be true so long as it is accepted as true. For example, a primitive tribe might say the sun rises in the morning because the Sun God has finished sleeping. The explanation satisfies them.

A Pygmy in the Ituri Forest might say that James Keenan had displeased the forest gods. As a result, the forest gods gave him emotional pain.

People in the Western world are taught that poor social relationships bring on emotional pain. Our conventional wisdom says that James Keenan felt troubled because he broke with his true love.

CONVENTIONAL PSYCHIATRISTS

The conventional psychiatrist in the western world accepts the conventional explanations of his world. Like the Pygmy, he has been taught explanations. Like the Pygmy, he believes them. James Keenan was depressed because of loss of love. It makes no difference whether the psychiatrist's explanations are true so long as they are accepted.

A conventional psychiatrist would give the patient a tranquilizer, an antidepressant, or both. He would then listen week after week as James Keenan told about the sadness that had dominated his life since losing his true love.

Then the psychiatrist would ask James about his childhood. They could have conversations about that sad subject until both the psychiatrist and the patient died of old age.

When the patient wept and talked about how sad breaking up with his girlfriend made him feel, he thought he was telling me about the cause of his unhappiness. He was not. He was reciting his symptoms.

SOCIAL PROBLEM OR BIOCHEMICAL PROBLEM?

True, the patient had a social problem, but it was a common social problem that many people face without becoming incapacitated. James had the pain of everyday life, which none of us can escape.

His social problem (breaking up with his girl friend) did not cause his incapacity. He had biochemical problems that resulted in an emotional breakdown. What biochemical problems?

James Went from This:

1. While living with his girlfriend James ate her solid, old-fashioned cooking.

2. His girlfriend kept several bottles of vitamins on the table and saw that he took them every day.

3. While living with his girlfriend, small amounts of wine had been his only alcoholic beverage.

To This:

1. James stopped taking vitamins.

2. After leaving his girlfriend, to avoid loneliness, James began hanging out in bars and drinking bourbon.

3. He sometimes ate a TV dinner, but most of the time he had a hot dog and ice cream. Gradually, he had fewer hot dogs and more ice cream and added cookies.

JAMES'S TWO BIOCHEMICAL PROBLEMS

1. He became vitamin deficient from living off of junk food and not taking his usual vitamins. (Laboratory tests proved me correct. He was deficient in three vitamins.)

2. He had overloaded his biochemistry with "new foods" to which he was allergic. My tests showed he was allergic to grains (as in the bourbon) to milk and sugar (as in ice cream.) The allergic reactions struck his brain, i.e., resulted in cerebral allergies. The allergic reaction disrupted the chemistry of his brain, made him depressed and unable to focus his mind.

His vitamin deficiencies intensified the reaction.

Once I removed the offending foods from his diet and got him on a proper vitamin-mineral program, he recovered.

As further indication that my diagnosis and suspicions were correct, I could produce tension, depression and disorganization by feeding the offending foods one by one.

Later we learned that his biochemistry could handle small amounts of grains, milk products, and sugar, but not the large amounts he began eating after separating from his girlfriend.

Proof

Psychiatrists will attempt to defend their turf by saying that I am only appealing to the patient's imagination, that I'm using the power of suggestion to heal the patient.

I once answered such criticism by saying that for one week I treated patients by allowing them to touch the hem of my garment and that no one improved!

Returning to the land of seriousness, I say to my critics: test and learn whether what I say is true. Isn't testing the scientific way to arrive at conclusions?

The method described below is not how I test.

If they want to be super scientific, however, here's how they can test their patients. Have them stop eating several highly allergenic foods (such as grains, milk and milk products, and table sugar) for five days. Then introduce a tube into the patient's stomach. Stand behind the patient and squirt a generous amount of the liquefied food into the patient's stomach and observe how the patient feels and acts.

If the psychiatrists want to be super-scientific, they should first perform objective psychological observations and tests on the patient and record baseline brain waves (EEG).

Do a placebo run with the stomach tube using water that has been boiled for ten minutes, then distilled under your supervision in a glass distiller and stored in a well-rinsed (with distilled water) glass container.

(It is possible that the patient will be allergic to the stomach tube and/or the carefully distilled water.)

After the placebo run, repeat observations, objective psychological tests and EEG.

Then administer the test food while standing behind the patient.

After 30 minutes, repeat observations about the patient, psychological tests, and EEG.

Repeat the tests each day for 2 more days. (Do not allow any of the test foods to be eaten during that time.)

The method described above is not how I test.

Further Proof

I'm allergic to many foods. If I eat certain cheeses, I will become depressed. If I eat a wheat product for dinner, the next day I find concentration difficult. It's impossible for me to properly integrate my thoughts. When I start to write, some of my thoughts are here and some over there. I cannot herd them all together to form a conception.

Having had a formal 900-hour Freudian psychoanalysis by a graduate of the Chicago Psychoanalytical Institute and a three-year residency in psychiatry, and having practiced psychiatry for many years, and being an old man given to thinking about what he reads and observes, you can hardly call me naive about matters regarding psychopathology, treatment, and suggestibility.

What Is an Allergy?

To me (but not to all allergists) allergy, untoward reaction, hypersensitivity, and incompatibility are all the same thing. I like the following definition of allergy:

Hypersensitive or pathological reaction to environmental factors or substances such as pollens, foods, dust, or microorganisms, in amounts that do not affect most people.
—*The American Heritage Dictionary of the English Language* (1981)

ALLERGISTS

Now and then I have a telephone call from Seattle or Tunisia. A patient will tell me about his mysterious illness that no one has been able to cure and ask whether I can help. Often I'll say yes, and add that it sounds like an allergy.

The patient doesn't call back for an appointment.

A year or two later the patient will show up in my office. "You said my trouble sounded like an allergy, but you must be wrong. I've been worked up by two allergists and both of them told me I'm not allergic."

The patients consulted allergists. I'm sorry to say this, but allergists don't understand allergies any better than psychiatrists understand emotional illnesses.

They don't understand how to diagnose allergies. They don't understand how to treat allergies. Especially do they not know how to diagnose food and environmental allergies.

I had my first allergy tests and "desensitization" in 1927. Since then I've taken and given thousands of tests and desensitization injections.

I wish I had the space to explore this subject in depth. For now you will have to take my word for it. Skin tests and blood tests for food and environmental allergies are of no value. They are of little value for other types of allergies. Challenge testing is the only valid test. Desensitization is rent-paying nonsense.

If desensitization were of value, I would desensitize myself to butter pecan ice cream and live off of it for the rest of my life.

OF ALLERGISTS, PSYCHIATRISTS, POPES, AND PETER PAN

Psychiatrists and allergists see me as a threat and call me all sorts of names. They mumble that my methods haven't been proven. They won't test their patients as I've outlined. They don't want to rock their boats. They just want to get through their days and stay out of the poorhouse, the crazy house, and the jailhouse.

What would happen if I gave the Pope absolute proof that Mohammed was a holier man than Jesus?

Do you think the Pope would change religions? Do you think he would surrender his entourage, his palace, his power and embrace the Muslim religion and start all over as low man on the totem pole?

You can bet your best blue bonnet he wouldn't. He wouldn't even listen to my arguments.

And that's why psychiatrists and allergists will not embrace what I know to be true.

They believe what they want to believe.

When I watch Mary Martin play Peter Pan, I want to believe that Peter Pan can fly. I could do a scientific experiment to prove that Peter Pan cannot fly. I won't do such an experiment because it would interfere with what I want to believe. It's fun for me to believe that Peter Pan can fly.

Self-styled psychotherapists, marriage counselors, psychiatric social workers, psychologists, psychiatrists and allergists want to believe what they believe. Their beliefs give them ego trips and put money in their pockets.

But, buddy—and sister—if you are having emotional troubles, you had better believe what I tell you. Otherwise, your most precious possession will gurgle down the drain and be gone forever.

THE FIVE O'CLOCK WHINES

Every mother knows that at five in the afternoon children become irritable and whiny. Nothing she can say or do pleases them. She can kiss them. She can tell them she loves them. She can make funny faces. She can stand on her head. Absolutely nothing pleases them.

Feed the little dears and right away they are transformed from little devils into little angels.

Why?

Because the children's brain chemistries were upset by hunger, nothing could make the dears happy. They suffered from scrambled brain chemistries. They had a chemical problem, not a social problem.

Those of you who are so great with placebos and the power of suggestion, so great with psychotherapy and tranquilizers and antidepressants, let me see you make Johnnie's five-o'clock whines disappear!

Almost everyone with emotional symptoms—from tension, insomnia, depression to anger—suffers because of a scrambled brain biochemistry, that cauldron of boiling and bubbling chemicals that burn 25% of the body's energy.

WITH THE IRRITABLE FIVE-O'CLOCK CHILDREN

You could have scolded and spanked your irritable five-o'clock children.

It wouldn't have helped.

You could ask them about their complaints and let them talk (whine) about them and call it psychotherapy. It wouldn't have helped.

You could give them a tranquilizer. It would have quieted them. They might change from whining to sitting stupidly in the corner. That would be third class treatment.

Why not correct the cause of their misery? Why not feed them?

WHY, OH WHY, DO PEOPLE ABANDON THEIR COMMON SENSE?

Instead of using their heads, people use what they've been taught and what they want to believe: emotional problems are caused by social problems: pills, love, and understanding cures all!

What nonsense! Try curing Johnnie's five-o'clock whines with pills and love and understanding and see how far you get!

After reading this far, are you now willing to grant that perhaps—just perhaps—I'm right. I should know. As a psychiatrist, I've worked both sides of the street.

I now use the vitamin-allergy approach because it almost always works—and quality of improvement is much better. It's usually quicker and less expensive, though in complicated cases we may need six months to a year.

Different allergens (foods, chemicals) strike different people different places. Which bodily organ a sugar allergy strikes, depends upon the biochemistry the patient inherited. Sugar may strike Jane's skin and give her eczema. It may strike Jill's lungs and give her asthma. Sugar may strike Tom's blood vessels and give him migraine headaches or high blood pressure.

In regard to James Keenan, sugar (along with grains and milk) struck his brain and gave him emotional symptoms.

The only difference between depression and arthritis is where the patient gets struck.

Inherited Factor + Precipitating Factor = Medical or "Psychological" Disorder

The *inherited factor* is a person's individual biochemical machinery. Basically, it's the biochemistry the patient inherited.

The *precipitating factor* (may be called "cofactor" by the profession) is something that reacts unfavorably with a patient's *inherited factor* and makes a person sick.

DIABETES

Let's speak about diabetes (diabetes mellitus, type II, formerly called adult onset diabetes).

Please allow me to repeat the definition of an allergy:

> Hypersensitive or pathological reaction to environmental factors or substances such as pollens, foods, dust, or microorganisms, in amounts that do not affect most people.
> —*The American Heritage Dictionary of the English Language* (1981)

By definition, diabetes can be called an allergy. People with diabetes react to foods (sugar) in amounts that do not affect most people.

Why do I speak of diabetes at this time? Because both you and those in the medical profession know that diabetes "runs in families," that people with diabetes have inherited a faulty biochemistry. (The *inherited factor*.)

And you and the medical profession know that diabetes is influenced by the amount of sugar eaten. (The *precipitating factor*.) If a person has inherited a tendency to diabetes (the *inherited factor*) and eats liberal amounts of sugar (the *precipitating factor*) the disease *diabetes* appears.

If the person reduces or removes the sugar from his diet (the *precipitating factor*), the diabetes lessens or disappears.

It's clear enough:

Inherited Factor + Precipitating Factor = Diabetes

OTHER EXAMPLES

The medical profession recognizes other diseases caused by the clash of an *inherited factor* + a *precipitating factor*.
For example:

Inherited factor + gluten = nontropical sprue

and

Inherited factor + milk = lactose intolerance syndrome

and

inherited factor + histidine = histidinemia, classic type

and

PKU, and others

The same formula (*inherited factor + precipitating factor = disease*) explains many other illnesses—including "emotional" illness—and points the way to curing them.

How do I know? I know the same way I know water runs downhill: I've repeatedly seen diseases brought on in certain people by certain foods or chemicals to which they were exposed.

Here's an example:

Sally Holmes, one of my lupus-recovered patients, promptly developed a 103 degree fever and a recurrence of her illness when she again started smoking cigarettes.

inherited factor + tobacco = lupus

Later we once again saw her lupus set off when she returned to smoking cigarettes.
We also learned that eating wheat would precipitate her lupus.

inherited factor + wheat and/or tobacco = lupus

Because we inherit different biochemistries, we have different *precipitating factor(s)* and suffer from different illnesses.
For example:

inherited (genetic) factor + precipitating factor = lupus

For Mrs. A. the formula may read:

inherited factor + table sugar = lupus

For Mr. B the formula may be:

inherited factor + wheat = lupus

And note this: in people with different inherited biochemistries:

inherited factor + precipitating factor = arthritis

inherited factor + precipitating factor = asthma

inherited factor + precipitating factor = depression

inherited factor + precipitating factor = chronic fatigue

inherited factor + precipitating factor = tension

inherited factor + precipitating factor = schizophrenia

inherited factor + precipitating factor = teenage suicide

et cetera

PRECIPITATING FACTORS

Precipitating factors are foods or chemicals that strike our body's biochemistry and harm it: most commonly what we eat, what we drink, or what we breathe. Here are some examples of precipitating factors and conditions they can cause:

automobile fumes = depression and fatigue

birth control pills = depression

canned tuna fish = hyperactive child syndrome

chlorine (from city water) = arthritis

formaldehyde (from pressed wood) = back pain

ink = depression

wheat = high blood pressure

wheat = paranoid schizophrenia

and on and on. . . .

SEVEN OBSERVATIONS

1. Usually, several insults (precipitating factors) join to bring on an illness.

Recently, I saw Lawrence Tilton, a former patient I had guided out of a depression by helping him find the foods and chemicals in his environment that caused his depression.

Like many people, he increased his intake of sugar, wheat and brandy during the Christmas season. In addition, he had "improved" his home for the holidays by adding new carpeting, which further injured his biochemical machinery with a heavy dose of formaldehyde.

The combination of insults pushed the patient back down into a depression.

inherited factor + sugar, wheat, brandy, and new carpeting = depression

2. Foods are the most common troublemakers (*precipitating factors*). What we eat stays in our bodies for three to five days. If the food cannot be properly used by our particular body chemistry, the food causes trouble for three or four days. If a patient eats the offending food twice a week, the patient is always sick from it.

Few people in the Western world fail to eat bread, pasta or some other wheat-containing food twice a week.

Few physicians in the Western world have ever seen a patient who has gone a week without eating wheat. Therefore, doctors do not know how their patients feel when they are wheat-free. Also, they do not know how patients react to medications when they are wheat-free.

3. Chemicals found where patients work or sleep are the second most important group of trouble makers (*precipitating factors*). Examples: an unventilated laser printer at work; an electric blanket on the bed that gives off chemical fumes when the plastic insulation around the wires becomes warm.

4. Exercise and nutritional supplements modify biochemical machinery and often make us more tolerant of foods and chemicals.

5. What I refer to as an *inherited factor* may not be purely an inherited factor. For example, people who are breast-fed as infants have more resistance to disease. Another example: biochemical machinery may be damaged by exposure to chemicals, lead, X rays, etc.

6. Usually young people, as opposed to older people, have more margin for error in their biochemical machinery.

7. Illness from any cause—flu for example—robs the biochemistry of its efficiency and leaves it less room for error. No matter what the illness, sick people do better if they are cross-matched for the foods that suit them best and are given extra amounts of vitamins, minerals and unsaturated fats.

DAWN

Gradually, it has dawned on me that civilization causes most of our illness. Civilization presents us with most of the *precipitating factors* that make us sick, physically and emotionally. (As far as I'm concerned there's no difference in the two.)

Foods

The foods that have entered our diet in large amounts during the past 5 to 10 thousand years are the biggest troublemakers (*precipitating factors*): grains, milk and milk products, table sugar.

Chemicals

Civilization has also blessed us with the chemicals that cause trouble: hydrocarbons (gas from the kitchen stove, automobile fumes, etc.), formaldehyde (carpet, pressed wood, plywood, etc.), polyesters (in pillows and clothes), et cetera.

CLEARLY. . . .

If *inherited factor* + *precipitating factor* = *disease*, then it would seem that we can cure the diseases mentioned in this book in one of two ways:
1. change the *inherited factor*; or
2. change the *precipitating factor*.

The first course is not practical. Some day we might be able to completely restructure the *hereditary factor*, the genetic factor, hence the biochemistry, but that time is far in the future.

Today, however, we can remove the *precipitating factor* and cure most disorders, including disorders that involve our emotions and our thought processes.

All over the Western world patients are lying on couches or sitting across a desk from social workers or psychologists or psychiatrists talking about their problems and often taking zombie pills.

What a waste!—a waste of money, a waste of time, a waste of lives.

> The mass distrusts controversy. Reluctant to reconsider its convictions, superstitions, and prejudices, it rarely withdraws support for those who are guiding its destinies, Thus inertia becomes an incumbent's accomplice. So does human reluctance to admit error. Those who backed the top man insist, against all evidence, that they made the right choice.
>
> —WILLIAM MANCHESTER

And Next . . .

In later chapters I'll give you details about how to crossmatch foods to learn exactly which foods are suitable for your particular biochemistry. Also, I'll let you in on the secret of how to test yourself for environmental insults to your biochemistry. You'll learn about nutritional supplements that you need to support and improve your biochemistry.

CHAPTER TWO

TO SAVE MYSELF, I HAD
TO LEARN MORE
ABOUT NUTRITION

Since you might not know me, let me take a few moments to introduce myself by sketching in my background and telling you how I became interested in nutrition.

My Medical Training

First, let me say that my ten years of medical training make me a solid member of the medical establishment. After receiving a B.S. in Medicine and an M.D. degree from Duke University School of Medicine, I completed a rotating internship at the University of Chicago and then took an internship in obstetrics and gynecology at the University of Minnesota.

That was followed by a residency in internal medicine at the Veterans Administration Hospital associated with Vanderbilt University. I then had a three-year psychiatric residency at the University of Illinois and its affiliated V.A. hospital. As a part of my training I had a 900-hour analysis by a graduate of the Chicago Institute of Psychoanalysis.

I was on the faculty at Northwestern University Medical School.

I published a number of scientific papers in medical journals, and am the author of a textbook on psychology that is used in universities around the world. In addition to the book you're now reading, I've had fourteen other books published.

I'm a member of the American Medical Association.

You'll find me listed in *Who's Who in the East* and *Who's Who in America*. More important, out of the 600,000 M.D.'s in the United States, I'm one of approximately 130 whose biography appears in Marquis' *Who's Who in the World*, the only M.D. in the field of nutrition to appear there.

How My World Turned Upside Down

If a particular event had not happened one morning in the 1960's, I might have continued practicing "cookbook" medicine the way most physicians do and, indeed, the way I myself had practiced it until then.

While jogging I got a sudden feeling of weakness and a discomfort in my chest.

I had allowed myself to become overweight. I checked my cholesterol and found it high.

I put myself on a complex-carbohydrate, moderate-protein, low-fat diet with the hope of reducing my cholesterol. Of course I restricted my total calories.

I had been on this diet for two days when suddenly I felt weak. I began sweating, and experienced a feeling of impending doom. Fearing a heart attack, I checked into a hospital where my physician did tests. He found no cause for the symptoms and discharged me.

After several days on my diet, the same frightening symptoms returned, and I went back to the hospital once more. This time I was checked by both my physician and his associate. Neither could find anything amiss, and I was again sent home.

WHEN FORCED TO, WE USE OUR HEADS

The next day, as if on cue, the symptoms of weakness, perspiration, and anxiety returned.

I decided that I'd exhausted my physician's diagnostic abilities.

Either I had to sign myself into a medical center for a complete workup—or find out myself what was wrong.

Perhaps none of us use our heads until forced to. As I lay sweating in bed and turning diagnostic possibilities over in my head, I remembered that while in the hospital I had awakened each morning at 4:30. The nurse had given me a glass of sweetened orange juice. After drinking the orange juice, I would drop off to sleep again for three more hours.

Could I be hypoglycemic? Could a drop in blood sugar have caused me to wake up at 4:30 every morning? Were my frightening symptoms the result of low blood sugar?

Proof wouldn't be hard to come by. I only needed to eat something sweet to raise my blood sugar. If I felt better after eating sweets, I would have my diagnosis.

I sent for a wedge of apple pie garnished with three scoops of ice cream. I propped my weak and cold-sweaty self upright in bed, and ate the delicious goo.

In less than five minutes all symptoms disappeared: the sweating, the weakness, the feeling of impending doom, the fear that I was about to die.

I had the big answer, but new questions began pouring in. The most pressing: What diet should I follow?

If I ate a moderate-protein, moderate-fat, low-carbohydrate diet—as indicated in the standard treatment for hypoglycemia— would it raise my cholesterol level? Would such a diet help my hypoglycemia but predispose me to a heart attack?

MY BACKGROUND IN NUTRITION

In one way I was fortunate. At Duke, more than at almost any other medical school, students were given considerable training in the field of nutrition. In fact, important diet and vitamin research has been carried out at Duke. As students, each of us had gone on special diets—mine had been heavy in spaghetti—and we performed blood and urine tests on ourselves to learn the biochemical effects of different foods.

As a medical student I had done research on the relationship of vitamin C to certain allergic reactions and had published the results in the *Journal of Allergy*. But as the years passed my interest had drifted away from the subjects of nutrition and allergy.

THE REIGN OF CONFUSION

The only suggestion my physician had was to eat "lean meats and complex carbohydrates."

On that diet I continued having attacks of hypoglycemia.

My physician gave me blood vessel dilators to keep my arteries open and medication to reduce my high cholesterol.

The medication made me tired and weak. I felt like an invalid.

My doctor was giving me standard treatment for hypoglycemia and the medications usually prescribed for keeping coronary arteries open.

You may be certain that when a physician becomes ill, he selects his attending physician with some care. The man I chose was a graduate of a prestigious university. He had taken his postgraduate training at a famous medical center in New York. I respected him both as a person and as a thoroughly competent specialist.

He had his limitations, however, when it came to treating nutritional disorders. This was not his fault, nor perhaps even the fault of the institutions where he studied. His lack of knowledge about nutrition merely reflected the almost universal neglect of matters nutritional by the medical profession. If I expected to feel better, I had to learn far more than I knew about nutrition.

My Re-education

I dived in to pick up all of the information I could about the nutritional side of medicine. It didn't take me long to find out that the nutritionists at universities knew a great deal about research and laboratory animals, but little about the nutritional treatment of sick people. Most university nutritionists spent their lives in laboratories, not in offices with sick people.

I then began visiting M.D.'s who specialized in the private practice of nutrition. I not only sat with them in their offices, but I read their papers and books and went to medical meetings with them in this country and in Europe.

Some of the things I learned turned out to be nonsense. Some of the information was very valuable.

ALLERGIES, VITAMINS AND BIG BUCKS

Very quickly I learned that the world of clinical nutrition was divided into several camps:

1. Those doctors who knew a great deal about food and environmental allergies.

2. Those doctors who had an in-depth knowledge of vitamins, minerals, and other nutrients.

3. Those doctors (and there are many) who practice nutrition mostly to make big bucks.

I learned all I could from the first two groups of doctors and vowed never to become one of those in the last group.

AND I LEARNED FROM MYSELF AND MY PATIENTS

Not only did I learn from manipulating my own diet, and changing my nutritional supplements and environment, but I also learned from studying how my patients reacted to nutritional treatment.

I learned to combine and integrate the knowledge of both the allergists and the nutritionists.

And I made a number of entirely new discoveries on my own.

I have used my new knowledge to help both myself and my patients.

Not only does my own medication-free life go smoothly, but I've helped hundreds of people completely change their lives—people who've come to me for many different complaints, from headaches, to emotional troubles to high blood pressure, asthma, arthritis, lupus . . . and dozens of other conditions that can be handled much better with nutritional approaches than with medication.

I have learned to correct the *cause* of illness.

The results are infinitely better than merely treating *symptoms* with medication.

If you have less than blooming good emotional health, if you follow the directions given in this book, your life too could be completely changed.

CHAPTER THREE

PLEASE DON'T EAT THE AVERAGE AMERICAN DIET

Unless—

You want to live the average American life—filled with fatigue, tension, depression, and insomnia.

And you want to die the average American way—of heart attack, stroke, or cancer.

"An apple a day keeps the doctor away." Right? Wrong.

We live in an age of elaborate controls, supervision, and expert advice. Having a baby requires a hospital, two doctors, and a brace of nurses. It takes a lawyer $900, and seven pages of single-spaced typing to write a will that says, "I leave everything to my wife." We need an examination, a test, and a license to drive a car or to practice a profession.

Certainly everything that affects your health is subjected to scrutiny and control by the government and/or a profession.

One of the few things left to the individual is what to eat. You don't need a license, a prescription, or a Ph.D. degree to get into a grocery store; therefore, most people assume that there can't be anything complicated about nutrition. We have absorbed a few hoary cliches about the subject from those noted scientific experts, our grandmothers. We certainly spend enough time and money on making our food taste good. So what could be wrong?

Plenty.

In many ways the medical profession is still in the Dark Ages. And the least illuminated of all the medical disciplines is the specialty of nutrition.

You can bet one thing for sure: Any doctor who says, "You'll get everything you need if you'll just eat the average American diet" doesn't know much about nutrition.

What would you think about a financial adviser who said, "Just spend the average American amount of money and everything will be all right?"

What would you say if an educator told your child, "You only need an eighth-grade education?"

Simplistic Answers Are for Simple People

The human body is a fantastically complicated collection of cells and chemical reactions. The more we learn about the diagnosis and cure of that system, the more we understand how extraordinarily complicated it is. And yet most of us assume that it is a relatively simple matter to nourish the human system properly.

Can that be right?

No. It can't and it isn't.

The "minimum daily requirement" of vitamins and minerals is a travesty—and a good example of what I mean.

The government and various medical groups setting standards persistently leave Americans with the impression that there is an average daily requirement of carbohydrates, fats, proteins, vitamins, and minerals that suits most adults perfectly well no matter what their age, medical history, size, sex or genetic make-up. They assure us that we can meet all our nutritional needs by eating "a normal, well-balanced American diet" without any nutritional supplements whatsoever.

This recommendation perpetuates four major fallacies:

1. That the American diet is normal, well-balanced, and nutrionally adequate. It is in fact inadequate on all these counts.

2. That there is some clear-cut, black-or-white difference between having a deficiency and not having one. It may be true that

an average diet prevents scurvy or beri-beri, but that doesn't mean there's no deficiency.

3. That there is an "average" person with "average" nutritional needs. There is only one average person in the United States.

4. That medical science has adequate information to establish nutritional standards, average or otherwise. It does not.

Because these notions are some of the most strongly held in the current myth of American nutrition, and because I believe them to be exceedingly misleading and potentially dangerous, let's examine each of them in turn.

CHAPTER FOUR

THE AMERICAN DIET BORDERS ON HORRIBLE

We are said to have one of the highest standards of living in the world. Americans hold on hard to that thesis; it seems to comfort us in the face of social and political confusion and disillusion, racial and sexual unrest, inflation, pollution, crime, terror, depression, frustration, and ennui. No matter how tough things seem, it improves our perspective to remember that so many people are worse off than us.

Shouldn't a high standard of living mean that we eat well? In fact, with more Americans concerned about overweight than any other aspect of nutrition, don't we eat too well?

Of course not. There is no such thing as eating too well. If you eat well, you are trim, fit and healthy, not obese. A great many of us eat too much, but that is definitely not the same thing as being well-nourished.

Most people in America assume that malnutrition is confined to the ghettos and poverty pockets in Appalachia, but the fact is that malnutrition, mild or acute, exists on all levels of our society. *America is the only country in the world where the average dog is better fed than the average person.* It is literally true that the nutritional requirements established for packaged dog food are far more stringent than those for the food we eat ourselves, *especially* processed convenience foods. If you doubt this, try comparing the label of a can of Alpo with a can of ravioli.

Clean and Good Is Not the Whole Story

To take a single example of the ways our attitudes about food are confused and manipulated, consider the case of "refined" wheat and wheat products. For centuries, wheat has been so central to the Western diet that bread is referred to as the staff of life. Taking into account bread, cakes, cookies, snacks, crackers, pasta, and cereal, Americans eat an enormous quantity of wheat; it forms a percentage of the diet that is by no means "balanced" for an animal with the basic enzyme system of a carnivore.

Up to the last century, most wheat products contained the whole grain, including the wheat germ, which is a rich source of B vitamins and certain essential minerals. Today, nearly all wheat flour and wheat products have been "refined." According to the dictionary, "refined" means "free of worthless matter and impurities." But refined wheat flour is so free of any nutrients, of the germ with all its vitamins and minerals, that the white flour that is left will not support even a weevil.

This is of great value to the manufacturer; it means that a product will last in the bin or on the shelf for weeks or perhaps months without growing rancid or buggy, because there is nothing in the flour for a bug or bacterium to live on. We have learned to like this fluff—even to prefer it—partly because it's called "refined." That sounds pure and modern and classy. In actuality it ought to be called "stripped."

As for "enriched" refined wheat products (sound delicious, don't they?) the enriching consists of taking out some twenty-three essential nutrients, and putting back six of the least expensive ones. That's like saying a mugger enriched you after he stole everything in your wallet and gave you back enough change for bus fare.

The same holds true for the refining of other grains. White rice is produced by removing the brown husk that surrounds the rice kernels. The husk is the part that contains the nutrients that sustain life, including large amounts of B vitamins and minerals. Chickens fed a diet of white rice develop beri-beri. The disease is cured by adding the rice polish removed by "refining" to the meal.

Some of my colleagues and I who are interested in relationships between food allergies and emotional illness have made a special study of bread and found its main constituent—wheat—to be highly allergenic. In all probability this is due not only to its relative newness in human nutrition but also to the particles of rat feces and cockroaches that it acquires during storage. Quite possibly, man's genetic makeup has not evolved sufficiently to handle grains efficiently and he is not able to metabolize them as efficiently as foods that his ancestors have eaten for millions of years like meats, vegetables, berries, and fruits.

Next time you feel like munching a chocolate bar, remember the following story told me at a recent meeting of the Society for Clinical Ecology. Food allergies are almost an obsession with members of the society. They are forever tracking down the sources of allergenic substances. One member recently visited a South American country to study the cocoa bean from which chocolate is made. He began at the site where it was grown and traced it all the way through the manufacturing process. At one point he went down to the docks where the beans stood on open wharves awaiting shipment. On opening one of the crates he found it alive with cockroaches. He estimates that about one-fourth of chocolate consists of dead, ground-up, melted-down cockroaches, and that this is one of the factors that makes it such a common allergen.

In the process of drying, storing, refining, freezing, and canning foods, many valuable nutrients are lost. In addition, most processed foods contain colorings, flavorings, and preservatives that can be dangerously allergenic. The additives may cause serious disorders, including cancer.

Even Unprocessed Food May Not Be Nutritious

Even if you eat mainly fresh foods, you're by no means assured of getting adequate vitamins and minerals from your diet alone. Fresh fruits and vegetables lose vitamins on the shelf. You rarely know how long a tomato has been sitting in a crate or on a truck between the time it gets from the vine to you; furthermore, minerals and many vitamins in fruits and vegetables come from the soil, and many of the elements have long since been depleted in farmlands that have been in constant production decade after decade.

Many more nutrients are lost during cooking. You can order charts from the government assuring you that there are X number of milligrams of calcium in a serving of cabbage. The figures, however, are virtually useless unless you grow and harvest your own produce and eat most of it raw—and even then you will lose nutrients if you smoke, or have alcoholic drinks.

In sum, it is extraordinary that a nation so obsessed with food knows so little about nourishment. Many people miss the notion that our diets are inadequate, saying that if we are so ill-nourished, why aren't people suffering from it all around us?

The answer is: they are.

We're too fat, too thin, depressed, angry, anxious, sickly. We have a million illnesses—from colds to a world record for heart attacks undreamed of a century ago. Does that sound like a society that is well-nourished? If we were to stop people on the street and test them at random for proteins, fats, carbohydrates, vitamins, hormones, and minerals, we would find an astounding number of deficiencies; and most (if not all) of these people could improve their health and well-being immeasurably by simply having their deficiencies corrected.

The Sweet Disaster

Even if none of the recent and dubious inventions of the food processors had come about, even if you forget for a moment about all the preservatives and additives and freeze-drying and refining that has changed the nutritional value of the food we eat, one other enormous change in eating habits has occurred in the last hundred years. The terrible significance of this one change for our mental and physical health is only beginning to be guessed at; this change is our yearly consumption of sugar.

Man first learned to produce a crude sort of sugar from the sap of sugar cane roughly 2,500 years ago. But between that time and the nineteenth century it was available only in tiny amounts and only to the wealthy. During the reign of Queen Elizabeth I, an

Englishman would buy sugar by the grain from a druggist. Queen Elizabeth herself was said to have been as fond of sugar as any modern teenager. Contemporary reports said that her teeth were quite black from decay.

When slave labor came to the Caribbean in the middle of the eighteenth century, the production of sugar increased greatly; but refined sugar has been commonly available for only a little over a hundred years. As in the case of grains, "refined" here means that what few trace vitamins and minerals occur naturally in sugar are removed, leaving a pure white powder that even bugs won't eat. Even with the recent rise in the price of sugar, it's one of today's least expensive foods—if, indeed, you can call it a food. When I say inexpensive, I refer to the purchase price per calorie. Its purchase price in terms of vitamins, minerals, proteins, and good health is higher than the price of platinum. If we take into consideration the incidence of diabetes and hypoglycemia, the obesity, malnutrition, rotted teeth, shortened lives, hardened arteries, depressions, and all the other medical liabilities for which it is wholly or partly responsible, sugar is the most expensive substance on earth.

In 1850, world production of sugar was only about one and one-half million tons per year. By 1890, it had risen to five million tons, and by the beginning of this century it stood at 11 million tons. In 1950 it reached 35 million tons, and is now well above 80 million tons. So there has been more than a fifty-fold increase in the total production of sugar over the past 140 years. The use of sugar has jumped from three pounds per person per year in 1850 to almost 45 pounds a year at present. But this average was arrived at by including the entire world population, including the inhabitants of underdeveloped countries. Taking the so-called civilized countries alone, the consumption of sugar averages about 100 pounds per citizen per year—or about one-sixth of a person's total caloric intake! The United Kingdom has the highest per capita consumption of sugar—120 pounds a year.

Tragically, the highest consumption of sugar is to be found among children and adolescents. Youngsters are more at the mercy of their appetites than older people who have learned some elements of nutrition. Also, it is only natural that mothers try to please their children and make them happy by giving in to their demands for sweets. In addition, the sugar industry has assiduously advertised its product as a source of quick energy; so mother has it in the back of her mind that she may be doing her child a favor by "giving him some quick energy." What she forgets—or doesn't know—is that she is also giving him a good start toward a long list of diseases.

Americans are obsessed with the idea of calories. Too many can make them fat, too few leave them listless and thin. But calories are not nourishment in themselves; a calorie is simply a unit of energy. For your body to be nourished you must provide it with proteins and fats and vitamins and minerals as well as calories. Your enzyme systems have evolved over millions of years to process (metabolize) certain kinds of foods. You can imagine, for example, that if you fed your dog nothing but pears, he would not thrive. Pears are food of a kind, and they provide plenty of calories, but they would not provide the protein and vitamins and minerals the dog's meat-oriented system calls for.

In the same way, sugars and massive amounts of starches do not make an adequate diet for the human body.

IF IT'S SO BAD FOR US, WHY DO WE LIKE IT SO MUCH?

I believe the answer lies in the story of our evolution. About 65 million years ago, man's ancestors lost the ability to manufacture their own vitamin C. Most animals have an enzyme in the liver that enables them to convert glucose into the ascorbic acid their bodies need. At some point in his evolution, man's ancestors began eating large quantities of fresh fruit, that supplied them with all the vitamin C they needed. When an enzyme is no longer necessary, nature eliminates it, since it is more efficient to use the chemical energy in other, more productive ways. Man's forebears lost the enzyme L-gulonolactone oxidase that helped them manufacture vitamin C, and became dependent on a steady intake of fruit to provide it instead. Gradually they developed a craving for the sweetness of fruit, which is, of course, full of fructose, or fruit sugar. This craving was a positive development, since our ancestors who ate plenty of vitamin C were more energetic, more efficient at hunting and fighting, and threw off disease more easily and healed more quickly than their cousins who craved sweets less and thus ate less fruit.

In the past hundred years, the positive genetic trait, the craving for sweet fruit, has been perverted into an addiction to sugar which is little short of grotesque. Our enzyme systems have not had the evolutionary time needed to evolve an efficient way to handle ordinary table sugar.

Our current body chemistry systems are makeshift at best, easily over-trained and driven haywire, leading to hypoglycemia and diabetes and numerous other diseases a great deal more serious than children's tooth decay. Studies by John Yudkin at the University of London strongly implicate sugar as the real killer behind heart disease and strokes.

Refined sugar does not simply fail to provide nutrients: it actually robs your system of nutrients vitally needed elsewhere, since the chemical systems mobilized to metabolize it have to take ingredients from somewhere.

Viewed in a historical context, in terms of what kind of animal man is, what his enzyme systems are designed to do, and what we ask them to do instead, it is clear that the average American diet is not normal, well-balanced or nutritionally adequate.

CHAPTER FIVE

EITHER YOU HAVE A NUTRITIONAL DEFICIENCY OR YOU DON'T?

Physicians tend to think of their patients' conditions in all-or-nothing terms. You have pneumonia or you don't. You are pregnant or you're not. Your appendix is inflamed or it isn't. This is appropriate when dealing with infectious diseases, but distinctly inappropriate when dealing with nutrition.

When the medical establishment says your diet is adequate, it generally means that it is adequate to prevent scurvy, beri-beri, kwashiorkor, or rickets. Preoccupied with acute clinical syndromes, few doctors have even begun to consider the possible shades of the nutritional gray area between someone being definitely well or definitely ill.

Consider the case of anemia. This condition is caused by a shortage of hemoglobin, the special protein in the bloodstream that carries oxygen to the cells. Physicians encounter anemia frequently; it is often caused by a nutritional deficiency. But the condition often remains undiagnosed and untreated because a patient is rarely clearly anemic or clearly not anemic. As his hemoglobin drops he may simply tire more easily, feeling neither completely well nor definitely ill. Such a state can continue for many years. The sufferer may never know that anemia is affecting the way he feels—unless he is given a nutritional supplement that wipes it out.

Nutritional Problems Are Different from Infectious Diseases Because They Tend to Develop Slowly

The patient ignores them, gets used to them, forgets what it was like to feel really well, if he ever knew. The doctor in turn tends to dismiss the complaints as "psychosomatic," by which he means that you must feel sick because you're neurotic, and he may never even consider that you may have become listless, depressed, angry, paranoid, or whatever because you are suffering from a nutritional disorder.

Physicians like to regard themselves as exact scientists, capable of quickly and accurately diagnosing an illness and prescribing medication that will cure it, or at least keep it within manageable bounds. The fact that so few doctors know much about nutrition tempts them to dismiss the whole subject as "unscientific," which amounts to saying, "I don't know for sure what's wrong with you, so it must be something else I do know about."

The disturbing truth is that most physicians don't even recognize a case of acute nutritional deficiency when they see it.

H.R. Follis, Jr., M.D., and his colleagues at Johns Hopkins University hospital reported that out of 69 cases of scurvy discovered at autopsy, the attending physicians had diagnosed that disease before death in only six cases. If the gifted and superbly trained physicians at Johns Hopkins miss this rather elementary diagnosis 91% of the time, how often must the disease go unrecognized in less sophisticated hospitals? And how much more often are milder deficiencies undiagnosed?

Deficiencies Often Show First As Emotional Symptoms

The average physician, indoctrinated at medical school with the belief that nutritional deficiencies only occur among alcoholics, on the dirt farms of Appalachia, or in Uganda, tends to assume that emotional symptoms have little to do with physical health. It will probably never occur to him that his own son's mood swings and bad grades might be caused by a nutritional disorder associated with a diet of potato chips and soda pop.

If the family doctor resists this notion, the psychiatrist resists it even harder. In one of my scientific publications, I once pointed out that one-third of my psychiatric patients from the New York area had low serum vitamin B_{12} levels, and that their symptoms usually disappeared when the deficiency was corrected. The paper was brought to the attention of a number of New York hospitals. Today many of them are ordering Vitamin B_{12} tests on their patients.

Why do physicians neglect this test?

When asked, they say, "Well, yours is only one study" or "The test is too expensive."

But I doubt that these are the real reasons. A more personal factor prevents physicians from adopting the test: they simply don't want to become involved in any nutritional problem. They wouldn't know how much vitamin to give, how often, the side effects, etc.

Psychiatrists (as well as psychologists, psychiatric social workers, and marriage counselors) tend to assume that anyone they see suffers, almost by definition, from an "emotional" problem, by which they mean a disorder brought about by a traumatic event.

These experts seem to have blocked out Freud's statement: "All our provisional ideas in psychology will some day be based on an organic structure. This makes it probable that special substances and special chemicals control the operation." In this instance, Freud's prediction was certainly correct. And when the day finally comes that his prediction is generally accepted, a principal key to psychological health will be found in the currently neglected chemistry of nutrition.

After the body chemistry is normalized, I find that few of my patients require psychotherapy. Others are so sick that they may require some supportive psychotherapy while the chemistry is being normalized. There is no reason not to use any psychiatric or medical technique along with proper nutrition.

For example, a patient with tuberculosis may be treated with surgery on the diseased lung or with chemotherapy to kill the tuberculous lesion; but this does not preclude the use of a proper diet and nutritional supplements.

CHAPTER SIX

THE "AVERAGE" PERSON WITH "AVERAGE" NUTRITIONAL NEEDS

If we hadn't been brought up with the idea of a "minimum daily requirement" of vitamins that the government and the manufacturers of grossly inadequate "fortified" cereals drum into our heads, we would see at once that the idea of an average person with average nutritional needs is irrational. People come in different sizes and shapes and with a vast range of different genetic characteristics. They can't possibly all be properly nourished by a single standard amount of anything. Larger bodies require more nutrients, and active people require more vitamins and minerals, just as they require a larger total amount of calories—and more vitamins.

As we will see in detail later, many people are born with physiological characteristics that cause them to need vastly more of some nutrients than the government presumes to standardize. Some people are missing crucial enzymes in their systems that prevent their absorbing the vitamins they eat. Others may lack a particular protein needed to carry the vitamin or mineral to the cells where they are needed. Such a person will require massive doses of the vitamin in order to finally get an adequate supply into the tissues. Some people's cell walls cannot be penetrated easily by certain substances. They too will need vastly more of that particular nutrient. Some have systems that "dump" or destroy certain vitamins and minerals.

This appears to be particularly true of many people with mental illness.

THE NEED FOR VITAMINS AND MINERALS INCREASES WITH AGE

Fifty thousand years ago our human ancestors lived to age 30. Our own chemistry was designed to last only about 30 years. Hence old age, the failure of our body chemistry, actually starts at about age 30. This is why after that age it is especially important that you get the best nutrition possible, the individual nutrition that is correct for you and you alone.

SOME PEOPLE ACQUIRE GREATER NEEDS FOR CERTAIN VITAMINS AND MINERALS

There is growing evidence that a period of malnutrition may cause a permanent enzyme change. The person who has been temporarily malnourished will require larger doses of certain vitamins for the rest of his life. The most acute, clear-cut cases of this occur in prisoners of war, who have been forced to live on a severely inadequate diet for months or years. When they return to society, their condition does not improve even when they are given fairly large doses of vitamins. They only feel well if they take what would be monstrous amounts of vitamins for a person with a more normal nutritional history. Usually large doses of vitamins must be continued indefinitely.

I believe that this syndrome occurs in milder forms throughout our society. Now that I am familiar with the symptoms of vitamin deficiencies, I believe I can pick out in retrospect several occasions in my life when I was suffering from a deficiency of one or more vitamins, even though I was raised on a perfectly "normal" American diet. Perhaps that explains why my system thrives on a quantity of vitamins that will no doubt seem large to you (more of that in Chapter 16).

I suspect the same thing is true of anyone who has lived for any length of time on an inadequate diet, be it an unwise reducing diet or a student's menu of potato chips and beer, a teenager's sugar binges or a young couple's early years on kisses, wine, and cheese. You may have felt fine on such a diet at the time, particularly if you were young, but when essential nutrients are missing, your elaborate system of enzymes and chemical responses has to compensate somehow, and the effects of those changes eventually show up in the form of altered nutritional needs.

MANY ENVIRONMENTAL STRESSES ELEVATE YOUR VITAMIN NEEDS

In addition to its many other dangers, tobacco destroys Vitamin A, B_6, B_{12}, and especially vitamin C.

Here's an example of an antimetabolite (something that destroys a substance that's required for the body's biochemical reactions). Hydrazine is the name of a chemical that may enter our bodies, then bind to and destroy its vitamin B_6. This chemical is becoming widely distributed in our environment. Not only is it found in tobacco smoke (do people smoke in the same room with you?), but it's left in the air when rocket fuel burns, as well as when fuel is burned by high performance aircraft such as the F-16 fighter plane.

Alcohol imposes stresses on the body, increasing its need for vitamins. Like sugar and refined grains, alcohol contains calories but virtually no nutrients, so it drains the body of vitamins and minerals in the course of being metabolized. The connection between nutrition and alcohol consumption is so important that the late Dr. Roger Williams of the University of Texas believed that it is impossible for a properly nourished person to become an alcoholic.

CERTAIN DRUGS AND MEDICINES, INCLUDING BIRTH CONTROL PILLS, ROB THE BODY OF VITAMINS

Your environment imposes other stresses as well, particularly air pollution and noise pollution. We all talk about these pressures but have you considered that these are not abstract emotional events but concrete physiological strains on the chemistry of your body? The same applies to emotional stress. Your emotions are not abstract, disembodied feelings; they possess chemical and physical components. When you feel a rush of fear or rage or anxiety, chemicals, minerals and electrical impulses undergo changes in your nervous system. If you are under emotional stress you must replenish the nutrients you need to keep the nervous system functioning properly. If you don't supply these nutrients the deficiency can cause further emotional symptoms of all kinds.

GOOD NEWS

For decades the government has championed a fixed figure for the amount of vitamins needed. For many years Roger Williams maintained that each person has a different vitamin and mineral need. For at least fifteen years I have been writing about the individual needs for nutrients.

At last a member of the U.S. government, M. Levine of the National Institutes of Health (NIH), has admitted that we do not know the optimal level of vitamin C. By implication, he is admitting that we do not know the correct amount of any vitamin or mineral for anyone.

My approach: give more than enough of each of the vitamins and depend upon the body to throw away what it doesn't need, and vary each vitamin separately and find the level at which the person feels his best.

CHAPTER SEVEN

DOES MEDICAL SCIENCE KNOW WHAT YOU SHOULD EAT?

Compared with other branches of medicine, the study of infectious diseases, or even of surgery, our knowledge of the chemistry of nutrition is in its infancy. The word vitamin was not even coined until 1911, and even then it was a misnomer.

Although scurvy had been a dread disease since the time of Hippocrates and had decimated the ranks of the Crusaders and seamen all over the world, it was not until 1753 that the Scottish physician James Lind discovered that it could be cured by adding fresh fruit to the diet.

It took forty years for the medical establishment to accept his findings. In 1795 the British navy (for the first time) ordered all ships to carry a supply of citrus fruit, which gave rise to the British nickname, Limey.

In the 1890's, Eijkman discovered that beri-beri occurred when pigeons were fed polished rice, and could be cured when unpolished rice was returned to the diet. But even then, people did not believe that there were special nutrients in the rice husk, but that there was poison in the germ or kernel of the rice, and that the husk contained some unknown natural antidote.

In 1911 Casimir Funk, a Polish chemist who worked at the Lister Institute in London, succeeded in isolating the nutrient in the rice polish that prevented beri-beri (it was thiamine, or vitamin B). He called it a "vital amine" because he believed that it was an amine, the generic name of the compound ammonia, which was incorrect. The great significance of his discovery was that he had proved at last that beri-beri was caused not by a germ, or a poison, but by the absence of an essential nutrient that must be present in every healthy human body but cannot be manufactured by the body itself. It must come from the diet.

Funk suspected, correctly, that if there were one such nutrient there must be more.

In the next twenty years vitamins, A, D and C were recognized. Research had continued through the century. Vitamin B_{12} was first synthesized shortly after World War II, and vitamin E, so significant in its interaction with hormone levels and its ability to decrease blood clotting and blood cholesterol levels, was not recognized by the FDA as essential to human nutrition until 1973.

Without doubt, there are more discoveries to come.

In a personal communication with me, William P. Murphy, who shared the Nobel Prize in Medicine in 1934, stated that he feels there are still vitamin-like substances in crude liver extract that have not yet been recognized.

In short, we are far from knowing everything there is to know about nutrition. More important, what we do know is not being widely taught, accepted, or even understood in the medical establishment or by the public. Thousands of practicing doctors went to medical school before Vitamin B_{12} was even heard of, and in many cases these established, illustrious figures are precisely the ones who maintain that only 0.3 mg of vitamin B_{12} is needed per month to maintain optimum human nutrition.

Not long ago I learned that only twenty-four percent of America's medical schools currently offer any courses on nutrition to their students. Although I was aware that the establishment neglects this subject, I was startled since my own school, Duke University, had given considerable instruction in nutrition.

Since I often walk past a world-famous medical school, I decided to drop in one day and check its curriculum. When I looked through this prestigious school's catalogue I could hardly believe what I saw: not a single required or elective course on nutrition! I studied the subheadings under biochemistry, physiology, and medicine, thinking the subject must be tucked away in another department. Still nothing. As a final check, I made inquiries at the bookstore run for medical students. It stocked exactly one book on nutrition—a rather naive volume written for nurses.

What a sad situation! Here we have a collection of modern medical skyscrapers, shiny with wealth and prestige, seemingly ignoring that most basic of life's realities—the fact that cells require proper nutrition to live.

Now every time I pass the institution, I think of all the patients I can help who are not helped by that multimillion-dollar collection of glass and concrete and scientific equipment.

There are many books and journals devoted to the field of nutrition. These publications could and should interest physicians, but they are usually ignored. And they are likely to continue being ignored unless you pressure not only your physician but also your political representative to learn the importance of nutrition.

This is no trivial issue. We are dealing with the welfare of individual cells that add up to be the most valuable thing in the universe—life.

SURGERY AND VITAMIN C

A twenty-five-year-old actress I know of suffered from a slipped vertebral disk, a painful back disorder. A surgeon operated to remove the disk. Because she remained in great pain, a second operation—a spinal fusion—was undertaken, but the bones did not knit properly and the pain continued. She returned to the hospital for a body cast and electrical stimulation to encourage the bones to fuse. When these measures failed, an anesthesiologist tried acupuncture. This, too, failed. She still remains in pain.

In this instance, a competent surgeon at one of the country's great hospitals apparently forgot the bone tissue, in order to thrive, requires generous quantities of calcium, magnesium, vitamin D, and especially vitamin C.

In fact, Houston neurosurgeon, J. Greenwood, Jr., M.D. found that massive doses of vitamin C benefited patients suffering from pain caused by slipped disks.

The New York surgeon, not thinking in nutritional terms, forgot that many actresses subsist on wretched diets. He made no tests to determine her vitamin level or magnesium levels of her tissues. Only hardware was considered: the scalpel, a cast, acupuncture needles.

I don't mean to imply that all back pain—or even her back pain—can be cured by proper nutrients. I do suggest that nutrition should have been among the first considerations in this and every other therapy. No matter how skillfully an orthopedic surgeon sets a broken bone, that bone will not heal if its cells are not given proper nutrition. Even the healing of fractures rests upon cellular chemistry, which in turn rests upon nutrition.

Had her surgeons been confronted with the questions of nutritional supplements, they would most likely have fallen back on the cliché that says the average American diet is nutritionally adequate.

EMOTIONAL SYMPTOMS ARE RARELY CONSIDERED AS NUTRITIONAL IN ORIGIN

Psychiatrists continue to think of emotions as separate from the human body, unconnected with the chemistry of the brain cells. Freud, misinterpreted, has so captured our society's imagination that even physicians forget that the brain is an organ in the body.

Unfortunately, a physical malfunction in the brain often does not signal its presence as obviously as do dysfunctions in other organs. If your liver fails to clear the bile from your bloodstream, you become jaundiced. Your yellow skin is there for all to see. Your physician takes one look and orders liver function tests. Neither he nor your friends consider your ocher complexion a moral, spiritual, or marital problem, an interpersonal relationship problem, or an unresolved childhood conflict brought about by Great-aunt Sarah's spanking you for pulling the cat's tail.

When the cells of your central nervous system malfunction, there may be no such telltale sign. The cause may be just as physical, though the resulting disorder may manifest itself in depression or elation, misinterpretation of other people's motives, perceptual distortions, or inability to concentrate.

But nervous symptoms of this kind continue to be regarded as mere results of environmental influences. When a patient tells his doctor that he is depressed, the doctor automatically asks what has been troubling him, and the patient will promptly recite a list of difficulties: His wife doesn't understand him, his colleagues are unfriendly, his boss expects too much, and life generally disagrees with him.

Some or all of these grievances may even be founded in fact. But think a moment: Aren't we all subject to such irritants? Life is hardly a bowl of cherries and each of us suffers losses, setbacks, and frustrations. It's called the "pain of everyday life." A healthy person is able to push his way through these difficulties without undue discomfort. A depressed individual is overwhelmed by the ordinary jolts of life.

In reality, the cause of the depression is usually some chemical disorder which affects the central nervous system—one that can often be traced to incorrect nutrition.

VITAMIN DEFICIENCIES ARE NOT THE ONLY SERIOUS NUTRITIONAL DISORDERS

Recently I saw a man in his twenties who suffers from schizophrenia. He spent many months at one of the most prestigious private psychiatric centers in the east, where his parents invested $42,000 in the most advanced psychotherapy, sophisticated tranquilizers, and even electric shock treatments. Instead of improving, his emotional state grew worse.

While in the hospital he gained 120 pounds. I asked how this incredible weight gain had come about, and learned that he was in the habit of eating large quantities of cake and candy at the institute. When I tested the patient, he turned out to be allergic to wheat, milk, and sugar, the basic ingredients of candy and cake. This is a prevalent finding, especially among schizophrenics, as we'll discuss in a later chapter.

ALLERGIES AND EMOTIONS ARE CLOSELY CONNECTED

I tested the patient's allergies by having him fast for five days and then fed him one food at a time as a "challenge feeding" to see what foods he could not tolerate. During the fast, his mental symptoms cleared up entirely. After the challenge feedings of wheat, milk, and sugar, his psychotic symptoms bloomed again.

Further tests also indicated deficiencies in the male hormone testosterone and in the vitamin B_6 and folic acid. Decreased levels of folic acid are suspected to cause brain damage.

This patient would not stay on the diet that we gave him. The last I heard he was still psychotic. His father was too lenient with him. He did not get testosterone as I suggested. If he had, it might have cut down the seriousness of his allergic condition, and made it easier for him to follow the diet.

Here, then, is a modern institution of high caliber and repute, which not only failed to test the patient for allergies and basic hormonal and nutritional deficiencies, but permitted the patient to gorge himself on foods that were demonstrably bad for him. If such gross neglect of basic nutritional values is practiced at so excellent and prestigious an institution, what can be expected of lesser ones?

Dr. F. C. Dohan at the University of Pennsylvania demonstrated in a state hospital setting that wheat products are toxic for many patients suffering from schizophrenia; those wards in which wheat products were forbidden had a much higher discharge rate.

WE MUST HELP OURSELVES

All of this underscores the physician's lack of training in nutrition and nutritional supplements, and brings us back to the fact that each one of us must establish his own optimum nutrient intake. This must be done with the advice of a physician, so you should do as much as you can to encourage your doctor to educate himself on the subject. But it is most important also to educate yourself, to know what clinical tests to ask your doctor for (and how to interpret the results better than he may be able to). In the coming chapters I'll show you, for instance, not only how to establish your own vitamin and mineral needs but how to recognize deficiencies or overdoses, and how to correct them.

You should not, of course, become your own physician, diagnosing and treating your own symptoms. It's dangerous for you to ignore persistent symptoms without seeking medical advice. By the time you discover—to mention only one possibility—that your illness is not related to nutrition, the delay may have done you serious harm.

But if you are one of the millions who are sometimes more nervous, angry, anxious, depressed, tired, or confused than is altogether necessary, then it is time for you to take an interest in your nutrition. To do this you will need to understand something of the general biochemical heritage you share with all mankind.

But you must also discover how your system differs from everyone else's.

CHAPTER EIGHT

NUTRITION AFFECTS THE NERVOUS SYSTEM

We tend to forget that we inherit an individual chemical makeup as well as a specific physical makeup. In fact, many physical characteristics are based on chemistry. We see the color of skin as being, say, either black or white. That physical fact is due to a chemical compound called melanin. If this chemical is present in large quantities, your skin is black; if present in lesser amounts, your skin appears pinkish white; if totally absent, you are an albino.

Similarly, we inherit our individual enzyme systems, those chemical carriers that help us use food for energy, repair bodily tissue, and remove waste products from the body.

If enough measurements were taken of everyone in the world, it would undoubtedly be discovered that each person has a different enzyme system.

Along with all the other bodily systems this book is concerned with the brain and central nervous system. The brain is a system of checks and balances, with one part checking as well as stimulating another.

In addition to different chemical (enzyme) makeup, each person has a different number of cells in different parts of the brain. As a result, each person needs a different number of enzyme parts to service each part of the brain. More cells require more enzymes to handle cellular metabolism.

The messages that go back and forth between the brain, spinal cord, and nerves do not flow like electricity in the copper wiring of a house. Each nerve cell in the brain and in other parts of the nervous system communicates with another set of nerves by sending out chemical substances called catecholamines. These act as chemical transmitters from cell to cell.

One of the most important transmitters is a chemical called norepinephrine. We know that sometimes this particular transmitter is not formed in normal amounts by the nerve cells, and therefore is not available to stimulate other nerve cells.

When proteins enter the digestive system, they are broken down by enzymes into amino acids. Norepinephrine has to be made from an amino acid called tyrosine; tyrosine, in turn is made from the amino acid phenylalanine.

If the diet lacks the simple protein phenylalanine, the nervous system will eventually lack norepinephrine, and transmission will be imperfect. A child born with a severe defect in the liver enzyme phenylalanine hydroxylase is doomed to be mentally defective—unless the defect is corrected by proper diet immediately after birth.

Other Nerve Cell Defects

For example, not only may a cell fail to make norepinephrine at a normal rate, but the cell membrane may not allow the chemical to pass out of the cell easily, thus preventing the chemical from stimulating the next nerve. The norepinephrine traveling from one nerve to the next may be destroyed too fast or not fast enough, depending upon the supply of an enzyme known as monoamine oxidase. Or the nerve cell which is touched by the chemical after it travels through the neural cleft (the space between the cells) may be relatively impervious to it and fail to respond properly to its stimulation. All these transmissions of signals in the nervous system depend in part upon a proper supply of vitamins and minerals.

Vitamins and Minerals Are Part of the Enzyme System That Runs the Nervous System

The way you think and feel about what happens in your life depends largely on whether the proper chemicals, including vitamins and minerals, are present to insure healthy transmission within the nervous system.

Suppose you suffer a disappointment. Let's say you didn't get a promotion that you felt you deserved. You may react by saying, "Well, that's a bum deal" and feel mildly annoyed or unhappy for a few days. On the other hand the rejection may make you wildly angry; or you may conclude that the world is totally mismanaged, that life is intolerably unjust, and that you had better kill yourself.

Much depends on how the information about your disappointment is flashed through your nervous system—whether it proceeds in a normal, orderly way, or is derailed or exploded by a chemical accident along the way.

The enzyme systems that control these operations differ from person to person. Each person's vitamins and minerals are different.

Are You Vitamin-Dependent?

Dr. Leon E. Rosenberg of Yale University has devoted much of his time to studying variations in individuals' needs for vitamins. He refers to people with large requirements for certain vitamins as "vitamin-dependent."

ONE TEST FOR VITAMIN NEEDS

One way to test for vitamin needs is to give a "loading test." Massive doses of a vitamin are administered. When a normal person is given a large dose of one of the water-soluble vitamins (C or the Bs, which cannot be stored in the body), his system will take what it needs of the vitamin and excrete the rest in the urine.

At California's Stanford University, Dr. Linus Pauling conducted a series of loading tests financed by the National Institutes of Health. He found that when massive doses of vitamin C—as much as 40 grams—were given to schizophrenics, little or none of it was discarded in urine. In other words, these seriously ill patients needed more than one thousand times the amount commonly recommended as the daily requirement. Similar loading tests with other vitamins produced similar results. Pauling concluded that many people suffering from schizophrenia require many times the normal amount of vitamins in their enzyme systems. My own clinical experience bears this out.

ABSORPTION COUNTS AS MUCH AS INTAKE

In addition to considering the amount of vitamin or mineral a person needs, we must take into consideration how well the vitamin or mineral is absorbed.

For example, some people are unable to absorb vitamin B_{12} because their stomachs do not produce what is called an "intrinsic factor." Such people eventually develop pernicious anemia, often accompanied by disorders of the nervous system, including emotional disorders such as depression and anxiety. These individuals cannot be effectively treated by any amount of orally administered vitamin B_{12}. They have to take it by injection.

Some people may have a normal blood level of vitamin B_{12}, but lack the protein (transcobalamin) that transports vitamin B_{12} from the bloodstream into the tissue where it's used. Such people must have massive amounts of vitamin B_{12} by injection in order to have normal tissue levels of the vitamin.

Somewhat similar mechanisms work with other vitamins. Over one thousand enzyme systems exist in the human liver and individual variations are almost infinite. Each enzyme system for each person will have a different amount of enzyme, which means each person will have a different need for vitamins and minerals.

For example, the enzyme phosphatase in a given person's system can vary from four to eighty-three units. To work properly, obviously eighty-three units of enzyme are going to need more vitamins and minerals than four.

What is true of vitamins is equally true of other nutrients. For example, the late Roger Williams, professor of biochemistry at the University of Texas and former president of the American Chemical Association, studied individual chemical differences in both laboratory animals and humans. He discovered that certain people require five times more calcium and amino acids (simple chains that build proteins) than others.

Your Brain Structure Makes a Difference

As mentioned earlier, there are variations in brain structure. We all have similar brain "compartments," but the number of cells in the various parts of the brain differs from person to person, as does the total number of brain cells. Obviously, people who have more brain cells than others are likely to have greater nutritive requirements.

As you may have guessed by now, we're dealing with a complicated subject that deserves everyone's careful attention.

CHAPTER NINE

WHEAT IS PURE WHAT?

Now and then a patient informs me that meat has chemicals and hormones in it.

Please, I'm not naive!

Everything in our modern world is more or less contaminated. The city of New York has some of the best drinking water in the country, yet it contains more than two hundred known chemicals, including some that are radioactive.

Mother's milk often has pesticides in it and is radioactive. I'm told that the level of radiation in mother's milk is so high that it's illegal for a wet nurse to travel from one state to another because her milk does not meet interstate commerce standards.

WHAT ABOUT WHEAT?

Recently I saw a patient from North Dakota who told me what happens to the wheat grown on her farm.

The wheat is sprayed with chemicals many times while growing, sprayed when it goes to the silo to keep away mice, sprayed to retard fungus growth, sprayed (with chemicals such as Tetrafume) yet again to keep out insects.

Last year's molded wheat is mixed with new wheat so it will get by inspectors (The mold *Aspergillus*—frequently found in wheat, grains, nuts, grapes, peanut butter, bread, cheese, apple juice—produces aflatoxins, which are among the most potent liver carcinogens known.)

Another patient of mine had a brother-in-law who ran a cookie factory. When the flour used to make the cookies arrived at his factory, it was sprayed three times to keep out mold, insects, and rats.

When flour is used to make bread, more chemicals are added to the wheat. Recently I checked the chemicals listed on the wrapper of a loaf of bread: lactylate, monoglycerides, biglycerides, polyglycerate 60, polysorbate 60, potassium bromide, artificial flavorings.

The words "artificial flavorings" may cover dozens of chemicals. For example, the artificial flavoring for apple may contain 183 different chemicals!

And remember, there is no requirement to list all of the chemicals used. Bread contains hundreds of other chemicals such as bleaches, dough strengtheners, firming agents, leavening agents . . . and on and on until bread appears to contain every chemical in the chemist's dictionary.

Pyrrolizidine alkaloids occur in thousands of plants. Often some of these plants find their way into wheat. Wheat containing pyrrolizidines has brought death in epidemic proportions to people who eat wheat products in Afghanistan and India, and has been linked to liver cancer among African blacks.

THE PHYTIC ACID FOUND IN WHEAT

Phytic acid, found in high concentrations in seeds and grains (including wheat), binds calcium, magnesium, zinc, and copper, and keeps the body from absorbing these important minerals.

Mellanby discovered that the binding of calcium by phytic acid in wheat contributed to rickets in children who ate wheat products (such as those found in cake, cookies, bread and breakfast cereals).

In the same way, the eating of grains (such as wheat) contributes toward the loss of calcium in bones (osteomalacia and osteoporosis).

Because phytic acid binds magnesium to keep it from being absorbed, it must contribute to irregular heartbeats, and all the other signs and symptoms commonly found associated with magnesium deficiencies such as poor appetite (anorexia), nausea, and alternating periods of overactivity and lack of energy.

Both laboratory animals and people have been found to have

deficiencies of both calcium and potassium when magnesium levels are reduced.

Other symptoms commonly found in magnesium deficiency: convulsions in infants, personality changes, and muscle spasms. Magnesium deficiencies (caused in part by eating wheat products) probably contribute to the restlessness, elevated suicide rate, anorexia nervosa, and bulimia that are becoming increasing problems, especially among teenagers and young adults.

Magnesium deficiencies are aggravated by the use of alcoholic beverages.

The low zinc levels encouraged by the binding of zinc into insoluble compounds in the gastrointestinal tract damage the body's immune system and thus make people more susceptible both to infections and cancer.

Because phytic acid from grains and other sources tends to lower copper levels, it may contribute to some forms of anemia. A copper deficiency was found to lower T-cell antigens in rats, which suggests that lower copper levels may contribute to some forms of arthritis, cancer, allergies and a host of other health problems.

A current report from the Memorial Sloan-Kettering Cancer Institute tells of a discovery that calcium added to the diet is protective against cancer of the bowel. Since the phytic acid in grains (including wheat and wheat products) reduces the body's ability to absorb calcium, in all probability the eating of wheat and other foods containing phytic acid increases the incidence of bowel cancer.

Dohan and others from the Medical College of Pennsylvania have repeatedly written papers agreeing with my finding that neuroactive peptides from the gluten in wheat and many other grains produce psychotic schizophrenic symptoms—especially paranoid symptoms—in people with certain commonly found genetic makeups.

In people sensitive to wheat—or its common contaminants—I have seen almost any symptom you can name, from nervousness, high blood pressure, depression, and paranoid ideation to arthritis and asthma.

There's no limit to the amount of dead insect bodies flour may contain. The number of dead insect wings, legs, heads and tails in a loaf of bread is astronomical.

And don't forget that insects are highly allergenic.

The wheat used to make your precious bread—even whole wheat

bread!—your breakfast cereals, your spaghetti and your cake is, by government regulation, allowed to have two *rat* pellets per 1000 grams of wheat, about a quart. (Bear in mind that rat pellets are considerably larger than mouse droppings.)

BON APPETIT!

Tomorrow morning when you're munching your breakfast cereal, don't forget ... somewhere a tribe of rats is rolling in a silo of wheat having belly laughs at the thought of what you're eating for breakfast!

SUMMARY ON WHEAT

I have nothing specific against wheat—other than it brings about vastly more illness than anyone dreams and costs all of us billions of dollars annually to treat and care for its victims. . . .

I only point out wheat's shortcomings to illustrate that meat is not the only food that presents problems.

TO LIVE IS TO COMPROMISE

The truth is, everything in life is a compromise, including food.

If you don't walk, you'll die from inactivity. If you do walk, you run the risk of being struck down by an intoxicated driver. Nevertheless, walking is the better compromise.

Even though mother's milk is radioactive, it is still the best food for human infants.

In spite of what meat has in it, meat might be the best food for your particular chemistry. You need to test and see what your body chemistry tells you about eating meat.

CHAPTER TEN

THE CHOLESTEROL MYTH

The fat-in-food cholesterol-in-the-bloodstream idea is dying hard. During the last decade it has become increasingly evident that the great hope of thirty years ago that heart disease could be controlled by limiting the intake of saturated fat (as in meat and butter) and cholesterol (in meat and eggs) and increasing that of unsaturated fat, especially polyunsaturated fat (margarine, certain vegetable oils) has failed.

LINUS PAULING

CLARK GABLE AND CHOLESTEROL

Things are seldom as they appear. Clark Gable had false teeth, drank heavily, stayed high on Dexedrine uppers and was described by many women as no good in bed.

The nice cereal people from Minneapolis who pay for the nice TV ads telling you their breakfast foods are free of cholesterol have no interest in your good health. They want to slip their hand into your pocket and extract money from you, as much and as often as possible.

The National Heart Association wants your money to pay for "research" that (remarkably!) always discovers what it says is true to be true.

THE PRINCES

Machiavelli wrote a book, *The Prince*, advising princes how to gain power and keep it. He might have written it for the princes of today, the leading pseudoscientists in the field of nutrition and the business leaders of the processed food industry.

> Machiavelli held that survival was the state's overriding aim; this consideration transcends any concern with moral or religious values and the interests of individual subjects.
> MARVIN PERRY AND GEORGE W. BOCK, *Western Civilization*

The princes of the food processing empires have poured forth so much false information about cholesterol that patients have consulted me with lives shattered by anxiety or dying from Crohn's disease or lupus who hesitated to eat red meat because it might raise their cholesterol levels!

What if the Pied Pipers of the food industry lead the human race into Evolution's bottomless pit?

That's not the princes' problem. The princes' problem is to stay in power. To stay in power, the money must keep rolling in.

The golden smiles of the food processing princes have lured scientists and politicians into their embraces.

Did you ever stop to think that the Jolly Green Giant rides to work in a chauffeured limousine?

People will happily die for an idea. If you don't believe me, ask Saint Sir Thomas More.

The two biggest scams in the 20th Century: communism and cholesterol.

Pinckney and Smith

Edward R. Pinckney, M.D., a former editor of the *Journal of the American Medical Association*, and Russell L. Smith, Ph.D., have written an important book about cholesterol, *Diet, Blood Cholesterol and Coronary Heart Disease: A Critical Review of the Literature.**

*(Vector Enterprises, Inc. 13601 Ventura Blvd., Suite 119, Sherman Oaks, CA 91423.)

These two responsible scientists undertook the gargantuan task of reading, reviewing, picking apart and analyzing 1700 scientific articles about cholesterol that appeared in peer-reviewed medical journals. They have given me permission to quote their important conclusions.

> The National Heart, Lung and Blood Institute (NHLBI) and the American Heart Association (AHA) are involved in a massive campaign to convince all Americans that diet is a major cause of high blood cholesterol levels and coronary heart disease (CHD). This report is a comprehensive and critical review of nearly 1700 medical research articles and reports, including food consumption trend studies, dietary cholesterol and fat experiments and clinical trials. In addition, literature relating CHD (coronary heart disease) with alcohol, exercise, aspirin and fish oils is also critically reviewed. Also, a detailed discussion of the effects and potential effects of cholesterol-lowering and cholesterol-lowering agents is presented.
>
> It is concluded that diet is, at best, only negligibly related to CHD (coronary heart disease), particularly for the vast majority of persons. Moreover, all the major epidemiological studies reveal an extremely weak relationship between blood cholesterol and CHD, often showing an increase in annual CHD (coronary heart disease) rate of less than 1% across most or all of the blood cholesterol range. This fact alone indicates that diet cannot possibly have more than a very minor influence on CHD (coronary heart disease).
>
> A major reason why diet and blood cholesterol *appear* to be important determinants of CHD (coronary heart disease) is because data are often presented in unorthodox ways, weak data are often interpreted as "powerful," and numerous reviews of the literature are invariably incomplete and strongly biased. In fact, the majority of relevant literature is either ignored or erroneously cited as supporting the diet-blood cholesterol-CHD (coronary heart disease) relationship. While NHLBI (The National Heart, Lung and Blood Institute) and AHA (American Heart Association) frequently state that the evidence "overwhelmingly" supports the relationship, clearly the reverse is true. It does not seem possible that objective scientists without vested interests could ever interpret the literature as supportive.

Translation: *The scientists who keep beating the drum about cholesterol have been bought off.*

Congressional Record

Read *Congressional Record, United States of America, Proceedings and debates of the 94th Congress, second session*, Vol. 122, no. 125, Aug. 24, 1975. The *Record* says that Frederick Stare, M.D., Ph.D., Professor and Chairman of the Department of Nutrition at Harvard, and many other professors of nutrition, get research money and personal money from food processors. When the government seeks advice, it consults the bought-off professors.

These professors would be the last to sit for a congressional committee hearing or a TV camera, smile and cut off their noses.

Various medical groups—like the American Heart Association—jump onto the shoulders of the cholesterol myth and ask the government and private citizens for money.

On and on the princes will push until eventually an accumulation of hard facts blasts the cholesterol myth and its princes back into Never-Never Land of mythology where they belong.

Already in the news we're hearing that oat products are not the great cholesterol reducers they have been touted. My conventional-thinking sister believed every ad she saw or heard. She died with a catastrophically low HDL of 11%—while clutching pills in one hand and an oatmeal bran muffin in the other!

Cherchez l'Argent

When looking for a criminal, the French police have a motto: *Cherchez la femme.* Translation: Look for the woman.

When trying to find who and what's behind messages about nutrition, I have a saying: *Cherchez l'argent.* Look for the money.

Once our ancestors crawled out of their cave in the morning to face obvious and comparatively harmless foes like saber toothed tigers or a gang of warriors from the other side of the mountain come to bash in their heads and carry off their women and their stone cutlery.

Such were our ancestors' good old-fashioned enemies. Our ancestors expected them. They took precautions against them.

Today, more dangerous enemies stalk us. Like computer viruses, today's unnoticed enemies secretly creep into our minds and deposit ideas that multiply and control us. The false information keeps us smiling as we happily hand over our money and our lives.

AMA

The *Journal of the American Medical Association* published a report on an experiment in which Vilhjalmur Stefansson ate nothing but meat for a year. The article noted that during the year of eating only meat, *Stefansson's cholesterol fell 50 points!*

The *Journal of the American Medical Association* published a study of 4,057 people in Tecumseh, Michigan which revealed no correlation between what people ate and their cholesterol levels.

Roger Williams

> *The evidence shows that high fat consumption, when accompanied by plenty of essential nutrients which all cells need, does not cause atherosclerosis or heart disease.*
>
> ROGER WILLIAMS, PH.D.
> Professor of Biochemistry, University of Texas

No one ever called the late Roger Williams an irresponsible researcher or reporter. No one ever bought him off. For more than a generation this Professor of Biochemistry at the University of Texas, Director of Clayton Foundation Biochemical Institute, University of Texas—President of the American Chemical Society, discoverer of the B vitamin pantothenic acid, pioneer in folic acid research, giver to folic acid the name "folic acid"—reigned as the Grand Old Man in the field of nutrition. In his internationally respected book, *Nutrition Against Disease*, Roger Williams also had this to say about cholesterol:

> How can this deposit of cholesterol be prevented? The most obvious answer is: consume less cholesterol. Superficially this sounds like a good suggestion; actually it is a poor one. Most of our good foods contain substantial amounts of cholesterol,

and if we try to eliminate cholesterol consumption we sacrifice good nutrition. In effect we would throw out the baby with the bath water. Anyone who deliberately avoids cholesterol in his diet may be inadvertently courting heart disease.

As we shall see later, the evidence points to the conclusion that good nutrition, if it is really good, prevents cholesterol deposits from forming, even when our cholesterol consumption is moderately high. We must remember that cholesterol is made within our bodies, and that this homemade cholesterol can be deposited in the arteries of a person who consumes no cholesterol at all. Furthermore, the rate of synthesis of cholesterol in the body is inversely influenced by the available supply of cholesterol from outside (feedback mechanism). Not consuming cholesterol may in effect open the valve which accelerates the production of cholesterol within the body thereby increasing cholesterol synthesis.

Yudkin

Professor John Yudkin of London University has demonstrated that the amount of sugar you eat is much more important in hardening your arteries than the amount of fat you eat.

Also, remember that the vitamins and minerals you will be taking will help lower your cholesterol. Especially important are ascorbic acid, and calcium-magnesium along with cod liver oil and an unsaturated vegetable oil.

Cholesterol is not a problem if you leave alcohol, processed foods, grains, table sugar, and milk products out of your diet.

Random House

Recently (1989) Random House published an important book exposing the cholesterol myth: *Heart Failure, A Critical Inquiry into American Medicine and the Revolution in Heart Care* by Thomas J. Moore.

Elliot Corday, M.D., Clinical Professor of Medicine, UCLA School of Medicine, Los Angeles had this to say about the book:

> This exciting new book should help create a much needed debate on the cholesterol controversy and clarify the legal issues

that are apt to follow. It is irresponsible to force the public
into a costly cholesterol-reducing program without firm scientific
evidence of its effectiveness.

Significantly, Random House published the book. Random
House not only holds a solid reputation as a responsible house but
brings out many books each year sponsored by the American Medical Association.

Atlantic

In the September 1989 *Atlantic*, a respected magazine for intellectu-
als that painstakingly vets its articles, printed an article by Thomas
J. Moore covering the same cholesterol debunking information
found in the book.

Reader's Digest

Even the April 1990 *Reader's Digest*, one of the most conservative magazines on the stands, began debunking the cholesterol
myth.

Pauling and Newbold

Linus Pauling and I agree that the 30.9% reduction of death from
cardiovascular diseases since 1977 comes not from people eating
less fat but from taking more vitamin C.

Linus Pauling in his recent book, *How to Live Longer and Feel
Better*, cites many scientific studies and goes to great length to
debunk the cholesterol myth.

Newbold

I've published two papers showing how cholesterol levels fall on a
meat, animal-fat, vegetable and fruit diet—if certain rules are followed. In 1986 and 1988, the results were published by two respected Medical-Index-listed, peer-reviewed medical journals, the

International Journal for Vitamin and Nutrition Research and the *Southern Medical Association Journal.*

Since 1929 no one else has published studies on patients who follow a diet anywhere near the one I have described.

I know of no other results showing such spectacular results lowering cholesterol levels and at the same time raising HDL levels. (HDL is the "good" fat in the blood, the higher the better.)

Here's the abstract of an article by me published in the *Southern Medical Journal*, January 1988. (For the full article see Appendix B.)

Reducing Serum Cholesterol by Feeding a High Animal Fat Diet

Abstract Multiple food allergies required a group of seven patients with higher than ideal serum cholesterol levels to follow a diet in which most of the calories came from beef fat. They were given nutritional supplements. Their diets contained no sucrose, milk, or grains. So far as the author has been able to learn, this is the only group of people in recent times to follow such a diet.

The triglyceride levels fell in the patients in the study group from an average of 113 mg/dl to 74 mg/dl.

At the same time, the patients in the group had a reduction of serum cholesterol from an average initial value of 263 mg/dl to an average of 189 mg/dl.

At the beginning of the study, patients had an average HDL% of 21. At the end of the study, the six patients retested had HDL% rise to an average of 32.

The findings raise an interesting question: are elevated serum cholesterol levels caused in part not by eating animal fat (an extremely "old food"), but by some factor in grains, sucrose or milk ("new foods") that interferes with cholesterol metabolism?

The *Journal of the American Heart Association* refused to accept the above article. It never takes articles that fail to agree with its thinking.

For Your Peace of Mind

You and your physician can easily test for yourselves and discover whether what I say is true.

Before taking any vitamins or minerals or any other nutritional supplements, and before you start testing or changing your diet in any way, have the following laboratory tests—and any other tests that your physician feels are appropriate:

CBC
routine urine
serum BUN
serum cholesterol
serum triglycerides
high-density lipoprotein (HDL)

Have nothing to eat or drink after 10 P.M. on the night before the tests and have the tests done first thing in the morning at a state approved laboratory.

By having your blood drawn first thing in the morning before you eat or drink, you will have a proper baseline and will later be able to repeat your cholesterol, triglycerides and HDL tests and learn whether they are improving. This will reassure you, your friends and relatives about what happens when you eat a diet high in saturated fat and leave off all grains, table sugar, and milk and milk products.

To calculate your percentage HDL (high density lipoproteins), divide the number for your HDL by the number given for your cholesterol. I prefer HDL percentages above 20. The higher the better. As long as your HDL percentage is high, your cholesterol level is unimportant.

As you follow the program, have your doctor repeat the tests for cholesterol and HDL. Don't forget: it's the percentage of HDL that's important.

FRIENDS AND FAMILY

If you learn eventually that you must eat meat to regain and keep your health, your friends and family will start saying negative things about meat. Have them read this chapter and appendix B several times.

Then ask them if they would like to take over and treat you.

CHAPTER ELEVEN

MEAT, FAT, AND CANCER

You hear and read that diets high in animal fats may give you bowel cancer.

In my view, epidemiologists who suggest this are not paying enough attention to details. For example, they dump all meats and fats together: aged meats, unaged meats, meats with preservatives such as hot dogs and salami, overly browned meats, smoked meats, etc.

They fail to state whether the meats were cooked with gas and thus have picked up hydrocarbons.

They do not measure the vitamin-mineral levels of the people studied, and they do not record the vitamin-mineral intake of their test subjects.

Much of their speculation is based on the positive Aimes test given by burned meats and fats. This test shows that burned fats and meats in high concentrations will cause bacterial cells to mutate. Whether this happens in the human body is not clear. Nevertheless, I strongly agree that burned meats and fats should not be eaten.

Many of the researchers who suggest that meats and fats may be harmful get their research—and sometimes their personal— money from processed food manufacturers who want to discourage meat eating and promote the eating of profitable grain products such as breakfast cereals.

HERE ARE THE FACTS

Statistics show that the diet commonly eaten in Finland is high in animal fat, yet the Finnish population has a low incidence of bowel cancer.

Years of clinical experience and a number of scientific facts have made me conclude that people need not fear a high-meat, high-animal-fat diet if the following facts are kept in mind.

1. Meat should be fresh, unaged, unpreserved; should not be smoked or have nitrates in it.

2. The possible risk from meat and animal fat comes not from the fresh meat and fat itself, but from *oxidized* meat and animal fat. Meat and fat are oxidized in two ways: by aging (exposure to the air) and by browning.

For years I have made the clinical observation that most patients feel best on marbleized fresh meat, such as beef rib steak. One of the reasons is that the central marbleized fat does not easily become oxidized.

For the same reason, meats should be cut thick.

The fat around the center (¼″) edge of the meat should not be eaten. Fats will oxidize if left in the refrigerator unfrozen.

BURNED FATS

The oxidized fat around the edges of meat is suspect if the fat has been burned. Fats (in red meat, chicken, eggs, etc.) oxidize even if refrigerated immediately after cooking. Cooking fats that are kept hot and used repeatedly for French frying—as is too often the case in restaurants—are especially suspect.

Boiling meat briefly gives the least oxidized meat and fat. Boiling is also the fastest—faster even than microwave cooking—and the least expensive. Most people react better to the meat if it is left pink in the center. Pork, however, must be well done.

Some people can tolerate meat only if it is boiled, hence not oxidized. Browned and non-browned fats and meats are two different chemical substances, just as rust and iron are two different chemicals.

Broiling, since it browns the meat, is the more likely to produce oxidized meat and fat. If broiled, meat should be only lightly browned. Any browned or burned sections should be cut away and not eaten.

Pan-frying is the most suspect way to cook meat. That's because the meat is subjected to a high temperature. If you eat pan-fried meat, fry it slowly so it's not burned. If burned, scrape and cut away the burned part.

Some people feel best on raw meat, steak tartare. If you do eat raw meat, it must first be frozen for three days if you want to be certain to avoid tapeworm.

3. Meat *must not* be cooked with gas. Gas is a hydrocarbon. Gas gets into meat, especially into the fat, if it is used in cooking. Hydrocarbons have long been known to cause cancer.

4. Much research indicates that adequate amounts of vitamins A, C, carotene, choline, E, folic acid, zinc and selenium are especially protective against cancer. Now vitamin B_6 has been added to the list. Scientific papers continue to stress this important fact, as evidenced, for example, by two current studies completed at Louisiana State University Medical Center and Massachusetts Institute of Technology. A recent study from Memorial Sloan-Kettering Cancer Institute showed that a generous intake of calcium also tends to protect against cancer.

CHAPTER TWELVE

FOOD INCOMPATIBILITIES AND YOUR NERVES

Suppose you walked into the office of a typically well-trained doctor and complained of vague symptoms like depression, listlessness, anxiety. (He's the one likely to call them "vague"; to you they're very concrete.)

Two centuries ago, the doctor would have bled you. One century ago, he would have doled out a laxative. Today, the physician is "more sophisticated": he'll prescribe a "tranquilizer" or an "antidepressant," or both.

Almost surely he will not ask about your diet or test you for allergies.

Although your physician may not be aware of it, the relationship between food allergies and emotional illness has been known for thousands years.

As with so many medical discoveries, Hippocrates—the "Father of Medicine"—led the way in the fourth century B.C. Here's his description of a classical attack of cyclic food allergy:

> Such persons, provided they take dinner when it is not their wont, immediately become heavy and inactive, both in the body and in the mind, and are weighed down with yawning, slumbering, and thirst; and if they take supper in addition, they are seized with flatulence, tormina, and diarrhea, and to many this has been the commencement of a serious disease, when they

have merely taken twice a day the same food which they have
been in the custom of taking once.

As early as 1621, the famous English savant Robert Burton, in
his classic, *The Anatomy of Melancholy*, flatly declared: "Milk and
all that comes from milk increases melancholy."

Since Burton's day, similar observations have been made by physicians of many nations. Reports of psychological reactions caused
by allergies began to proliferate in the 1870s and continue to this
day. Yet the psychological symptoms produced by allergies are
largely ignored by our medical schools. Even the best physicians
instantly think of allergies in terms of "pollen" when you sneeze
in summer, "dust" when you wheeze, or "shellfish allergy" when
they see your face pops out with hives after a lobster dinner. Allergists do not understand food allergies.

Not many physicians consider allergies when you slump into a
depression or threaten to punch your mate without apparent
reason.

I myself thought little about the link between allergies and emotions until a quarter of a century ago. That was when I saw a film
made by Dr. Theron Randolph in a patient's room at Chicago's
Wesley Memorial Hospital, one of the teaching hospitals associated
with the Northwestern University School of Medicine where I once
taught. Since seeing the film, I've tested every new patient for allergic reactions to learn what role allergies play in his or her life. The
results have been dramatic and usually very helpful.

The film I saw showed a doctor talking with a young woman
who appeared calm, poised, and thoroughly in control of herself.
The doctor then inserted a tube through her nose into her stomach.
Standing behind her, he could introduce solutions of foods through
the tube. This method ruled out any possibility that visual suggestion could influence her reactions.

I watched the doctor squirt in the first food. He then returned
to the front of the bed and chatted with the patient for a few
minutes. She remained composed.

After enough time had passed to be certain no reaction would
occur, the doctor again walked around to the other side of the bed.
Out of the patient's sight, he injected a solution of corn through
the stomach tube.

Within minutes, the woman began striking at him. She threw herself off the bed. Struggling with the nurse and attendants, she tried to force her way out of the room. She shouted and argued. No one could reason with her. In short, she displayed psychotic behavior.

This anger and loss of control continued for four days, then ended as quickly as it began. The woman snapped out of her confused state. She had no idea that most of a week had passed since she lost contact with reality.

The history revealed that the woman had consulted the doctor because she suffered periodic psychotic spells.

After the diagnostic workup, part of which I saw in the movie, the patient was taken off the foods to which she was allergic. She was completely freed of her attacks, and able to live a normal life.

Another film showed a patient who could be thrown into convulsions simply by introducing certain common foods into her body.

Like all physicians, I had known something about food allergies, but the subject had not particularly interested me. The field of allergy is complex and full of controversy. Most physicians push the subject to the back of their minds. After seeing these films, however, I could no longer ignore allergic reactions, nor could I allow my patients to ignore them.

I Carry Out My Own Tests

To learn more about the relationship between allergies and emotional symptoms, I did a study in which I examined my patients for multiple food and chemical sensitivities by giving provocative tests after a four-day fast. Later, when I learned more about provocative allergy testing, I tested non-fasting patients by feeding them one food at a time.

The symptoms induced by these tests varied from arthritis to high blood pressure to a slight itching of the skin to depression to full-blown psychotic attacks. One patient cried all afternoon after a test for milk sensitivity. Another, when tested for tobacco, suddenly turned on her mother with a savage verbal attack that lasted half an hour.

A young man, discovered to be sensitive to sugar and wheat, cheated on his diet by eating a piece of apple pie à la mode. Shortly, he began to hallucinate. He turned delusional and went into an uncontrollable rage. A strong tranquilizer was needed to calm him down. After sleeping for eight hours, he awoke composed.

The next chapter will be devoted to discussing allergy testing techniques.

Resistance

Sometimes patients resist treatment because the foods to which they are allergic are the ones they like best. These foods actually give the patient a lift, or a "rush," a feeling of well-being not experienced with other foods. After some time they slide off the "lift" and plunge into a depression or some other emotional symptom such as nervousness or irritability. The eventual result is a vicious cycle: the hills and valleys of allergic addictions.

ALLERGIES AND ORDINARY TENSION AND DEPRESSION

With food and environmental allergies, patients' reactions need not be ones in which they become uncontrollably angry, or begin hallucinating. They may have none of the rashes or trouble breathing that we ordinarily associate with allergic reactions. The patient may only feel tired or depressed, or be unable to sleep. Possibly he will only get in a "bad mood" or want to be alone. Patients may have any of a number of other symptoms often labeled "neurotic" for lack of proper understanding.

As a rule, the general allergic reactivity level becomes milder or disappears after patients are given a diet free of items to which they're allergic and placed on adequate vitamins and other nutritional supplements.

But the reverse is also often true: Poor nutrition (a diet containing much sugar and wheat and other items to which the patient is allergic, a diet low in minerals and vitamins) leads to more and more allergic reactions.

Poor nutrition often contributes to the serious condition known as allergic addictions.

Food Addictions

What's your very favorite food: ice cream, chocolate, coffee, bread, cheesecake, milk?

Decide which is your absolute favorite, then ask yourself how often you eat it—every day, every second or third day? And now here's the clincher: What happens when you don't have it? Do you become nervous, irritable, or depressed?

If the answer is yes, you suffer from a food addiction. You may be every bit as hooked as an alcoholic or heroin addict.

Betty Does Cake

To help you understand food addictions, let me tell you about an advanced case, a patient we'll call Betty. Betty was a nurse with a long history of depression and unsatisfactory love relationships. She had been in continual psychoanalytical therapy for nine years. Her current analyst, whom she had been seeing for five years, sent her to me because she was not making progress. He wondered whether I had anything to offer her. (For an "orthodox" psychoanalyst to consider the possibility of contributory physical factors was once an unusual feat of open mindedness but gradually analysts are recognizing that biochemistry can strongly influence emotional illnesses.)

Betty was a bright, intelligent woman with a master's degree in her field. Despite her obesity, she was quite attractive. Like many well-read people, she was certain that Freudian analysis had the answer to her problems. She saw symptoms as being totally separate from body chemistry. This inappropriate dichotomy of mind and body is a concept many people find difficult to set aside. For some reason it becomes a religion, a keystone in their personal philosophy and approach to life.

Her basic complaints were obesity, the inability to form meaningful relationships, a great deal of suppressed anger, and chronic depression. In short, she was a lonely, withdrawn woman trying to keep the lid on the seething cauldron of her rage over being unable to get the things she felt she deserved from life.

Every waking hour of every day, she waged an unceasing battle to control her voracious hunger. On Saturday nights, for example, she would be determined to stick with her diet. She would have a modest dinner, and sip tea while watching TV.

By eleven or twelve, however, she found herself growing uncontrollably restless and irritable.

She intentionally kept everything out of her apartment that could make her gain weight. Eventually, after a vain struggle with herself, she'd grab up her dog, rush out of the building, and try to make it to the neighborhood delicatessen before it closed.

As often as not, she got there too late. She would then take a cab and set off across the city, feverishly trying to locate two or three chocolate cakes. Sometimes she was desperate enough to drive from one restaurant to another, buying whole chocolate cakes, but having to pay for them by the slice.

On the way home she would begin eating. Often she had finished a cake and a half by the time she reached her apartment. Once there, she poured herself a glass of wine and polished off the remainder of the cake.

During this process her restlessness gradually subsided, until, some $145 lighter and 15,000 calories heavier, she was once more the kindly social worker whom everyone admired at the clinic where she worked. After watching a few minutes of a late TV movie, she would go to bed and practically pass out in a coma.

The Morning After

When she awakened late Sunday morning, she would invariably be in what she described as her "black sack of depression." She felt as if her apartment had turned into a black plastic bag into which no ray of light could penetrate. She would be stifling hot, and filled with a sense of utter hopelessness, a feeling that she had been totally abandoned and was no longer a member of the human race. Sensitive and cultivated person that she was, she could only abhor the memory of the cake-gorging tub of lard she had been the night before.

Only half-conscious, she would drag through the day, locate another chocolate cake, eat dinner, and have a second cake afterwards. Slowly the black depression gave way as the familiar state of hazy well-being enveloped her once again, enabling her to spend a few peaceful hours watching TV with her dog.

Of course by the next morning the depression was sitting on her chest smothering her again, but now it was Monday. She had to face a full working day. To get herself together, she downed a cup of thick hot chocolate fortified with milk and sugar. On the way to the clinic she wolfed down several chocolate cookies. These gave her enough of a lift (a large enough "fix") to enable her to function until the midmorning break, during which she ate half a package of—you guessed it—chocolate cookies.

A CLASSIC

Betty is a pitiful example of someone suffering from an advanced case of food addiction. Food addictions are quite common. Fortunately most of them haven't advanced this far. Betty, in case the parallel has escaped you, would be a full-blown alcoholic if her addiction were to alcohol rather than to specific foods.

Tests

Betty was instructed about how to perform a series of allergy tests at home. In Betty's case symptoms weren't long in coming. She responded violently to milk, sugar, chocolate, and wheat.

The test for milk gave her a reaction that almost reached the stage of hallucination. She felt she had left her body and was floating around the room, bobbing against the ceiling.

Because the reaction frightened her, she asked that we do the remaining tests in our office.

The test for chocolate produced a marked lift. She began babbling nonstop, punctuated by inappropriate giggling. After about ten minutes she came crashing down into a depression. She began weeping and, between sobs, bemoaned the desolation of her life.

While testing for wheat sensitivity, she was leafing through a magazine. Moments after she ate wheat, she was no longer able to follow the story she had been reading. She felt confused, disoriented, unable to think clearly.

Does Betty Turn Into a Cinderella?

You might think that the results of the tests would convince anyone to avoid the offending foods.

Unfortunately, breaking addictions isn't that simple.

Addictions are among the strongest forces in the universe. They rank up there with gravity and atomic power. Addictive forces are often stronger than the desire for beauty or good health, stronger than the drive for sex, stronger than the need for security and honor, even stronger than the will to live.

My first discussion with Betty about the results of her tests appeared to be productive. She agreed that she suffered from multiple food allergies, that she craved precisely those foods to which she was allergic and that she craved them to the point of addiction.

She understood that basically her problem with food addictions was the same as those of alcoholics and heroin addicts.

Betty made the same resolutions we hear from people addicted to alcohol or heroin.

When I told her that she could only beat the addictions by absolutely cutting out the food to which she had allergic addictions, she argued that she couldn't cut them out all at once.

She *absolutely* promised, however, to gradually cut down on those foods and to gradually cut them off entirely.

She sounded exactly like the alcoholic who vows to have only a couple of drinks an evening from now on, or the three-pack-a-day smoker who's going to reduce his cigarettes to two packs, then one, then none.

Those of us engaged in clinical medicine know that such plans guarantee disaster.

The alcoholic follows the regime for perhaps a week or two. The tensions build up. Then some little things goes wrong, and in his overwrought state his problem becomes the straw that breaks the camel's back. He says to hell with it and drinks a whole bottle of whiskey, practically in one gulp.

The same thing happens to the chain smoker. We all know him—the guy who gives up smoking on the first of every month.

And So It Goes . . .

After two weeks Betty returned to tell her story. She had drastically cut down on chocolate cake for a week. Then she went to her parents' home for a holiday. Her mother welcomed her with the usual huge chocolate cake, and insisted that her little girl have a nice big helping of her favorite homemade ice cream along with it.

The milk in the ice cream plus the wheat, sugar, and chocolate in the cake jettisoned Betty into orbit. After a few agonizingly restless hours with her parents, she gave an excuse to leave, jumped into a cab, and began one of her frantic cake hunts. By the time she returned to her apartment, she had gorged herself until she was nearly out of her head. In a stupor, she collapsed across the bed.

A New Start

Betty and I had a long talk about her addictions. She agreed that I had been right. SImply cutting down on addictive foods wouldn't work. She would simply have to do as I said and absolutely cut them out.

She got through two days, then took off on another monumental eating spree.

At the time of her next visit, she again tried to argue that her problems were really psychological, not allergies at all. She was going to make an appointment with a new therapist.

They Also Serve Who Stand and Wait

The new therapist would probably be telling Betty that her eating orgies were an outlet for her aggressions, plus a symbolic representation of her wish to be nurtured by a loving mother.

Sadly, I had no choice but to wait for Betty to fail again.

After several weeks Betty telephoned to say that the new therapist wasn't helping her. She was going to a highly recommended psychiatrist to be put on medication.

I tried to talk her out of it, but of course I got nowhere. The psychiatrist would give her antidepressants, and/or tranquilizers. They wouldn't solve her problem.

The Return of the Prodigal

Two months later, Betty returned to see me. In tears she told me about her new failure. Would I give her another chance?

She agreed to use the method most frequently successful in breaking food addictions. A five- to seven-day fast.

FASTS CAN BE TOUGH

In view of the hardships involved in fasting, and the strength of her addictions, I wasn't too optimistic about the outcome in Betty's case, but it had to be tried.

People like Betty are physically (biochemically) addicted to foods. When they stop eating the foods to which they're addicted, they become just as sick as a drug addict who stops taking his drug. They have withdrawal symptoms. Profound chemical changes take place in the body's cells.

Experiments have shown that if you deliberately addict artificially grown tissue to hard narcotics, then cut off the narcotic supply, under the microscope you can actually see the cells change. Withdrawal can cause any symptoms you can imagine—all the way from confusion and hallucinations to back pain and headache, to diarrhea and vomiting.

Betty Fasted

As expected, the moment the withdrawal symptoms surfaced Betty became extremely restless and depressed and had a strong sense of impending doom. These symptoms continued almost unabated through the second day of the fast. The third day was not quite so bad. By the fourth day she felt a great deal better. When I saw her on the fifth day, she was cheerful and pleasant and had regained her energy.

Once more I urged Betty to stay away entirely from foods that were so clearly disastrous for her. She promised. I crossed my fingers.

Final Chapter

At first, Betty kept her word. But, like so many addicts, after a few weeks she began experimenting with small amounts of the forbidden foods.

After a fast, as I have mentioned, many patients' general sensitivity levels are reduced, so that for a while they may get away with eating some of the addictive foods in small quantities.

Eventually, however—like the heroin addict who starts back with "only a Saturday night fix"—such piecemeal return to the addictive substances is always disastrous. Inevitably the patient increases the quantity, begins to experience small elevations in mood and as a result continues to increase the intake of the foods to achieve the desired high.

And that, as you may have guessed, is what happened to Betty. Gradually, the unfortunate woman returned to her former eating habits, and was soon back at her midnight rambles to buy chocolate cake. Once more she became submerged in the vicious cycle of depression, elation, anxiety, and withdrawal.

Only after a near-fatal suicide attempt did Betty finally face the facts: either she would have to follow her diet, or die. Happily, when the cards were finally down, she chose to live.

MILDER REACTIONS

To make a point, I've been writing about a patient with a severe emotional illness. A vast range of lesser emotional symptoms, however, is also caused by allergies. Ninety-nine percent of my patients suffer from simple depressions, anxiety, phobias, asthma, backache, high blood pressure, migraine headaches, and dozens of other such troubles. Those symptoms are usually the result of food and/or environmental allergies and those patients recover just as dramatically as those with more serious conditions.

AND REMEMBER

Food allergies are by no means the only dangers. You can also be allergic to alcohol, tobacco, drugs, air pollution, plastics, fluorescent lights, and a variety of other common things that surround you.

THE RUSH

Don't forget that you can get a "rush," a "high" from foods to which you are allergic. I'm reminded of one patient—a well-known TV star—who knew that eating candy would give him a high for approximately two hours. If at the end of that period he ate a wheat product, he not only forestalled the letdown, but added a boost to his high. Two hours later he had to smoke at least three cigarettes to keep the high going. He continued that way throughout the day, day after day, riding the crest of his allergies.

There was only one problem; finally he would crash and his allergies would no longer give him a high. At that point he tailspun into a depression. Once we got him away from the things to which he was allergic, he lost his depression—and learned that he could "psych" himself into a high before going on the air. He gets along very well without his allergic highs.

Winston Churchill drank a quart of brandy a day to keep going, and of course his addiction to cigars became a hallmark. Obviously he rode his addictions a long way, but I've been told by those who knew him that he often lost his highs and plunged into the blackest of depressions.

But the Churchills of the world are few. For most allergic people, there comes a point when they can no longer control their addictions.

TWO MORE SHORT HISTORIES OF ALLERGIC PATIENTS

Mrs. Bradley was a forty-three-year-old woman who consulted me after visiting a psychiatrist twice a week for six years. The psychiatrist had not been able to relieve her nearly disabling symptoms: bouts of palpitations. She had also consulted a cardiologist, who agreed that she was prone to attacks of excessively fast heartbeats. The cardiologist told her she was "nervous," and prescribed a tranquilizer. The tranquilizer only made her sleepy.

My routine tests showed her to be deficient in vitamin B_{12}, a condition rather frequently seen in people with severe allergies. (Because the inability to absorb vitamin B_{12} is often an inherited disorder, I make it a policy to test blood relatives of any patient with a lower serum B_{12} level. Each of Mrs. Bradley's three children had low serum B_{12} levels—one at 0!)

A careful history established that her palpitation attacks were especially troublesome at three locations: when she went into her basement, where the gas-burning furnace was located; when she was in her kitchen, cooking on a gas stove, and when she was in her car, driving in heavy, slow-moving traffic.

On each of these occasions she was exposed to high levels of hydrocarbons: from the gas-burning furnace, from the gas stove in the kitchen as well as the smoke of frying foods, and from automobile exhausts so common in slow, dense traffic.

With a patient such as this, it's sometimes impractical if not impossible to do everything necessary to avoid hydrocarbons. But at least the exposure to them can be greatly reduced. An offending gas furnace can be vented by a special fan, or relocated in the garage. In Mrs. Bradley's case, her symptoms were greatly reduced by simply having her avoid the basement as much as possible, and opening the basement windows to improve the ventilation there.

Her gas stove was replaced by an electric range, and a hood was installed to ventilate the stove area. She was told to avoid frying foods, and advised to get an air purifier for her car.

This regimen (together with injections of vitamin B_{12}) resulted in a disappearance of Mrs. Bradley's attacks of palpitations.

As a bonus, she also became more energetic, and lost much of her former tension and depression.

Need I tell you that she dropped her psychiatrist?

AND THESE WAS HAROLD

Harold was a thirty-year-old who for nine months had been suffering from a fluttering in his chest, from lightheadedness, numbness in his left arm, and from periods of great anxiety. He feared he was about to have a heart attack.

Several cardiologists had given him extensive tests and told him that he was "only nervous."

His dietary habits left a good deal to be desired. It turned out that because he was divorced and didn't like to cook, he had been living on canned junk foods and TV dinners.

I gave him a computerized psychological test—the Minnesota Multiple Personality Inventory (MMPI). The printout stated:

> This patient appears to be tense, anxious, and chronically worried. He may complain of physical symptoms which are closely related to his tension. He attempts to control his anxiety by compulsive orderliness and by overconcern with his physical complaints. Although these complaints are more frequently imagined than real, frequent demands for reassurance and medical care may be anticipated. This personality pattern is likely to remain stable and be quite resistant to charge.

The computer interpreted the patient's symptoms as being "functional" in nature. That is, the computer said that Harold's physical symptoms were caused by psychological problems.

Of course the computer made the same mistake made by the rest of the medical profession. That's because the computer was programmed by a psychologist who knows little about vitamin deficiencies, or hypoglycemia or food allergies.

I don't mean to say that the test is of no value; it's quite useful in illustrating the degree of a patient's suffering. The computer simply fails to point out the real cause of the patient's suffering.

A six-hour glucose tolerance test revealed that Harold had marked hypoglycemia. At the end of three hours his blood sugar fell to 40 mg percent (55 mg percent is normal). At that time many of his symptoms surfaced.

Allergy tests revealed him to be sensitive to wheat, milk, and corn. (I might add that corn is in the same food family as cane sugar. Often there is a cross sensitivity. This sensitivity may make the blood sugar go down even if there is nothing wrong with insulin metabolism.)

Harold was put on vitamins, mineral supplements, and a diet free of the foods to which he was sensitive.

When he returned for his next check-up, he reported a change for the worse during the three or four days following the change in his diet. After that his symptoms rapidly disappeared. He was pleased with his progress.

ALLERGIES AND HYPOGLYCEMIA

Hypoglycemia and food allergies always go hand in hand, and both these conditions as a rule are accompanied by mineral and vitamin deficiencies.

It is my strong impression that the whole complex of allergies, emotional disorders, and hypoglycemia constitutes a syndrome caused by a defect or breakdown of enzyme systems, a failure of the body's cellular chemistry.

Basically, such disorders are hereditary. Harold, for example, reported a strong family history of allergy and diabetes. Hypoglycemia often precedes diabetes. However, the fact that it is an inherited disorder does not mean that nothing can be done for those who suffer from it. Such patients need special diets and vitamin and mineral supplements. Sometimes they also need hormones, as indicated by the individual tests.

With this kind of support they can usually lead normal lives, indeed, more than normal lives. Many of these people are unusually intelligent and creative, and have the capacity to contribute a great deal to our world.

IN SUMMARY

Vitamin and mineral deficiencies, allergies and allergic food addictions cause almost all of the emotional (and the majority of physical) troubles seen in our society.

Sadly, their diagnosis is almost universally missed even by well trained physicians.

Do you wonder that I feel duty-bound to write books about it?

In my opinion any psychiatrist—any physician—who does not test for vitamins and minerals, and test for food and environmental allergies is badly neglecting his patients.

He is fighting illness with one and a half hands tied behind his back.

There's a place for medication, but only after the cells are given ideal nutrition and an ideal, allergy-free environment and still fail to recover—and that rarely happens.

CHAPTER THIRTEEN

THE ART AND SCIENCE OF ALLERGY TESTING

EVERYBODY LIKES TESTS

Patients like tests. Tests sound so modern, so scientific, so definitive. A doctor who does tests must be up-to-date. He gives the patient confidence. When some naive, potential new patients call for an appointment to see me and learn that I don't perform the usual type of allergy tests, they may decline to see me.

Insurance companies like tests. The clerks who decide on whether to make payments can look tests up on a chart and know exactly what's been done and how much to pay.

When I tell an insurance company that I only talked with a patient, they're left confused.

Doctors like tests. Tests help pay their rent and get their children through college. I can well understand why my colleagues turn red in the face with fury when they hear me say that tests for allergies are nonsense. When I stopped doing allergy tests in the office, my income fell 50%.

And test reports give doctors something definite to hold onto in the complex and uncertain world of biology. Then too, if the doctor gets sued, he can take the tests to court and show them to the jury. They'll help prove his case.

THE TRUTH ABOUT TESTS

Few tests are definitive. You can perform a simple test on the blood and learn whether or not a patient is anemic. No question about it.

What if, however, you test the blood for calcium? The laboratory does the test and reports a number. But in terms of helping the patient, what does it mean? Certainly the test tells whether the blood has a normal amount of calcium in it, but that's about all.

For example, the test doesn't say whether the calcium is normal because the blood is stealing calcium from the bones and leaving them depleted.

ALLERGY TESTS ARE EVEN MORE INDEFINITE

The other day I saw a patient who can eat peaches and not have an allergic reaction so long as the peaches are not quite ripe. If a peach is fully ripe, she gets a headache.

Red delicious apples put me to sleep, but I have no trouble with yellow delicious apples—unless they've been stored too long and the chemical preservatives used on them have penetrated too deep.

At the moment I get a stomach ache from the Granny Smith apples I buy at a Korean fruit market on Third Avenue; however, I do well on the Granny Smith apples I buy at the Food Emporium on Lexington Avenue.

Some patients can eat potatoes grown in Maine, but not those grown in Idaho—or the other way around.

I have a patient in Philadelphia who can eat nothing but pork—but if she eats short ribs of pork her face and hands swell from an allergic reaction.

SHOW BIZ

Can you understand why I say allergy tests are great show biz, but have little to do with helping a patient get well?

You can forget about skin tests and blood tests for allergies. They hide the diagnosis more than they reveal it.

Skin tests are not an accurate way to diagnose food allergies—a fact you can verify by consulting most textbooks on allergy.

Even if the skin does react abnormally to a substance, this does not necessarily mean that the central nervous system, or the joints, or the blood vessels, or any other part of the body will react the same way. For example, the skin on your hands may be sensitive to a brand of soap and break out in a rash. But that doesn't mean you will necessarily also become depressed as a reaction to the soap.

I introduce the food (or other substances that I suspect of being allergenic) directly into the body itself. Then I observe the reaction of the whole system; I don't merely look for a local reaction such as a rash. Especially I look for a reaction in the central nervous system—such as unusual behavior, cluttered thinking, or changes in mood. Other reactions may include abdominal pain, headache, joint pains, a rise in blood pressure, muscular pain—almost any symptom you can name.

THE TWO STEPS IN DIAGNOSING AN ALLERGY

A careful history is the essential first step in diagnosing an allergy.

The trouble with taking a good history is that it uses up the doctor's time, his most precious commodity. Isn't it obvious that the doctor will make more money if he employs three technicians to give allergy tests? He will not pay the technicians as much as they charge the patients. Some of the extra money goes to pay overhead and some of it goes into the doctor's pocket.

My second step in diagnosing an allergy is to expose the patient to the questionable substances and observe what happens.

If you suspect that a patient is allergic to red delicious apples, have the patient eat a red delicious apple and see if he gets hives or becomes depressed.

If you suspect a patient is allergic to molds, have the patient visit a mold-smelly basement and find out if the patient develops symptoms.

(Admittedly, to give the maximum information, exposures must be made in certain controlled ways. More about that shortly.)

IS IT POSSIBLE TO TEST YOURSELF FOR ALLERGIES?

Yes, but first check with your doctor and get his permission. If you're suffering from tuberculosis or diabetes, or taking certain medications—to give only several examples—you must have your doctor's permission and must have your tests supervised by your physician.

If he's not familiar with food challenges, your doctor will probably try to talk you into using a different method.

Don't allow him to.

Feeding one food at a time is the Rolls-Royce of food tests.

Your doctor may try to talk you out of fasting or testing foods one by one. Unless he has a very compelling reason why you shouldn't, then stick by your guns. Tell him you want his help, not his ridicule.

CELERY?

If you discover you tolerated celery, you will have made a discovery of little importance. Eating only celery, you will fade away and die of starvation. If, however, you discover that you tolerate a red meat, you have made an important discovery. A rib steak, and/or other red meats, will satisfy your hunger and take you far down the day's road. Thus rib steaks can keep you going while you test other foods at your leisure.

Also, in my experience, after eating rib steaks for a short time, people found rib steaks acceptable to eat day after day. In addition, people's biochemistries tend to tolerate meats well even if eaten frequently. When people eat a vegetable or fruit repeatedly, they often begin to react unfavorably to it. If you can find a meat that you tolerate well, the entire process of testing moves along faster and easier.

LEAST REACTIVE FOODS

Patients often say, "Why test beef rib steaks? I never eat beef rib steaks."

If you suffer from tension or depression or unpleasant thoughts or any other emotional difficulty, something has been injuring your biochemistry. Probably it's an ordinary food that you eat frequently that makes you ill. You need to test foods that you commonly avoid; then, if they pass the test, put those foods into your diet and take out those foods which you usually eat.

After your symptoms disappear, you can start returning the old foods one by one and record how your body chemistry votes.

Write everything in a notebook so you can refer back to it.

Beef is not beef

Of the patients I see in my office, the highest percentage have bio-chemistries that tolerate mid-rib beef steak the best. Most people in the field of medicine think beef is beef. Not so. Different cuts of beef taste different. That means that the different cuts are biochemically different. The body chemistry handles each cut in an individual way. Beef deckle is only half an inch from the rib steak, yet most people become ill if they eat the deckle. Some of the inner fat on the steak must be eaten along with the lean. People eating a large amount of meat and fat must drink at least a quart and a half of water a day.

About 85% of the people I see thrive on beef rib steaks, but 15% of them find they contribute to their illness. I had one patient who could only eat a common brand of chicken, and, as if some Cossacks had once climbed into his family tree, I once had a patient a nice Jewish man from Staten Island who could only tolerate pork.

None of us knows what genes may have sneaked into our family tree in the year 5351 B.C. or 1281 A.D. Your grandmothers weren't always sweet old ladies. No one can know all about the biochemistry he has inherited. That's why foods, one by one, must be cross-matched against your particular biochemistry.

Here is a list of meats that my patients *tend* to tolerate. The first on the list is tolerated best, by about 85% of my patients. We go down the list and end with chicken. Only about 40% of my patients can eat chicken and remain symptom-free.

Best tolerated meats

beef rib steak
filet mignon (problem: not much fat on it.)
porterhouse steak
chuck steak
breast of veal
veal chops

veal kidney
pork loin
pork chops
buffalo rib steaks
rabbit
lamb shoulder
oily fish, such as salmon, halibut, cod, etc.
rock cornish hens
chicken (dark meat)
chicken (white meat)
turkey
duck

Poorly tolerated meats

calf liver
beef liver
beef short ribs
pork short ribs
sirloin steak
non-center cut rib steak
strip steak
preserved meats such as ham and bacon
luncheon meats
sausage

Poorly tolerated other foods

wheat, wheat, wheat!
other grains except rice
table sugar
milk and milk products (except sweet butter)
all seasonings
rice
fructose (fruit sugar)
nuts
beans
all canned, frozen, processed foods

BUYING MEATS

When you buy meats for testing—or, later, for eating—you should accept only fresh meat. The beef must be pink—not red—and look and smell fresh. When you shake the meat it should be limber, not stiff. Do not buy meat packaged in plastic.

Get all the information possible about the meat. Ask the butcher whether he sells hung or cryovaced beef.

"Hung meat" is skewered on hooks and taken to the wholesaler in refrigerated trucks, where it's cut up and delivered to butchers.

At the point of origin, they cut "cryovaced meat" into sections, place it in plastic sacks, seal the sacks and remove the air. They then chill the meat, pack it in cardboard boxes and ship it to the wholesaler in refrigerated trucks.

Some people do well on hung beef. Others are happy only when eating cryovaced beef.

Ask about the origin of the beef. Some patients do best on New Jersey beef, others feel miserable on it and can only manage mid-western IBP beef. Many feel best on Colorado beef. Sometimes the breed of cattle makes a difference. For example, my biochemistry's at its best when I eat mid rib steaks from Black Angus cattle. Surprisingly, most patients who consult me react poorly to "organic beef," beef grown without the use of hormones and chemicals. I suspect patients do not thrive on "organic beef" because the beef has little fat in it and it's aged to make it more tender.

If you plan to keep meat for more than a day, wrap it in a heavy duty aluminum foil (dull side against the meat) and freeze it. To keep the meat from aging and oxidizing, cook the meat while it's still frozen. Remove the foil before cooking. Heated foil sometimes causes trouble. Do not use foil to catch the drippings.

Some people react poorly to beef if it's too young, i.e., the meat is only a day or two old. Such people need to wrap the meat in aluminum foil (dull side against the meat) and leave it in the refrigerator for a day or two before freezing it, or eating it.

COOKING MEATS

Although evidence that mankind's association with fire goes back 600,000 years, anthropologists believe that cooking became fashionable only 40 to 50 thousand years ago, during the Würm glaciation when our European ancestors needed fire to keep warm.

For a time I wondered why we prefer cooked meat. Gradually it dawned on me that browned meats have been caramelized: they are sweeter and hence appeal to our inborn desire for sweets.

Foods that must be cooked—such as grains and beans—are new foods and thus tend to be among those that cause many biochemical incompatibilities and much sickness. Our bodies cannot use "new foods" for growth, repair or energy unless they are cooked. Eating raw wheat or rice will only give you abdominal distress.

Our biochemistry can easily use raw meats, fish and fowl. Sushi (raw fish) bars are popular here in New York. Steak tartar (raw ground beef) graces menus at the most expensive restaurants. People who say that they would never eat raw beef have eaten steaks cooked medium or rare. The pink meat in the center of steaks cooked medium or rare means that the meat in the center is in fact raw.

Like everything else in nutrition, people vary in the way their individual biochemistries react to different amounts of cooking. The highest percentage of people have biochemistries compatible with raw meat or meat cooked rare or medium.

CROSSMATCHING MEATS

Blood tests, skin tests and other laboratory tests will not tell veterinarians what to feed a giant panda. Also, such tests will not tell you which foods to eat and which to avoid. Laboratory tests will not tell you which food will give you gas, diarrhea, hives or insomnia. Blood tests, skin tests and other laboratory tests for food intolerance are glitzy, but only pseudoscientific medical show biz. We have more than a hundred thousand genes in our bodies and each gene may influence multiple biochemical combinations. Most of our biochemistry is far too complicated to test in the laboratory. Only specific trials can tell us which foods we can thrive on and thus how to cure our illnesses.

Often crossmatching is just going forward with great care to find compatible foods. Probably pandas do not breed successfully in this country because the soil where we grow bamboo has a different chemical composition from the soil in China. Our bodies, and undoubtedly the bodies of pandas, can discover differences that laboratories cannot identify. I have one patient who tested more than 75 different waters before finding one she could drink without reacting to it. I've seen patients who thrive on potatoes grown in Maine, but do poorly on Idaho-grown potatoes, and vice versa.

To Speed Testing

Testing moves along faster and more successfully if patients first test meats, the meats least likely to give an unfavorable reaction.

Do not take or do anything or test anything without your physician's approval

---

When testing meats, eat about one part of the center fat to six parts of lean. People should avoid luncheon meats, preserved meats (like bacon) and old meats such as that found in hot dogs and salami.

Test (crossmatch) meats first by eating one meat at a time. Test only once a day, either at lunch or dinner. The rest of the day have the foods you usually eat. Do not test at breakfast or near bedtime.

Have nothing to eat for 2 hours before or 2 hours after the test meal. You should have no flavoring on the meat, not even salt. You may drink water with the test meal. Do not drink the water you use to boil the meat.

If the test meal gives you no side effects, or if you have only mild side effects, test the same meat once again the next day. Do not reheat meat. Reheating oxidizes fat. Oxidized fat gives multiple problems.

People unaccustomed to eating a meat-only meal usually do not know how to judge when they've had enough. You know the nice solid, full feeling you get after a spaghetti meal, or after eating apple pie à la mode. You don't get that feeling after meat. You can easily eat too much meat and later feel nauseated.

Best solution: eat half of the rib steak at the first test meal. Wrap the other half in heavy duty aluminum foil (dull side against the meat) and refrigerate it. Then on the next day for the second test meal, eat the meat cold.

Do not eat the beef deckle, a tough outer part next to the rib. (Ask your butcher to point it out to you.) Most people react poorly to it. Later, much later after you have regained your health and have become a sophisticated tester and observer, test the deckle if you wish. (Incidentally, it's not a good idea to feed the deckle to your pet. I've had patients with dogs that become sick from eating deckle.)

THE MATHEMATICS OF TESTING

Because it's compatible with the highest percentage of biochemistries, first test a mid-rib rib steak. Have it cut 1¼ inches thick. Thickly cut meat is tolerated best because less surface area per pound is exposed to the air and therefore it's less oxidized. Thick-cut meat works best. Trust me. I know. Cook the steak medium. Broil it in an *electric heated oven* or *boil* it in spring water. If you boil the meat, cut into it frequently to make sure it's left pink in the center.

Repeat: do not cook the meat in foil and do not catch the drippings in foil.

After testing beef rib steak, test beef porterhouse steak and chuck steak.

Then test chops or breast of veal. Always remember that you need fatty meat (unless you are vastly overweight). Eating red meat without carbohydrates and without eating some of the fat will give you diarrhea and make you ill in other ways.

Next, test fish, fresh fatty fish such as salmon or halibut. After testing fish, because of contaminants in fish, it's better to eat fish no more than once a week.

About 60% of the patients I see react poorly to chicken, but if you wish, you may test it. People react differently to different brands of chicken. Buy whole chickens, not cut up chicken parts. When chicken is cut up, more air reaches it, hence it's more oxidized. Sometimes packagers paint antibiotics on cut up chicken to keep it from spoiling. The least reactive chickens are fresh kosher chickens or fresh range-fed chickens. The dark meat is less reactive. You must eat the skin, otherwise you will have no fat.

Details on Testing

Depending upon your biochemistry, testing foods may move along quickly. Rarely, testing takes months. You can't force testing or complete it all at once. You will be learning about your relationship with Nature. That always takes time, just as it takes time to learn about your less complicated relationship with your mate. Look upon the time you spend testing as a hobby to play along with.

Step 1. As mentioned, make either lunch or dinner your test meal. Except for your test meal, follow your usual food habits. To test a food, eat nothing for two hours before the test meal. At the test meal, eat only the food you want to eat. Do not eat or drink anything else. Use no seasoning on the food. Water is permitted, but no other liquids. Wait two hours before eating anything else.

Step 2. Eat only a modest amount of the test food. If you have a strong reaction to the food, don't test it a second time. If you have no reaction, a questionable reaction or a mild reaction, test the food again the next day.

Step 3. After testing beef rib steak, move down the list of best tolerated meats, fish and fowl, and continue testing until you find, I hope, four or five items that you can eat without having a reaction. If at all possible find at least 3 red meats. Rarely, people will find only one or two meats they can tolerate.

The meats that you tolerate will become the backbone of your diet while you test other foods.

Do not change your diet yet. Making a change in diet is complicated. If you aren't careful and knowledgeable you'll make mistakes and fail.

I know this sounds complicated. Anything new sounds complicated. If I wrote out directions for making love or driving a car, you'd say it sounded too difficult. Take heart. Many people learn how to drive a car and/or how to make love.

Remember, we're doing the impossible: we're curing incurable diseases.

In biblical times, miracles were instantaneous. Today miracles require a bit of blood, sweat and tears.

Take it easy.
Go slowly.
Read.
Think.
Rest.
Reread this book. (I don't know about you, but I must read a book a couple dozen times to make it a part of me.)
Retest.
Gradually learn and understand.

Your emotional health, your happiness, the rest of your life depend upon what you learn.

Crossmatching Other Foods

Next test fresh, raw, non-root vegetables (root vegetables include potatoes, carrots, etc.) and fruits.

As when testing meats, test only one food at a time. Eat nothing for two hours before your test meal and eat nothing for two hours after it. Peel everything possible. Wash well and rinse extra well any fruit or vegetable which you cannot peel.

Test no more than one half a cup of vegetable and no more than one cup of fruit.

Each variety of fruit or vegetable is a separate test. Red Delicious apple is one test. Yellow Delicious apple is another test.

Unlike the meats, test the fruits and vegetables in rotation. That means test a fruit or vegetable once, then wait 72 hours before repeating the test.

If you react to many fruits and vegetables (often people do), wait three days and test the fruits and vegetables again one by one immediately after eating a meat that you have tested and found to be compatible with your biochemistry. The meat and the fat will slow down the entrance of the fruit or vegetable into your body and your body chemistry will then have a better chance to adjust to it without reacting.

Fixed and Cyclic Food Allergies

The main reason the general public, physicians and—especially—allergists don't understand food incompatibilities is that they fail to grasp the *dynamics* of food incompatibilities. They know a few things about *fixed* food incompatibilities, but they do not understand *cyclic* food allergies.

FIXED FOOD ALLERGIES

If you have a *fixed food allergy*, you have an *absolute* deficiency in the biochemical pathway that handles that particular food.

How to Discover Fixed Allergies

If you eat only one food at a time, you'll find the answer. For a week do not eat the test food, say grapefruit. On the test day, for 2 hours before the test meal do not eat or drink anything (except water). Then eat a meal made of nothing but grapefruit. Eat nothing for 2 hours after the meal.

Observe how you feel. Do you become hungry, or do you experience a headache? Do you have gas, or develop other symptoms—anxiety, depression, confusion, unpleasant thoughts? If you react unfavorably in any way to the food, you have a fixed food incompatibility to the test food. To double check for a fixed food incompatibility, wait for a month and repeat the test on exactly the same food. If you react again, then clearly you have a *fixed* food incompatibility. You always react to grapefruit every time you eat it because you have a *fixed* food incompatibility with that food.

In the body, each food and each variety of food, is metabolized by a separate biochemical pathway.

If you have a fixed food allergy, you have an *absolute* deficiency in the biochemical pathway needed to metabolize that food. You may as well be eating axle grease.

During the time it takes your body to destroy and excrete the incompatible food, you will continue to react to it. Food reactions usually last 3 days, but sometimes go on for a week.

Don't forget that an allergic reaction to a food may strike any organ in the body, give any symptom known to mankind.

CYCLIC FOOD ALLERGIES

Cyclic food allergies confuse most people, especially allergists.

If you do not react the first time you test a food, you may still have an allergy to the food. You might have a cyclic rather than a fixed food allergy. To check whether you have a cyclic food allergy, test the food again the next day. Then test it again on the third day. An unfavorable reaction will not show up until the second or third time you test the food.

How Cyclic Food Allergies Trick You

In working out food allergies, people often eat (test) a food such as grapefruit. They have no reaction. They conclude that food is compatible with their biochemistry. They mistakenly believe they can eat the food without harm. They begin eating the food every day or two. After a few days they have an unpleasant reaction to the food—and don't understand what's happening and do not know what they're reacting to.

"It couldn't be the grapefruit," they tell themselves. "I tested the grapefruit and had no reaction to it."

They are allergic to grapefruit, however. *The reaction didn't show itself until they ate the food several times at close intervals.*

Biochemical Pathways and Cyclic Food Allergies (Incompatibilities)

As noted, people with *fixed* allergies have an *absolute deficiency* in the biochemical pathway need to turn the food into energy or flesh.

With *cyclic* food allergies, however, the person has only a *relative deficiency* in the needed biochemical pathway.

The biochemical machinery is there, but it's weak.

We must allow it to "rest" between the times we use it.

Important Note!

We can eat a food to which we have a cyclic food allergy without harm if:

We eat limited amounts of the food and eat it at three day plus intervals. That way our body's chemistry has had time to recover between the times we use it.

I have a cyclic food allergy to grapefruit. If I eat one grapefruit every week, it makes me depressed and sleepy. If I eat one grapefruit every two weeks, it doesn't bother me.

Instead of feeling sleepy as a result of an allergy, you may become hungry—or depressed, tense, obsessive, or angry.

I also have a cyclic food allergy to certain flavors and brands of ice cream. I can eat a small amount about once a month without reacting. I don't bother with it, however. It's less trouble for me—and probably will be for you—to let sleeping dogs sleep.

MARY, MARY QUITE CONTRARY

Mary, an attractive 42-year-old who looks ten years younger, is allergic to fruit, all fruit. If she behaves herself and stays on her rather strict—largely rib steak diet—she has no significant emotional difficulties.

Now and then she goes wild and eats fruit. She then feel miserable for three days. During those three days she has obsessive thoughts that nearly drive her wild. Over and over again she thinks about her mother's death and keep asking herself whether she did all she could to save her.

Ordinarily—when she doesn't eat fruit—she thinks about her work, her husband, what she's going to do on her vacation—and other non-painful topics.

HEAR THIS

Everyone understands that the kidney's full-time job is clearing the blood of waste products and excreting them in the form of urine. That's the kidney's full-time job.

One of the brain's full-time jobs is producing thoughts and feelings. It does this automatically. Just as the kidney secrets urine, the brain secretes thoughts and feelings.

If the brain is made toxic (by eating a food that causes a cerebral allergic reaction—like Mary's fruit) then the brain puts out toxic thoughts and feelings. You don't need to go looking for the "stinking thinking." It simply appears.

If I eat certain cheeses, I become toxic. I experience an allergic reaction, a cerebral allergic reaction. Automatically, toxic thoughts appear. I think that I should have stayed in Chicago and become a professor. I should take more vacation and not work so hard. The world doesn't appreciate me, and on and on. . . .

On the other hand, if I stay away from things which give me cerebral allergic reactions my thoughts are pleasant. I think about the book I'm writing and the next book I want to write. I feel satisfied about the many books I have had published. I think about a patient with a particularly difficult illness I cured and realize that I am probably the only doctor in the world who could have changed his life around. In short, my brain secretes nontoxic thoughts.

DREAMS

If you cannot remember your dreams, it means you are in biochemical difficulty. You may be toxic from something to eat, toxic from sleeping on a non-cotton pillow, be short on a vitamin or mineral you need.

If your dreams are unpleasant or frightening, it means you are having toxic dreams. You are allergic to something or you have a vitamin and/or mineral problem.

TESTING WATER

"Test water!" you say. "Come on, are you kidding?"

For some people water causes no reaction. For others, it's critical. I had a patient from Cleveland with arthritis caused only by chlorine in the drinking water. Certain brands of spring water make me tired or depressed.

Test plain (unflavored) bottled spring water. To test waters, drink one water for three days, then switch to another water for three days and on and on. Repeat the test if you're not sure. The answer will come to you.

If, when you change brands of water, the new water causes symptoms, stop drinking it at once and either go back to a water that agreed with you or start testing a new water.

I have one patient who can drink only a certain brand of bottled club soda. One other very unusual patient could not tolerate any water but could drink a certain brand of prepackaged orange juice without symptoms. (Don't try it. She's probably the only person in the world with such a biochemistry!)

THE SYMPTOMS AND SIGNS OF FOOD AND WATER INTOLERANCE

You can have any symptom or sign of emotional or physical illness known to mankind, such as aches in any part of the body, anxiety, asthma, depression, fever, gas, headache, hunger, hyperactivity, insomnia, nasal discharge, paranoid thinking, rash, swollen glands . . . The list would stretch on and on if I listed everything.

And remember that an incompatibility may cause a flare up of your illness, any illness.

Meats give the longest and most severe reactions. For example, a meat reaction may make you feel as if the inside of your head turned to hot, sewage-contaminated oil that bogged down your muscles and irreparably damaged your liver and stained your soul.

That's bad, isn't it?

You can also die from an allergic reaction if your illness happens to be something like asthma or pemphigus.

Milk and milk products give the second worst reactions.

Reactions are dose-related. Test a small amount of a food and your reaction will be less and will not last as long.

Do not take or do anything without your physician's approval.

Reactions can often be lessened and shortened by taking two Bufferin tablets and two Alka-Seltzer tablets. (Take only the Alka-Seltzer tablets in the gold box, the Alka-Seltzer tablets that contain *no* aspirin.)

People with high blood pressure and certain other disease should not take Alka-Seltzer

Do not take or do anything without your physician's approval.

Alka-Seltzer tablets should be dissolved in a full glass of water. Ascorbic acid (vitamin C) 2 to 4 thousand milligrams is often helpful.

Do not take or do anything without your physician's approval.

An hour's walk also reduces the symptoms from a reaction.

"Why am I reacting to so many foods?" patients often ask me. "I've never had any reaction from foods before."

Most people are always reacting but don't know it. They're reacting from the wheat in the roll they had for breakfast when they eat the wheat in the bread used to make a sandwich at lunch, and are still reacting from that when they have cake for desert at dinner.

Also, when you separate foods and eat them one at a time, reactions are sharper and more distinct.

After a few months have passed and the immune system has begun to recover, people become less reactive.

In the next chapter we'll talk about hypoglycemia, which is only another manifestation of an allergy. Either a marked raising or lowering of the blood sugar level can be a manifestation of an allergic reaction.

CHAPTER FOURTEEN

HYPOGLYCEMIA IS A FORM OF ALLERGIC REACTION

IF you press me to the wall, I'll admit that "hypoglycemia" is an antiquated diagnosis. Hypoglycemia—low blood sugar— is only one of many biochemical changes that can take place in the body during an allergy attack. It happens that blood sugar is easy to measure, so it gets all the attention.

It also happens that table sugar is one of the most allergenic of foods, so it gets all the blame for causing low blood sugar attacks.

LAMB AND HYPOGLYCEMIA

Traditionally, patients with hypoglycemia are taken off sweets and given diets high in proteins and fat.

However—and this is going to blow your mind—I've seen a patient develop a hypoglycemic attack from eating lamb. He happened to be allergic to lamb.

I've seen a number of patients get hypoglycemic after eating cheese—they were allergic to cheese.

I'm sure you can get hypoglycemia from breathing perfume odors or gas from your kitchen stove—if you happen to be allergic to them.

So, please remember: hypoglycemia = allergy.

Ideally everyone with hypoglycemia will find exactly what he's allergic to and avoid it, regardless of whether the food is a fat, carbohydrate or protein.

If such is done—and the environment is cleaned up and the patient takes the right supplements—then the hypoglycemia will take care of itself.

Now Hear This

It happens that more people are allergic to carbohydrates—starches (like potatoes), fruits, grains—much more often than they are to fats and proteins (with the exception of cheese). That explains why people who are put on a "hypoglycemia" diet often feel better.

Many times I see patients who are no better—sometimes they're actually worse—after some doctor has put them on a "hypoglycemic" diet. Usually such patients are eating cheese because the doctor told them cheese was good for patients with hypoglycemia. The patient, unfortunately, is allergic to milk products and gets low blood sugar attacks after eating cheese.

Doctors tell patients to have frequent small meals. That's nonsense—unless the patient's eating things he's allergic to and trying to prevent withdrawal reactions. The truth is if you're eating a proper diet, one that does not contain things to which you're allergic, you should do perfectly well on three meals a day. Many people do well on two meals—if they're staying away from foods to which they're allergic.

LET'S PRETEND

Because the term "hypoglycemia" has become so fixed in people's minds, and because everyone doesn't want to go to the trouble of working out all of his food allergies, I'm going to write the rest of this chapter from a classical viewpoint, i.e., I'm going to pretend that hypoglycemia is not simply an allergy reaction, and that it only comes from eating sweets.

IT'S EVERYWHERE

Even though public awareness of hypoglycemia has increased in the last few years, this condition is still one of the most frequently undiagnosed diseases in the civilized world. It's been estimated that 20 to 40 million Americans have it; I suspect the figure to be two or three times that.

Most people who have heard of hypoglycemia assume it to be the opposite of diabetes—i.e., diabetes means high blood sugar, and hypoglycemia means low blood sugar. But it's possible to have both hypoglycemia and diabetes at the same time, and hypoglycemia is often one stage on the way to diabetes.

Medical students are taught almost nothing about functional hypoglycemia, that is the common type of hypoglycemia that's not brought on by an overdose of insulin or liver damage.

Almost all emotionally upset people have hypoglycemia. Almost all obese people have hypoglycemia. In addition, millions of people suffer occasional hypoglycemic attacks brought on by food and other allergies.

It's So Important that I'm Repeating

Although sugar is the most common offender, anything to which a person is allergic can bring on a hypoglycemic attack, anything from perfume, to gas from the kitchen stove, to wheat, to lamb— so long as the patient is allergic to it.

THE BRAIN CELLS AND SUGAR

Because the cells of the central nervous system mainly use glucose (sugar) in their metabolism, any malfunction in the blood sugar level will almost surely produce a malfunction in the nervous system. Low blood sugar produces emotional symptoms ranging from temporary depression or anxiety to acute insanity.

It can also produce any physical symptom.

As a critical connector between nutrition and the state of your nerves, the importance of hypoglycemia cannot be overstated. Since everyone's personality and biochemical make-up are different, the ways in which individual brains may react to hypoglycemia are so numerous that they can hardly be described. Symptoms include just about every complaint imaginable. Hardly a month goes by that I don't see a hypoglycemic patient with a new symptom. That's why I call hypoglycemia the great impersonator.

A partial list of possible symptoms includes depression, fatigue, anxiety, thoughts of suicide, all kinds of allergies, headaches, drug abuse, fainting spells, nightmares, insomnia, forgetfulness, confusion, anger, palpitations, some forms of arthritis, and alcoholism. I have seen such physical symptoms as post-nasal drip, asthma, hay fever, eczema, dizziness, and sweating. In effect, what I am saying is that if you feel bad in any way for more than a few days, hypoglycemia is at least a possibility.

The Psychologist with Hypoglycemia

Recently I was consulted by a psychologist who had begun to have such severe symptoms of weakness and depression that she was forced to stop working. First she had herself examined at what is probably the most important medical center in New York, where they were unable to establish a definite diagnosis. They told her that she *might* have an unusual type of liver disease.

Next, she went to a medical center in Connecticut where, to their great credit and my great surprise, they diagnosed hydrocarbon sensitivity. That is to say, they told her that she was allergic to such substances as automobile exhaust fumes and gas from the kitchen stove.

Removing hydrocarbons from her environment only provided slight relief. She continued to work, but she was still so anxious and depressed that she eventually became addicted to illegal drugs.

After a valiant effort to hold herself together enough to practice her profession, she finally had herself admitted to a clinic in New Jersey.

The doctors there performed a three-hour glucose tolerance test, apparently because they suspected diabetes. The patient had a long-standing craving for sweets, as well as strong family history of diabetes. Her glucose tolerance test showed a fasting blood sugar of 100 mg/dl. One-half hour after being fed the usual test dose of sugar, her blood sugar had risen to 236 mg/dl, and at one hour it stood at 300 mg/dl; in two hours it had fallen to 210 mg/dl, and in three hours to 79 mg/dl.

These are quite abnormal figures. Most doctors confronted with them would say that the blood sugar went too high and stayed high too long. They would conclude that the patient was predisposed toward diabetes, which was, in fact, the interpretation made at the clinic.

The patient was told to cut down on sweets. That was good advice and she soon improved enough to return to work—with the added aid of antidepressant drugs and tranquilizers.

Her condition was better, but far from good. Because she felt very depressed in the mornings, she would stay in bed until 11 or 12 o'clock. She saw patients in the afternoon, went home to sit in front of the TV until 10:30, and then took her bedtime medication and retreated into sleep.

When she consulted me I ordered a number of additional tests. I discovered two interesting abnormalities which were missed at the three institutions where she had been hospitalized. The first was a low level of sex hormones—not too surprising in a forty-five-year-old woman. (Male sex hormones, tend to stay at a higher level longer.) The second, far more important, finding which had been missed was her serum B_{12} level, reported as 59 pg/m by one laboratory and as 104 pg/m by another. By any standard, both these levels are abnormally low. I don't think any physician would take the stand that an abnormally low serum B_{12} level is a desirable condition; but most physicians associate it only with pernicious anemia, and don't realize the emotional problems caused by such a deficiency may precede pernicious anemia by many years.

Low serum B_{12} levels are dangerous and can result in damage to the central nervous system. Also, they are often associated with hypoglycemia.

It's unfortunate that the clinic did not perform a five- or six-hour glucose tolerance test on the patient. (To properly diagnose hypoglycemia, I prefer a six-hour test though a number of physicians experienced in the field are satisfied with a five-hour one.) The three-hour test done on my patient is useful for diagnosing borderline or potential diabetes, but it may or may not show hypoglycemia.

Missed the Diagnosis

It so happens that her tolerance test did clearly indicate hypoglycemia, but such a diagnosis was not made by the clinic staff. This is not unusual. I would guess that only one physician in five thousand can properly interpret a glucose tolerance test.

Most of them think in terms of absolute blood sugar levels, instead of looking at the curve, or pattern of blood levels taken throughout the test.

Since your doctor is not likely to know how to interpret your glucose tolerance curve I advise you to have him give you the figures from your test so you can review them yourself and draw your own conclusions in accordance with the guidelines I'm about to give you.

Hypoglycemia is indicated:

1. When the fasting blood sugar is lower than 85.
2. When the blood sugar level fails to rise more than 50% above the fasting level.
3. When during a glucose tolerance test the blood sugar falls 50 points or more during any one hour of the test.
4. When the blood sugar level during a six-hour glucose tolerance test falls in the range of 50 or lower (anything below 65 is suspicious).
5. When clinical symptoms such as dizziness, headache, confusion, palpitations, depression, etc., appear during the course of a glucose tolerance test—regardless of what the blood sugar readings may be.

The last criterion is important, because glucose levels may fluctuate quickly in the course of a tolerance test. The low point may occur between the blood sugar levels measured at one-hour intervals. You should, therefore, take into account any symptoms you exhibit during the test. Ideally, if any clinical symptoms make their appearance, extra blood should be drawn at once, to find out what the sugar level is at that point.

The clinic doctors failed to make the diagnosis because they fell into the common error of looking at the glucose tolerance curve in terms of absolute values. The blood sugar level did not fall below 79 mg/dl. If you ask the average physician whether 79 mg/dl represents hypoglycemia, he will reply that it does not. However, if you examine this patient's test figures again, you will note that the blood sugar level fell from 300 mg/dl to 210 mg/dl between the first and second hour—a drop of 90 mg/dl. Between the second and third hour it dropped from 210 mg/dl to 79 mg/dl—a drop of 121 mg/dl in one hour. This fall is much more than the 50 mg/dl which is considered abnormal by physicians experienced with hypoglycemia.

In addition, the patient had severe emotional symptoms—depression, restlessness, and a sense of impending doom during the course of the test.

As noted, brain cells rely heavily on glucose for their metabolism. Also, brain cells, unlike others, are not able to store glucose. This makes blood sugar levels all the more important to the functioning of the nervous system. If the cell metabolism becomes conditioned, over a period of time, to functioning with a blood sugar supply between 80 and 120 mg/dl, the cell will accommodate itself to this sugar level. However, if the blood sugar level changes radically, the whole chemistry of the nerve cell is thrown off balance. That usually results in marked emotional symptoms.

INSTANTLY PARANOID

Once a patient consulted me because of a depression. I did a glucose tolerance test, and between the third and fourth hour she became paranoid and suspicious of the laboratory technicians, believing that they were going to harm her. Checking back, we found that during this period there had been a rapid fall in her blood sugar level. This was the first and only time this woman had ever had paranoid symptoms.

Strange as it may seem, a startling number of physicians still don't know that sugar is the last thing a person with hypoglycemia should eat. Like a lay person, many physicians falsely conclude that if the blood sugar is low, sugar should make it go up. They base their conclusions on experience with diabetics who have taken an overdose of insulin which makes their blood sugar levels dive down to dangerously low levels. In the case of diabetics who are having hypoglycemia due to an overdose of insulin, eating sugar is the proper treatment.

Not so with people suffering from functional hypoglycemia. Such a patient's blood sugar also rises after eating sugar. But the relief will be quite temporary, and soon the patient is in real trouble. Whenever sugar enters the bloodstream, the insulin-producing glands are activated. The insulin in the bloodstream causes the sugar to be stored in the liver. This lowers the level of sugar in the blood, making less sugar available to the central nervous system. This process takes place in all so-called normal people. But people with fuctional hypoglycemia overreact to stimulation by sugar. They may produce too much insulin and their blood sugar is driven down too far too fast.

Other Factors besides Excessive Insulin May Be Involved

In describing how to interpret your glucose tolerance curve, I mentioned a "flat" curve, which sounds like a contradiction in terms. This refers to a line on a graph recording the rise of sugar in the blood. If the line fails to rise 50 mg/dl above the fasting level, the line forms a shallow, or flat curve. This may indicate excessive and rapid insulin production. Or it may indicate that the person cannot absorb sugar. Or it may indicate low thyroid levels, and the thyroid should certainly be tested at once. If thyroid gland tests are normal, many patients with flat glucose tolerance tests do better when given thyroid tablets (60-120 mg daily).

As Mentioned Earlier, Many Hypoglycemics are Allergic to Sugar

Hypoglycemics do not, ordinarily, have hives, asthma, or other classical allergy symptoms. Their allergic response may take the form of a lowering of blood sugar, with all the myriad symptoms that syndrome can produce.

Allergic reaction to foods other than sugar may also cause blood sugar to drop. In fact, it is even possible that allergies other than food allergies may also drive blood sugar levels down. In turn, a low blood sugar level tends to aggravate allergic reactions—so you can see how quickly the patient can be enmeshed in a vicious cycle.

In my opinion, no patient with hypoglycemia can be properly treated without an allergy workup as outlined in this book. People with functional hypoglycemia also have food allergies.

I urge my patients to treat sugar as if it were arsenic.

SHOULD EVERYONE HAVE A GLUCOSE TOLERANCE TEST?

When I first became interested in hypoglycemia, I ran glucose tolerance tests on all my new patients. After a while, I grew so dismayed
at the prevalence of hypoglycemia that I rarely did glucose tolerance
tests because I began to realize that absolutely no one should eat
sugar.

As I've mentioned earlier, our enzyme systems have simply not
evolved a capacity for handling sugar. Sugar has been widely available to the mass of mankind only during the past one hundred and
fifty years—far too short a time for Mother Nature to adapt our
systems to adjust properly to using it.

In addition, sugar contains no minerals, vitamins, or proteins.
To metabolize it, one must receive nutrients from other sources,
and the "average American diet" simply does not include enough
excess nutrients to handle the job.

As if this were not enough reason to stay away from sugar, Dr.
John Yudkin, professor emeritus of nutrition at London University,
convincingly explains how sugar increases hardening of the arteries,
contributes to heart attacks and strokes, destroys teeth and joints,
and may even be a contributing factor in the development of cancer.

IS RAW SUGAR BETTER THAN REFINED SUGAR?

Raw sugar, or turbinado, is white table sugar before being stripped
of all nutrients. It does contain a few vitamins and minerals, and
therefore does not drain your system of nutrients quite as much as
white sugar. But it still hits your bloodstream as sucrose, and it
still triggers the same insulin and/or allergic response as white
sugar. Light- and dark-brown sugar such as you buy at the super-
market (raw or turbinado sugar is more likely to be found in a
health food store) is the sugar equivalent of "enriched" bread. It's
sugar that has been stripped or "refined" and then treated with
molasses to make it look dark again. True, molasses has some
nutrients that white sugar does not; but it is still sucrose.

Honey contains a few—very few—nutrients and it consists of
fructose or fruit sugar, and glucose. In my view, honey is just as
bad as plain table sugar. People who use it in place of table sugar
are only fooling themselves—not their biochemistry. Honey, like

plain sugar, also causes obesity, tooth decay, heart disease, and the rest.

As far as I'm concerned the difference among these sweeteners is insignificant. I repeat: DON'T EAT SUGAR.

And let me add, DON'T EAT WHEAT. I know that wheat's complex carbohydrate and complex carbohydrates are supposed to be better for hypoglycemics than simple carbohydrates like sugar. Sometimes yes, sometimes no.

This will startle you

MORE HYPOGLYCEMICS HAVE TROUBLE WITH WHEAT THAN WITH SUGAR.

HYPOGLYCEMICS SHOULD ALSO AVOID ALCOHOL

A Texas physician who consulted me because of hypoglycemia told me the following story.

One afternoon he came home from the office, had a cocktail, and spent the next hour mowing the lawn. Then he showered and went to a cocktail party, where he had one more drink—and passed out.

At the hospital emergency room they tested his blood sugar level, found it low and gave him intravenous glucose. Within an hour he was back at the party. That's not the best way to discover that you have hypoglycemia.

One of my patients, a business executive, had two drinks before a lunch conference. After leaving he got in an argument with a man on the street, then at the insistence of his associates, took a taxi home. When he arrived at his apartment building, he was confused and went to the wrong door, which his key wouldn't open.

He began banging on the door and eventually succeeded in actually breaking down the door. Police officers arrived. He mauled two of them so badly that five more were called to help subdue him.

Some hours later he woke up in the hospital, surprised to find himself in a somewhat battered condition. He had no memory whatever of anything that happened after he left the meeting.

Because of this experience he came to see me. I ordered a six-hour glucose tolerance test, during which he nearly passed out. As I expected, the test showed him to be severely hypoglycemic.

Alcohol, Allergy, and Hypoglycemia: The Triple Whammy

When a person with hypoglycemia has a drink and then eats something he's allergic to, he can more easily develop emotional symptoms including confusion, depression, fatigue, restlessness, irritability, or even outright psychosis.

You get an allergic reaction from food when tiny particles of the toxic substance move from the intestinal tract into the bloodstream. You get a blood sugar drop from alcohol because, like sugar, it is a pure, empty carbohydrate and is metabolized very fast—too fast for your body. Also, alcohol has small quantities of the substance from which it was made—corn or wheat for example.

And This is Important

When you drink and eat something you're allergic to, the alcohol carries much greater than usual amounts of the toxic food into your bloodstream, and it does so with great rapidity. As a result, the alcohol drives down the blood sugar, and the allergic reaction drives it down still faster and further.

My Friend

I once had lunch with a friend at the Plaza Hotel. After a glass of sherry she began her appetizer of oysters, remarking that she was slightly allergic to them but couldn't resist eating them once or twice a year. Before the main course had arrived she was in such a state of confusion that I had to lead her out of the dining room.

Several years ago I was walking past the Brasserie restaurant in New York when I saw a man struggling in an attempt to lift a limp woman from the sidewalk into a waiting taxi. She was in her mid-thirties, rather obese, and practically unconscious.

"She only had two drinks, for God's sake," the man kept saying over and over, while I helped him as best I could with his limp burden.

"What did she have to eat?" I asked.

"Smoked halibut," he replied. "She loves it, but she hardly ever has a chance to eat it."

I suggested that he take her to a hospital emergency room and tell the doctors there that she was probably having an attack of hypoglycemia brought on by the combination of alcohol and smoked halibut.

"She has hypoglycemia," he told me, "but I thought that was only caused by sugar."

"Anything that she's allergic to can bring on an attack. It was probably the combination of alcohol and smoke halibut."

A VICIOUS CIRCLE

Hypoglycemics are often tense, depressed people. Tension and depression can make hypoglycemia worse, and hypoglycemia can make tension and anger worse. It's a chicken-and-egg problem.

Want To Be Like Hitler?—Then Eat Sugar

Adolf Hitler, the world's most famous vegetarian, ate toast and chocolate for breakfast, was a candy bar freak, and undoubtedly suffered from hypoglycemia and sugar allergy. When blood sugar is low, the brain becomes irritable and hyperactive. This irritability can stimulate a rush of adrenalin which will in turn very likely exaggerate your excited or furious feelings. At the same time the brain stimulates insulin production as a reaction to the blood sugar elevation produced by the adrenalin. The insulin causes a sizable amount of blood sugar to be stored in the liver, leaving you with lower blood sugar than ever—and feeling more tense and angry than ever.

TENSION AND HYPOGLYCEMIA

Hypoglycemics should avoid tense situations as much as possible, just as they should avoid fatigue and the foods that radically alter their blood levels.

IF YOU SUSPECT HYPOGLYCEMIA

If you suspect hypoglycemia, what should you do about it? One obvious answer is simply to assume you have it, and put yourself on the diet I am about to describe. For many reasons, I feel it is the healthful, well-balanced diet that most humans should eat anyway. But if you want proof that you have hypoglycemia, ask your doctor for a six-hour glucose tolerance test.

IF YOU HAVE HYPOGLYCEMIA, THERE'S GOOD NEWS AND BAD NEWS

First the bad news. It would be better not to have it.

Now the good news. A great many people can improve their mental and physical well-being tremendously simply by changing the way they eat.

Most people with hypoglycemia require extra vitamins and minerals. See chapters 15, 16, and 17 for guidance.

EAT PROTEINS AND FATS FOR HYPOGLYCEMIA, AND LIMIT CARBOHYDRATES

Different foods are absorbed by the body at different rates and affect blood sugar in different ways. For example, sugar is absorbed directly and quickly. The blood sugar rises rapidly and then falls rapidly, and the person is soon hungry again. In the case of a hypoglycemic, the system overreacts to the rapid flood of sugar into the system, then the body overreacts by squirting out too much insulin and the blood sugar falls.

THE BODY MAY PRODUCE TOO MUCH INSULIN

As a rule, however, the reaction is not that simple. Many times during an attack of low blood sugar, the measured insulin level of the body is quite normal. We blame insulin, but the chemistry is much more complex than: too much insulin = low blood sugar.

Sugar, as you know, is a simple carbohydrate. More complex carbohydrates, like potatoes and grains, are also converted by the body into sugar. They get into the bloodstream a bit more slowly than sugar, but even complex carbohydrates show up rather quickly in the blood stream in the form of sugar. The sugar then quickly fades away, leaving you hungry or worse.

BREAKFAST CEREAL

Nutritionist Adelle Davis once wrote that when you sit down to a bowl of cereal in the morning, you should imagine that you are about to eat a bowl of pure sugar, because that is how it will affect your blood sugar level.

Proteins and fats, by contrast, are digested much more slowly than carbohydrates. The blood sugar rises slowly and steadily, remains sustained for a longer period of time, and falls slowly. To avoid low blood sugar attacks, simply avoid large amounts of carbohydrates, eat more protein and fat instead, and your body will do the rest. Naturally, you must avoid food to which you are allergic.

Here's a Pearl

Many people put milk on their cereal. In my experience, most people should not eat cereals, but I know many people are going to eat them regardless of what I say: they have long standing addictions that they aren't ready to give up.

Do yourself a favor: instead of putting milk on your cereal, use cream.

Now I know this goes against your religion, but please hear me out.

Cream has less sugar per spoonful than skimmed milk. Cream (fat) slows down the entry of carbohydrates into the body. Ice cream, for example, eaten after a meal of prime ribs, will cause a milder reaction than ice cream eaten after a meal of crepe suzettes.

You worry about the calories in cream?

Pray do not. Fats may have several times as many calories per unit weight as carbohydrates, but they satisfy four or five times as much, so in the long run you will eat less.

You worry about the cholesterol?

Pray do not! Read my article on cholesterol that appears in Appendix Two at the end of the book.

How Much Protein and Fat Should You Eat?

To answer the first question first—eat as much as you need to avoid hunger.

If you are overweight, as so many hypoglycemics are, don't worry about total calories on this diet.

People with deranged carbohydrate metabolism grow fat because their appetite control is knocked out by the wildly fluctuating blood sugar levels. Half the time they don't know whether they're hungry or not, so they eat constantly just to cover all bases. When you change over to a high-protein diet, you may still eat constantly at first, just out of habit, but eventually your appetite control will regain its equilibrium and you will probably lose weight without consciously trying to. Most weight problems, whether obesity or thinness, correct themselves when you begin to eat a diet that actually nourishes your particular body adequately.

What Kind of Protein and Fat Should You Eat?

Beef, lamb, and pork satisfy best. Glandular meats such as liver and kidneys are nourishing, though somewhat lean. You will find yourself feeling hungry less often if you deliberately eat fat as well as lean, no matter how you have been conditioned against it. Fish and poultry are excellent sources of protein, though again, they are mostly too lean to sustain you as a steady diet. By all means eat the fat on steaks. Rib steaks are great. (But avoid aged fat, fat cooked with gas, fat that's burned or browned.)

Cholesterol on a Hypoglycemic Diet

You may be wondering what the high animal fat content of my diet would do to your cholesterol level. Reread chapter 10, on cholesterol.

But What Can I Eat for Breakfast

If you eat a high-carbohydrate breakfast—things like ceral or toast, and fruit juice, let alone donuts, sweet rolls or pancakes or waffles—your blood sugar will rise and then swoop down so that two or three hours later you are feeling dragged out, let down, and in need of another lift. This syndrome is so common among devotees of the normal American diet that its corollary, the mid-morning coffee break, has become an American institution. Also, the mid-morning low blood sugar attack is part of the American way of life. Coffee, tea sweet rolls, and cigarettes, all of which temporarily elevate blood sugar levels, are used every morning around 10:30 by millions of Americans to correct the effect of their high-sugar breakfasts, just as diabetics use insulin at regular intervals to correct their blood sugar levels.

I know of one coffee-addicted executive who considers non-stop coffee consumption so normal that he regularly orders coffee for himself and any visitor without even asking if his visitor wants any. He thought it passing strange when a health-conscious insurance salesman declined coffee at eleven one morning, saying, "No, thank you, I've finished my breakfast."

Tests have shown that if you eat a significant amount of carbohydrate at breakfast your blood sugar levels will remain erratic for the rest of the day, no matter what you eat at lunch and dinner. And you tend to feel hungry even when you have consumed more than your share of calories, because hunger is felt when the blood sugar drops below a certain level (about 70 mg/dl), not when the stomach is empty. If you've ever tried to diet keeping yourself bloated with celery, lettuce, water, and diet soft drinks, you know that you feel as grouchy and hungry as ever even while you're stuffed like a sausage. Now you know why.

Breakfast for Hypoglycemics

Most people with hypoglycemia do best if they eat fresh meat (with some of the fat), or an oily fish, plus a cup of non-sweet fresh fruit for breakfast. Also, consider eggs (careful, many people are allergic to them), lamb chops, pork chops, or a steak with a small amount of potatoes cooked any way you like. The meat and fat are digested slowly, releasing a steady supply of sugar into the blood so that your blood sugar stays elevated until lunch time, and falls much more slowly than usual because you have not triggered insulin over-kill by filling your empty stomach with carbohydrates.

Most people with hypoglycemia should have no more than one

piece of fruit a day—as a dessert, not eaten alone on an empty stomach.

Fruit juice contains much too concentrated a source of fructose, so I do not recommend it, particularly at breakfast. Eating the whole fruit will give you roughage. (For a complete rundown of what I usually eat, meal by meal, see chapter 14.)

What to Eat for the Rest of the Day

As with breakfast, each meal should consist mainly of protein and fat. You might try including a small amount of brown rice or potatoes every third day. Feel free to eat a salad or a leafy green vegetable. These provide essential roughage, and are mainly water and minerals, with few carbohydrates.

Dressing is fine, as long as it is safflower oil and lemon juice. Avoid ketchup and other prepared condiments. Most of them contain sugar, or are loaded with artificial preservatives to which many people are allergic. And remember: a hypoglycemic is allergic.

If you are overweight you should cut down on fruits. Do not eat more than a cup of vegetables at a meal. Try to avoid all nuts and grains. Drink only water. Eat all the fresh meat and fresh fatty fish you desire. If you never make any exceptions to this diet, your weight loss should be slow but steady. Vitamin supplements and mineral supplements should be taken, as later outlined.

Most people do best on beef rib steaks, or porterhouse steaks. These should be fresh (unaged) and cooked with electricity, *not* cooked with gas. By unaged, I mean the steaks should be no more than five or six days old. If they are too "young" many patients are allergic to them. They may be wrapped in aluminum foil (dull side against the meat) and frozen by you. Frozen steaks are not considered aged so long as you freeze them. Before cooking the meat you freeze, remove the foil and cook the meat while still frozen. Do not leave cooked meat in the refrigerator and eat it later.

Do not eat the deckle on rib steaks. Most people are allergic to it.

REMEMBER

Hypoglycemia = allergy.

Repeat: If you have hypoglycemia, wheat (in any form) is usually as bad or worse for you than sugar.

Most hypoglycemics do not do well on cheese. I see a number of patients with hypoglycemia who eat cheese and feel worse because they're sensitive to milk products.

WHAT'S LEFT?

Meat with fat, a few fresh vegetables, a few fresh fruits. *Please read chapter 12 to learn why you need not fear the meat-cancer goblin. Please read chapter 13 to learn that no food is perfect, especially wheat.*

You should always keep in mind which foods are the most likely to cause allergic reactions. Once more, they are: eggs, milk, all grains (including corn), sugar, sweets, and chocolate.

Also, beware of peanuts and lettuce. In the chapter on food allergies you'll learn how to test foods for allergic reactions.

N.B. People with hypoglycemia should avoid milk (too much sugar) and milk products such as cheese and yogurt (too many people have subtle, hidden, unsuspected allergies to them).

BEDTIME SNACKS

The bedtime snack is particularly important for people who tend to awaken during the night or early in the morning—often because their blood sugar has gone down. The same is true of people who awaken in the middle of the night with attacks of allergic asthma. If their blood sugar can be kept up during the night, their condition often improves.

Eat a piece of meat, or eggs if you can tolerate them. Don't eat a bowl of cereal, or cookies and milk as the commercials urge you to do! Milk is a taboo with me anyway (see chapter 15).

AVOID COFFEE, TEA, AND TOBACCO

Coffee, tea, and tobacco are stimulants—the square American's legal "speed." They give you a lift by stimulating your adrenalin production which raises your blood sugar. This triggers an insulin reaction, knocking your blood sugar down again, and soon you're in a familiar spiral. Whether you call this an allergic reaction, an addiction, or a chronic low blood sugar syndrome makes little difference. The effect is that you're hooked, and the only way to break the cycle is to avoid it in the first place.

AVOID ALL CANDIES, SOFT DRINKS, AND BAKED GOODS

And while we're on the subject, it is not a good idea to use artificial sweeteners either. Some people become so conditioned to the release of insulin as a response to the intake of anything sweet that the body reacts to artificial sweeteners as if they were real sugar, and releases excessive amounts of insulin just as if it were real sugar.

Also, if you use artificial sweeteners you tend to keep on desiring sweets, because the flavor constitutes a perpetual reminder of the forbidden taste, and becomes a constant temptation.

Altogether in my view, food should be nourishing and adequate, but preferably not particularly appetizing. This may not be very popular advice—but believe me, it is good advice, and can add years to your life.

When food becomes too important an element of pleasure in life we tend to indulge in too much of it, become overweight, and from that we go on to all the complications of heart attacks, strokes, diabetes, and even cancer.

Since I have advised you against sweets, tobacco, alcohol, coffee, tea, and milk, you might well ask what pleasures are left to you.

I'm happy to report that sexual activity does not bring on hypoglycemic attacks—if perfumes and polyester pillows are avoided!

In fact, physical activity is often good for the hypoglycemia sufferer.

I strongly advise everyone to get outdoors and walk vigorously every day for an hour—at a good fast pace—unless some medical contraindication exists.

You can also make money, go to the movies, read (or write!) good books.

Some Tests to Ask Your Doctor For

When a doctor works up a patient to check for hypoglycemia it is always a good idea to get a thyroid profile. Many patients with hypoglycemia need extra thyroid. Even if the tests come back normal, it's often a good idea for the doctor to place a patient on a trial dose of thyroid hormone. This is especially important if the patient often feels chilly when other people do not.

Your doctor should also order an SMA 24, a complete blood count, a routine urine examination, a serum vitamin B_{12} level and folic acid determination. These are the mineral tests.

VITAMINS AND MINERALS

People with hypoglycemia usually do better with extra vitamins, minerals, and unsaturated oils. Read chapters 16, 17 and 18.

People with hypoglycemia often have an abnormal desire for sweets. They eat a lot of "empty calorie" foods that not only supply no nutrients, but actually drain the body of vitamins and minerals. As we have seen, an inadequate diet of this kind can, over a period of time, result in chronic vitamin and mineral deficiencies. Correcting the diet, removing sweets, and lowering carbohydrates stops the damage from going further.

Adding vitamin and mineral supplements begins to correct the damage that has already been done.

You need not worry about roughage if you eat plenty of animal fat. Like roughage, fat helps prevent constipation. Also helpful: vitamin C and magnesium.

Never eat burned or browned fat, or fat in preserved meats such as smoked meat and salami. These fats are toxic, will make you feel bad, and may well encourage cancer.

You can have too much unsaturated vegetable fat.

Never have more than one teaspoon daily and never have any made from corn oil. Be doubly sure to take vitamin E if vegetable fats are used. Also, do have some vegetable fats. Vegetable fats are needed by the body just as vitamins are needed. Every cell in the body is surrounded by a fatty membrane. Without that fatty membrane life would not be possible.

Do not eat meat without also eating some of the fat. Lean meat without fat will make you sick.

Too Expensive?

You may feel that the diet I have outlined is too expensive since it contains so much meat and so little of the cheaper carbohydrates. You will save some money by not using processed foods, but this diet will take a bigger slice out of your budget. Yet consider the compensations: the improvement in health that comes from proper diet usually results in greater well-being, greater energy, and greater efficiency at work.

On this diet everyone earns more money.

Even if you don't, you should lose your depression, fatigue, nervousness, insomnia—surely those are worth a lot.

By decreasing your susceptibility to colds, emotional illnesses, and serious diseases, including ailments like cancers, you cut down on what you pay out for doctor bills and drugs.

By following this diet and generally improving your nutrition you may increase your life span by many years.

Before you dismiss this diet as not worth the money, under your doctor's supervision, try it for a month. A fair trial will probably add less to your normal expenses than one visit to your doctor for a flu shot. I'm sure you've gambled more before, with less promise of reward.

WARNING: People frequently feel less well the first week on a new diet. This happens because they may be experiencing withdrawal symptoms by getting away from foods to which they had an allergic addiction. Also, the bacterial make-up of the gut will gradually change.

WHAT IF YOU CHEAT?

Since people are not machines, I realize that you will probably not follow all the directions I have given you, at least not all the time. My patients don't. Even I don't. The lure of our addictions is strong, and sometimes life's pleasures seem too few and far between to allow our missing any. The "consume now, pay later" attitude is an American way of life. So being a realist, I am going to give you some tips on how to cheat in ways that will cause the least havoc.

Please don't assume that I advise cheating; you will be much better off if you follow my diet to the letter.

For example, if you can't, or won't, give up smoking I suggest that you smoke only after eating; this will cause less disturbance in your metabolism. Also you might buy—and use—one of the cigarette holders now on the market that can be twisted to gradually reduce the amount of smoke you take in. These are useful, and so are the cigarette holders with filters that reduce the amount of tar you inhale.

If you must use alcohol, stay off beer, cordials, and sweet wines. Have an occasional glass of dry wine or champagne (French champagne, for some reason I don't understand, is tolerated better.)

White wines are tolerated much better than red wines. Cheap wines cause less trouble than expensive wines (exception: champagne.)

Whiskeys are a big problem.

Gin is usually better tolerated, but not nearly as well tolerated as cheap, dry, white wine.

If you use a mix, use seltzer, water, or club soda.

All sodas (except club soda) are prohibited. Also, have your drink with or after a meal, especially a fat-and-protein-rich meal. Drinking on an empty stomach is particularly bad for you.

If you are going to cheat by eating sweets, you would again be well advised to eat them only after a meal generous in fats and proteins. Then the sugar will cause fewer fluctuations in your blood sugar level because your blood sugar will be sustained by the fat and protein.

Abram Hoffer, M. D., Ph.D. advocates a clever method of cheating. He says that if you must cheat on your diet, you should select one day of the week to do all your cheating. That way you will receive a dramatic illustration of how rotten you feel when you go off your diet, and eventually this may cause you to give up your forbidden drinks, smokes, and foods. I have found this an effective method.

If you take two Bufferin before cheating, it will lessen the toxic effects. Also, a shot of vitamin B_{12b} or a good dose of ascorbic acid is helpful both before and after.

In summary, if you feel sick for any length of time and your physician can find no explanation, it is likely that you have hypoglycemia. Have a six-hour glucose tolerance test and have it interpreted according to the criteria I have laid down. If you cannot get a six-hour glucose tolerance test, it would be safe to assume that you have hypoglycemia. If your physician approves, go on the diet I recommend, and take multiple vitamins. Frankly, the hypoglycemic diet is nothing but a well-balanced, nutritious diet which almost everyone would be well advised to follow. Nutritional supplements are indicated as well.

NOTE WELL

Everyone with hypoglycemia has food allergies. No food should be eaten by people with hypoglycemia unless, with their physician's approval, they first test the food. Remember that any food can cause hypoglycemia if you are allergic to it.

Foods should be tested as outlined in this book, by isolating foods and feeding them one at a time.

EAT ONLY FRESH MEAT. MEAT SHOULD BE PINK, NOT RED.

CHAPTER FIFTEEN

THE NEWBOLD DIET

I have news for you: Many of our fellow travelers through time experience periods of anxiety, insecurity, insomnia, depression, withdrawal, shyness, rage, aggression, suspiciousness, and all the other symptoms we label neurotic or psychotic. They also suffer from abdominal pains, arthritis, high blood pressure, and a thousand other disorders.

If you find this hard to believe, it's because you, like most people, are simply unaware of how much your neighbor suffers. You meet someone in the elevator on your way to work and exchange pleasantries about the weather. You marvel at the other fellow's serenity, wishing your problems were as few and innocuous as his.

But you only see him on stage. You are not present when he gnashes his teeth in rage, sobs in agony, curses the world, and wonders how many sleeping pills it'll take to get him out of it.

You see Frank Sinatra on stage and marvel at his serenity and control, but on several occasions he became so distraught that he attempted suicide.

The truth is, most people are more or less twisted up, and could well use more tranquility. One reason people are often a bit on guard in the presence of psychiatrists—even in the neutral territory of a dinner party—is because they suspect that they, too, harbor a small but dangerous seed of madness.

Such suspicion is well-founded. Sanity and insanity are not two discrete entities, but two points along the same continuum.

LET'S LOOK AT ENZYME SYSTEMS

If you're ill or simply not feeling great, the chances are that you've inherited enzyme systems (and other biochemistry) not suited to metabolize the heavy grain-milk-sugar diet eaten by Europeans and Americans. Your chemistry may be out of synch with your times.

If this is so, then you must change your diet or you will remain ill or semi-ill for the rest of your life.

Perhaps the enzyme systems you have inherited are exactly right for caveman times. Maybe you will do great on a diet high in meat, fish, or fowl along with limited amounts of vegetables and fruits.

If that's true, don't fight it. You can't win a fight against natural force, whether it be a earthquake or biochemistry.

I'm Not Putting You Down

Please understand that by saying you may have primitive enzyme systems, I'm not putting you down. My enzyme systems are straight out of the cave. I eat a fish-fowl-meat and limited-vegetable-fruit diet and feel great.

That doesn't make either of us bad people, or even make us primitive people. We can still go to concerts and plays and read great books. Indeed, we can have the best of the caveman world and the best of the modern world. But only if we feel good can we enjoy the fruits of civilization.

Exactly What Are Enzymes?

When I speak of enzymes, I'm not talking about simple digestive enzymes, but rather those and all the other enzyme systems in the body that help bring about the chemical reactions that make life possible.

In the laboratory when we want to make a chemical reaction take place, we run some water in a test tube, add chemicals, then hold the mixture over the flame from a Bunsen burner.

The heat makes the chemical reaction happen.

Obviously, the living body cannot use heat from a flame to bring about a chemical reaction.

Instead of using heat to cause the reaction to happen, living creatures use enzymes.

As you see, the body is a skin full of chemicals and everything that happens in it happens because of enzyme systems.

Enzymes are made of proteins, vitamins, and minerals. Now you understand why these things are so vital to the body.

My clinical observations lead me to believe that every different food uses a different enzyme system. For example, Red Delicious apples put me to sleep because my body lacks the enzyme systems needed to help metabolize Red Delicious apples. Because I lack the enzymes needed to use Red Delicious apples, Red Delicious apples are toxic for me. I might just as well be eating axle grease.

Until my body gradually excretes the "food" that my body cannot use, the unused food is floating around in my body making me feel ill.

People who have enzyme systems that can handle Red Delicious apples do perfectly well on them.

On the other hand, I happen to have enzyme systems that can handle Yellow Delicious apples and Granny Smith apples.

And so it goes. . . .

The most important tricks in the world of nutrition are to furnish your enzyme systems with all the proteins, vitamins and minerals they need to function at their full capacity . . . and to eat only those foods that match your enzyme systems.

This takes work, work that must be done for each person. No two people have exactly the same set of enzyme systems.

FOOD AND PHILOSOPHY

That's why it's not wise to choose your diet from a philosophical viewpoint: choose to be a vegetarian, or a lacto-vegetarian, etc. It's not a philosophical question. Do you ask your priest what fuel to put in your car? It's all a question of giving your body only foods that can be handled by your enzyme systems.

To do so requires much knowledge and much hard work on your part and the part of your doctor. That's one of the reasons why most doctors and the government reject this approach.

MEDICATION

Let's face it: it is easier to take a pill to treat your ulcer rather than find out which foods you are eating that your body cannot handle.

To take a pill is to stick your finger in a crumbling dyke. Pills may control your ulcer, but the toxic food will start giving you an irritable bowel, or make you depressed or tired, or give you high blood pressure and insomnia. Taking medication is usually an exercise in futility.

WHAT IS ALLERGY?

When a food or substance is not compatible with your enzyme systems, we say that you are "allergic" to that food. You could just as well say that you are "sensitive" to the food, or that you have an "incompatibility" with that food.

WE UNDERSTAND THAT ALLIGATORS EAT FISH

We humans see ourselves as built in the image of God. I don't know much about that, but I do know that like the alligator, the horse and the tiger, we humans have a biochemistry and unless our biochemistry is working properly, we don't feel well.

If you bought a pet alligator and kept him in the closet away from the sunlight, warmth, and good juicy mud that was his natural environment, you would expect him to become ill.

If you stopped feeding him fish and instead fed him a diet of cola drinks, potato chips, doughnuts and ice cream you would expect the alligator to become ill.

Why not you?

Do you really think you are above biology, above the laws of nature?

If you do think the laws of nature do not apply to you, try going without oxygen (but only with your doctor's approval!) for two minutes and see how you feel.

Did you learn that your chemistry needs a supply of oxygen to function properly?

It also needs vitamins and minerals and all the other nutrients—and it must have food that it can utilize.

Give your body nitrogen instead of oxygen and it will become sick and die.

Give it the wrong foods and it will become sick and die—perhaps not as quickly as it does when nitrogen replaces oxygen, but just as surely.

Alligators Eat Fish; Humans Eat Fish-Fowl-Meat and Limited-Vegetable-Fruit

For 2.2 million years man's ancestors lived on a diet of meat, fish, occasional eggs, roots (such as potatoes and carrots), fruits, nuts, and vegetables; he ate what he could kill or gather.

During that 2.2 million years, evolution tailor made mankind's enzyme systems to handle those foods.

About 10,000 years ago, man learned to cultivate such grains as wheat, barley, millet, rice, and legumes.

In a mere 10,000 years, evolution cannot change enzyme systems that were fixed over a period of 2,200,000 years.

EVOLUTION WANTS YOU

Evolution is trying to eliminate those of us who do not feel well on the "modern" diet of grains, milk products, and sugar.

Personally, I don't care to have evolution eliminate me.

If you don't care about yourself, then lie down and die.

If you do care . . . read on and learn how to fight back.

Life Changed

Gradually, man's life changed from that of a wandering hunter to that of a farmer. When he began to stay settled in villages instead of roaming from place to place, he learned to domesticate animals. He kept sheep, goats, and chickens. For the first time, he could add milk and cheese to his regular diet.

If you think of the evolution of man from his beginning to the present as being one day long, grains and dairy products enter the picture only fifteen minutes before midnight. Sugar appears as dietary staple just as the bell begins to toll.

Man is an adaptable animal.

Some people have a chemistry that can handle grains, sugar, and dairy products, although I contend that many of them would feel better if they avoided these "new" foods.

Many young people, whose enzyme systems have not yet broken down from age and cumulative abuse, can handle the new foods more efficiently than older people. The drastic upsurge of reactive hypoglycemia and diabetes in middle age lends support to such a theory.

A great many people have enzyme systems that have not yet adapted to mankind's new diet.

Much aging, heart disease, hardening of the arteries, depression, anxiety, insomnia, delinquency, alcoholism, and schizophrenia are caused by taxing less well-adaptive enzyme systems with the new foods.

More to the point: How much sickness or half-sickness do the new foods bring to your home? To find out, try the Back-to-Nature diet that I am about to describe, the diet I myself follow. You will note that it is not really different from the diet that I have discussed for hypoglycemics. This is perfectly appropriate because hypoglycemia, food allergies and associated conditions are all part of the same syndrome.

WE RESIST CHANGE—ESPECIALLY CHANGES IN OUR DIETS

People tend to like what we grow up with. The French children grow up eating snails and adult Frenchmen enjoy eating snails. Chinese like rotten eggs. Eskimos enjoy eating rotten (ripe) fish, upper class rural English enjoy eating spoiled (ripe) venison. And so it goes.

That explains, in part, why Europeans and Americans like ice cream and doughnuts and potato chips.

WHY DO WE RESIST CHANGE?

Clinging to the familiar is an inherited trait in higher primates.

In nature, the animal who refuses to venture into the unknown avoids trouble. The animal that does not sample every odd-looking nut or berry has a better chance of surviving than one who routinely gets lost in the woods, hasn't the sense to avoid snakes and lions, or poisons himself out of curiosity.

Professor Irvin Devore of Harvard did an experiment with modern baboons to find out which was stronger—the animals' fear of an enemy they knew was deadly, or the fear of the unknown.

A group of anthropologists, driving jeeps and firing rifles, chased a baboon troop across the veld. The baboons, who had been hunted by man before, ran at breakneck speed until they reached the invisible line that marked the edge of their territory; then, rather than cross the line, they stopped and waited to be shot.

People tend to resist the unfamiliar—especially changes in food— in much the same way. "People" includes scientists, even professors of nutrition. People may stop short of waiting to be shot, but they scorn what they don't know—and make fun of it because they fear it!

PEER PRESSURE TELLS US NOT TO ROCK THE BOAT

Our society acts as if people who are concerned about eating properly are drug-crazed hippies, or strange old ladies in tennis shoes. They call them "health nuts." Isn't that an interesting concept— that to be concerned with health is to be crazy.

It's pointless to protest that you are sane. You are different, therefore, by definition, you are crazy. The truth is that a person who rejects a diet of pizza and "toastem popups" makes others uncomfortable, like a teetotaler in a roomful of drinkers. And few of us like to be set apart, or to make others uncomfortable, so we resist changing our eating habits.

BESIDES, WE OFTEN BECOME ADDICTED TO WHAT WE EAT

Most allergic people easily become addicted to the new foods. For example, I saw a patient the other day who must have some form of wheat and sugar each morning for breakfast, otherwise she gets a headache and feels nervous. She gets withdrawal symptoms. Once she eats the sweet roll for breakfast, she feels better. She concludes there's something in sweet rolls that is good for her.

It's exactly like the heroin addict. If the heroin addict doesn't get his "fix," he feels bad. Once he gets it, he feels better.

Withdrawal symptoms usually last 3 or 4 days. No wonder people don't change diets. They don't want to feel bad for 4 days . . . and for all they know they will feel bad forever.

FOOD AND FREEDOM

In spite of what the government keeps telling us, modern man has few freedoms left. And the freedoms he does have are not very palatable.

For example, you are free to pay your taxes or go to jail. Do you like either of those freedoms?

You are free to put up with your husband's alcoholism or take your three children and leave home and try to make it on your own.

The truth is that all of us live bound and gagged.

About the only true freedom we have left is choosing what we put in our mouths. Many people don't want to learn what they "should" eat or "shouldn't" eat. They don't want to lose their last freedom.

AND LASTLY, SOME PEOPLE WANT TO BE SICK

As Freud pointed out, two conflicting impulses work within all of us: one urging us toward life, the other toward death. And it is this conflict, I believe, that leads so many of us to make self-destructive habits a way of life.

The other day I saw a young girl in my office whom I had earlier diagnosed as extremely sensitive to wheat and sugar. After a stormy period of recovery from an emotional illness, she had begun to feel almost normal again. She had improved to the point where she was ready to re-enter the community by doing some volunteer work. The Sunday before she was to begin, she ate a plateful of macaroni, which she knew contained wheat. She followed this up with two hefty slices of cake. The predictable result was a two-week period of extreme emotional stress.

This girl was terrified of being propelled into health so fast, of losing the attention (and security) of her childlike dependency, of having to meet the demands society would place on her as a healthy adult.

She was also angry. Often when you feel anger or resentment at people you love, or upon whom you are dependent, you take out your hostility on yourself. This accounts in part for the furious self-inflicted wounds a psychiatrist sees so often, the slashes on the wrists of rebellious teenagers, as well as the self-destructive drinking, smoking, and drug use.

The Milk Controversy

Before I describe in more detail the way to design a Back-to-Nature diet, I want to discuss the question of milk and dairy products, since so many people labor under the delusion that milk is "a natural," "nature's perfect food," as the milk industry constantly tells us in its commercials.

If you are a white, middle-class American, the chances are you didn't even know a milk controversy exists. Americans have been bombarded with advertisements from the dairy industry stating flatly that "adults need at least three glasses daily" and children need a quart of milk a day or more. Perhaps it will come as a shock to you to learn that the great majority of the earth's adult population have enzyme systems that cannot handle milk properly. Milk gives them gas, cramps, indigestion and often causes emotional side effects such as depression and confusion.

In My Practice: Schools, Blacks, Chinese

Most children at about age two experience a gradual reduction of the body supply of lactase which is an enzyme essential for utilizing lactose, or milk sugar. In evolutionary terms this was probably one of nature's survival measures, insuring that older children would stop nursing in time for a new baby to receive all the mother's supply of milk.

In Oriental, African, and American Indian cultures adults drink little milk. Studies at Johns Hopkins University revealed that up to 70% of Afro-Americans cannot metabolize milk properly, a fact that gives rise to a good deal of well-justified rancor in the black community, because ethnocentric government agencies continue to waste money on milk for school lunch programs in areas where the children badly need nutritional supplements and are only made sick by being fed milk.

It is currently admitted that inability to metabolize milk and dairy products runs as high as 40% even among adult Caucasians. I believe that our current tests for milk intolerance are incomplete, so that the actual figure is much higher. No one over the age of two should drink milk.

I am aware that being against milk is like being against the American flag and motherhood, but I want to emphasize that our feelings about milk have been dangerously manipulated by expensive ad campaigns from those who have most to gain by perpetuating the milk myth, just as we have been tricked by cleverly worded misinformation about "refined" sugar and grain products.

It is true that milk is a fair source of protein, calcium, and vitamins for those who can handle it. But I have seen great damage to infants, children and adults who are unable to metabolize milk, who are allergic to it and who have suffered for years without even dreaming that milk could be causing trouble.

Another Overlooked Fact About Milk

Calcium and magnesium work as a team in the human body. For this team to work properly, our bodies must have about half as much magnesium and calcium. If you take calcium without getting magnesium, you throw this team into confusion.

Milk is not a good source of magnesium.

When you drink milk and get calcium *without* getting magnesium, you throw the body's chemistry into confusion.

Another Problem With Milk

If it were up to me, I would recommend that babies be given mother's milk up to the age of two, and that after that their milk intake should be eliminated. (If for any reason an infant must be given a formula, it should be made *without* cane sugar. It is entirely possible that the baby whose formula is laced with sucrose may grow up to be an adult with hypoglycemia or diabetes.) (Of course after age 2, children must be given minerals.)

Having raised my objections to milk as forcefully as possible, I must concede that a great many people will be unwilling to forego milk and dairy products. Indeed, many people probably can tolerate dairy products especially in small amounts. And while I believe that many more are allergic to milk than suspect it, surely some are not.

The milk product best tolerated: sweet butter. Most of my patients do well on it. Those patients who cannot tolerate butter may tolerate it well if they "clarify" it before eating it.

The milk industry will be relieved to know that I advise against eating margarine. We don't know enough about margarine's long term biological effects.

MORE OF THE BACK-TO-NATURE DIET

To start with, you should be careful that whatever you eat is in the most natural condition possible.

That means foods that are fresh, unprocessed, uncanned, unfrozen, uncolored, unflavored, and free of chemical additives. Processing destroys vital nutrients. More important, additives in processed foods can cause (or contribute to) a range of dangerous physical and mental diseases. Some 2,000 additives are currently allowed by the FDA. Few have been adequately tested. Of the ones that have, many continue in use because of pressure from wealthy food processors, even though there is strong evidence that the chemicals are dangerous. Several have been found to cause cancer in laboratory animals; many others speed up the growth of cancers already present. Equally important, they cause emotional disorders in many people.

To give one example, Dr. Ben Feingold, director emeritus of the department of allergy, Kaiser-Permanente Medical Center in San Francisco, has been studying hyperkinetic children. Hyperkinesis affects hundreds of thousands of children and adolescents. The symptoms are extreme hyperactivity, aggressive behavior, short attention span, insomnia, a low frustration threshold, and other forms of behavior so disruptive that many of these children have to be put in special schools.

When it was discovered that, unlike adults, hyperkinetic children calmed down when given amphetamines (or "speed"), a furor developed over the practice in many schools of urging the parents to put their children on permanent doses of speed to make the youngsters easier to handle.

Dr. Feingold took the opposite approach by prescribing a diet that contained no preservatives, flavorings, colorings, pesticides, or hormones. Within one week, many of the children in his study were completely symptom-free. But their hyperkinesis could be reactivated in some cases by as little as a single commercially-baked doughnut.

My experience tells me that Fiengold didn't go far enough. He would have gotten much better results if he had also taken the children off milk, sugar, and all grains.

Organic

I have not been impressed with the feeding of "organic" fruits and vegetables that have not been sprayed. For one thing they are difficult to find. For another, you have no way of knowing what chemicals were used on them.

You see yellow and green and red photographs of great heaps of "health giving" fruits and vegetables.

No longer.

What you see are great heaps of chemically treated fruits and vegetables that are still loaded with chemicals.

Here's the Best Solution

Peel everything possible. What you can't peel, wash.

Eat very few fruits and vegetables. That way you will get less chemicals. Eat not "heaps of health-giving salads," but rather eat no more than 1/2 cup of vegetables three times a day, or more than 1 cup of fruit three times a day.

That's the best, most practical way to reduce your chemical intake.

It's far better to eat them raw. If you must cook them, steam them lightly. In no case drink the water they were cooked in.

If you can grow your own fruits and vegetables, that's ideal.

Chicken

People react very differently to different sources of chicken.

I had one patient who could eat no chicken bought in the New York area. She moved to Lexington, Kentucky and found she could eat the chicken sold there.

I have two patients in Pennsylvania who can only tolerate chicken grown on their own farm.

Many of my patients do well on Kosher chicken or Holly Farms chicken. Most of my patients do poorly on the most widely advertised brand of chicken in the New York area.

Many people tolerate whole chicken and do not tolerate cut up chicken. I suspect they paint antibiotics on the chicken parts when they cut them up to keep them "fresh"!

If you wonder what could be wrong with a nice, fresh, nationally advertised brand of chicken, consider that a commercially grown chicken goes from egg to butcher block in six weeks—six weeks! What if you fed the same growth hormones to your own children? They would grow up in two years instead of twenty and you'd save a fortune in groceries.

Unfortunately, in addition to making chickens grow faster, the chemicals in ordinary commercial chicken can also make cancers grow faster. During butchering, these chickens are often found to have abnormal growths and tumors.

It is common practice for cancerous parts to be thrown away (or used in pet food) while the rest is packaged and sold as "cut up chicken parts."

Always stay away from processed meats such as canned meats, bologna, commercial sausage, bacon, and ham. They are often loaded with sodium nitrate, among other chemicals, one of the most dangerous of the common food additives. I know firsthand that sodium nitrate produces many emotional symptoms in adults as well as children and cancer.

WHAT I EAT, MEAT BY MEAL

I have already described the many differences in individual nutritional needs. Obviously, then, I am not going to turn around and give you a rigid diet and assure you that it will be just right for you.

Even though I find many ill people recover when eating a diet high in meats and animal fats, I have some patients who must totally avoid all animal products.

In the chapter on allergy I help you establish your own proper diet.

First, a little introduction. Assume you have hypoglycemia. It's very common, especially among people who think enough about food to buy a book such as this. The same goes for people who have allergies to foods.

Unless proved otherwise, your diet should be based mostly on meats and animal fats, laced with 1/2 cup of fresh raw vegetable 3 times a day. Many people can also tolerate one cup of fruit 1 to 3 times a day.

To reemphasize: our ancestors ate the foods I have mentioned for many millions of years, so evolution has equipped most of us with enzyme systems to handle these foods. We weren't designed to live in a zoo and eat over-engineered food. Some hardy souls thrive on such treatment, but many fail to bloom under such adverse conditions.

Now I am going to describe what I eat and why, and what I don't eat and why. From this you will be able to form guidelines for your own diet. You should, as I've said, start with the most natural diet you can manage. In this chapter I will deal with foods, but you should keep in mind that this diet is only part of a nutritional program that includes vitamin and mineral supplements as well. Those will be dealt with in subsequent chapters.

MY BREAKFAST

I hate to disillusion you, but like every other person in the world, I lack perfection. (Please don't tell anyone!) I have a cup of black coffee first thing in the morning. My particular allergies will allow me to get away with it. Yours may or may not.

Pearls About Coffee

While we're talking about coffee, you should learn a few things about it.

For one thing, most of my patients who drink coffee do better on regular coffee than on "decaffeinated" coffee. Why, I'm not sure. Possibly it's because there are fewer chemicals in it.

"Decaffeinated" coffee is 97% caffeine free.

Regular coffee is 95% caffeine free.

Like most advertised products in the world of food, "decaffeinated" coffee is only a figment of an advertising executive's imagination.

Point number two: Some people tolerate ice coffee much better than hot coffee.

Next important point: People vary widely in their reactions to different brands of coffee. The other day I sampled a cup of coffee grown in Hawaii. It made me sleepy. Some coffees will give me eczema. Some brands are just right for me, though they might not be for you.

In the world of allergy, everything that's different is different.

BACK TO BREAKFAST

First let me say that I don't eat the minute I get up. This morning, for example, I got up at 5:30. As I write this line it's nearly 8:30. My breakfast is now cooking. (I use electrical timers for all cooking.) It will be ready to eat in about 30 minutes, some 3½ hours after I got up.

The first rule is: eat only when you're hungry.

Every morning I eat a beef rib steak. This is usually hung IBP beef that is only a few days old when I get it from the wholesaler. I wrap it in aluminum foil (dull side against the meat), then place it in the freezer. I removed the foil before putting it in my toaster broiler. I cook it while still frozen. This 1¼ inch thick steak will cook for 20 minutes on one side, then 20 minutes on the other side.

I'll peel and eat a Granny Smith apple. That's my breakfast.

Sometimes I have Yellow Delicious apples, but this time of year they have a chemical taste, so I wait until they taste right.

Then I have my vitamins, minerals, oils, etc.

Cook in the Morning!

Many people would rather starve than cook in the morning. But don't use that as an excuse to eat toast and corn flakes! You can cook the meat the night before and eat it cold in the morning, or you can use timers the way I do.

I cook almost all of my food, yet spend less than 20 minutes a week at it. The secret is the use of timers that actually cut off the electrical current to the broiler after a certain length of time.

I have a hot plate, a toaster broiler, and a microwave oven. About 50% of the time I boil my steak (leave pink in center!).

My Lunch

I only eat lunch if hungry. Often I'm not hungry and skip it. Often I don't have time to eat lunch.

At lunch, I may have some cold leftover steak from breakfast and a piece of fruit, perhaps a fresh, but not fully ripe, papaya. Incidentally, most allergic people tolerate fresh, but not fully ripe, papaya. (Don't eat the seeds.) Why people tolerate papaya is a mystery to me. It's one of those quirks of nature.

Never Cook with Gas

You should never eat anything—especially meat—broiled under gas. The meat picks up the hydrocarbons and may give you an allergic reaction. Hydrocarbons have also been found to cause cancer.

Browned and Burned Fats

Never eat fats that are browned or burned. Such fats are very likely to give you an allergic reaction—tiredness is the most likely allergic reaction from browned and burned fats—and such fats are probably carcinogenic. Suggestion: Reread what I've already said about fats in chapter 12.

You will not get enough to eat unless you eat some of the fat. Also, you will become ill if you eat a heavy meat diet and do not eat some of the fat. You will have to learn by trial and error how much fat to eat.

But That's Too Heavy for Me!

Wait until you get hungry before eating.

If it's too heavy, eat less.

People eating spaghetti and pizza and ice cream and such are used to a certain pleasant feeling of fullness they get following a meal. If you eat enough meat and fat to reach that stage, you'll probably make yourself ill.

Easy does it, especially at first.

But Meat Doesn't Satisfy Me!

True, it won't—until you get past the withdrawal stage that lasts for 3 or 4 days when you leave off grains, sugar and milk products.

After four days, the meat will satisfy you. Keep working at it. Things will settle down. And don't forget, beef might not be right for you.

I mentioned a Jewish patient on Staten Island who can only eat pork. I have another patient whose ancestors come from a seaport in Norway. He can tolerate no beef. He does beautifully, however, on plates full of oily fish. He has to be careful to keep from drinking too much cod liver oil!

If You Work in an Office

It's much better to carry your lunch. Cook a steak ahead of time freeze it and take it to work. By lunch time it will be thawed enough to eat.

Several years ago I went to Iceland to give some speeches. I took enough frozen steaks to last for several days. It worked beautifully.

Do not reheat meat—or anything else.

MY DINNER

For dinner I almost always eat another rib steak. Note: Eat what likes you, not what you like.

The rest of my dinner is the same as lunch. Once or twice a week I have a small piece of non-sweet vegetable such as endive.

On the weekend I sometimes eat out at a restaurant that I know cooks the food as I ask them to and I know I don't react to it. I seldom eat at an unknown restaurant. Usually I eat beef or veal.

Now and then on a weekend I have my big treat—pork chops and fried bananas. For some reason I can eat the pork chops from this restaurant. If I cook my own pork chops, they make me tired. Same if I fry my own bananas. It's a cheap Spanish restaurant on 8th Avenue. They don't like gringos and treat me like dirt.

But so it goes. . . .

COOKING

Some people have fewer reactions to meat that is well done, whereas others can only thrive on meat that is cooked rare. A few people only react well to raw meat!

Again with vegetables, some people react well to them only if they are cooked. Other people thrive only on raw vegetables. Test yourself and decide!

If you eat your fruits and vegetables raw, you will probably be healthier six months from now than you would be if you cooked them.

WHAT TO DRINK

You will not be surprised that I suggest that milk be omitted. Also, omit soft drinks, since sugar and sugar substitutes both cause problems. Diet sodas are full of chemicals that cause problems. Fruit juices are not recommended. Vegetable juices also give trouble.

Hypoglycemics should cut out tea and coffee. Decaffeinated coffee is even worse than regular coffee because of the added chemical impurities. Herbal teas usually cause reactions. Sassafras tea has been found to be carcinogenic.

Water

Anyone following a heavy fish-fowl-meat diet must drink at least 1½ quarts of water daily, otherwise he will be ill.

Since you may be allergic to fluorine and chlorine and other additives and impurities that turn up increasingly in public water supplies, I urge caution. Even if you are not allergic to it, you should avoid chemically treated water.

I prefilter my water, then distill it. Do not drink store-bought distilled water.

To find the right bottled water for you, drink one brand for three days straight, then drink another brand for three days, then another. It will dawn on you which one is best for you.

Some people react well to all sources of water. Some people have a great deal of trouble finding the right water. I had one patient who moved to Hawaii because that was the only place she could find water that agreed with her.

If you buy bottled water, buy it in glass if possible. If you buy it in plastic, boil it in a glass pot for five minutes, then put it in a new glass bottle. Do not use an old apple juice bottle. Everybody seems to have old apple juice bottles at home. The trouble is you never get all the old apple juice out of them. If you do, then you never get all the detergent out of them.

Horror Story

I have a million horror stories. Want to hear one?

I once visited a bar with a friend and very virtuously had a glass of city water. (I can drink a glass of it now and then without reacting to it.)

This glass of water, however, made me so sleepy I almost put my head down on the bar and passed out.

I finally figured out what happened. The barman washed the glasses in a chemical to sterilize them. The glasses were not adequately rinsed. As a result I had some sterilizing chemical along with my water.

IS IT WORTH IT?

We are all constantly making choices.

If longevity is not among your overriding ambitions, if you don't much care whether you grow senile or spend your most productive years feeling less than your best, by all means follow your own dietary inclinations.

If you are considering trying my way, the first decision you must make is not whether you want to feel your best. The question is: Do you want it badly enough to make some sacrifice for it—not a day, a week, or a month, but for good?

Always Remember: The body goes through a period of adjustment on a new diet. As a result, you may feel worse during the first seven or eight days on a different diet. So a bit of extra patience is valuable.

DO NOT BUY MEAT WRAPPED IN PLASTIC. PUT THE PLASTIC ON YOUR TONGUE AND TASTE IT. YOU'll UNDERSTAND.

EAT ONLY FRESH MEAT. BUY MEAT THAT'S PINK, NOT RED.

NEVER REHEAT MEAT.

CHAPTER SIXTEEN

YOU NEED TO KNOW THIS ABOUT VITAMINS

(Also see Chapter 18, *How to Establish Your Ideal Vitamin and Mineral Program*)

Vitamins are organic compounds that are needed in small amounts (along with minerals and proteins) to form enzymes. For example, the enzyme called carboxylase is made up of thiamine (vitamin B_1) and magnesium (a mineral) and a protein.

As pointed out earlier, enzymes are essential agents that speed up the chemical reactions that take place in the body. Without them we could not grow and reproduce. In fact, we couldn't live without them. Enzymes, for example, help the cells of your body turn a steak (a collection of chemicals) into energy so you can breathe and walk and shake your fist at a baseball umpire.

Our bodies are unable to make most vitamins. We must either take them by mouth or have them interjected.

Natural vs. Synthetic Vitamins

We have learned to recreate in the laboratory the vitamins that occur in nature. These are called synthetic vitamins.

Most chemists maintain that for biological purposes no difference exists between manufactured vitamins and these occurring in na-

145

ture. I'm not so sure. Some of our foremost scientists, perhaps secure enough to be able to admit ignorance, stress that we have not yet worked out the entire vitamin puzzle.

For example, one evening before dinner I was talking with Albert Szent-György, the 1937 Nobel Prize winner for discovering ascorbic acid. He remarked that Vitamin C needs substances to work with it, substances still unknown to us.

"Whatever the unknown substance might be, it's not in those," he remarked as he pointed at a table heavy with French pastries. "It's something in there," and he indicated a salad bowl.

GROWTH RATE

An article in the *Journal of Nutrition* reported the results of a research project carried out at the Agricultural Research Center in Beltsville, Maryland. It was found that rats' growth rates were greatly impaired while they were on an artificial diet that contained all the known substances needed for rat nutrition. When natural food was added to their diet, proper growth promptly resumed. The inference is that the natural food contained substances not present in the artificial product.

Several studies have established that natural vitamins A and D are much less toxic than the artificially produced variety. It has been reported that synthetic vitamin D in the recommended dosage to prevent rickets, has caused toxicity in children, while there have been no such reports about natural vitamins A and D taken in normal dosage.

The Canadian Medical Association reported on fifteen cases of skin disease which were treated by injections of synthetic vitamin B with no improvement. When yeast or liver extract (both rich sources of vitamin B) were given to these patients, the benefits became quickly manifest.

The Vitamin Research News of the Soviet Union reported on vitamin C-deficient guinea pigs which recovered much more quickly on doses of natural vitamin C than on the synthetic form.

It was reported in the *American Review of Tuberculosis* that patients suffering from tuberculosis responded much better when given natural vitamins A and D in the form of cod liver oil than when the same substances were administered in synthetic form.

MURPHY'S WORD

In 1934, William P. Murphy, George R. Minot, and George H. Whipple shared a Nobel Prize for discovering that pernicious anemia could be controlled by injections of liver extract. During the late 1940's, Murphy began to switch from crude liver extracts (which contain a wide spectrum of the B-complex vitamins) to purified vitamin B_{12} which had been demonstrated to control pernicious anemia as well as the crude liver product. Murphy found that purified B_{12} did indeed prevent and control pernicious anemia. Many of his patients insisted, nonetheless, on going back to the crude extract because they had lost the sense of well-being it had provided. These patients were receiving benefits from the natural substance that were missing from the synthetic product.

In conversation with me, Dr. Murphy, one of the great heroes of the medical world, said that crude liver probably contains a vitamin or some other similar substance that we have not yet discovered.

My own case provides an interesting example of the desirability of taking natural vitamins. A number of years ago I developed an allergic dermatitis on my hands. The two dermatologists I consulted recommended cortisone and superficial X-ray therapy. Neither inquired into my dietary habits or vitamin intake.

An injection of cortisone did almost completely heal my hands for a week, but when the cortisone wore off the inflammation promptly returned. Other preparations were tried, with similar results.

It became more and more obvious to me that these two specialists were concentrating exclusively on the local disease process while ignoring possibly underlying nutritional and metabolic factors. On my own, I decided to give myself an injection of crude liver extract. Though I was already taking large amounts of all the known B-complex vitamins by pill, the effect of the crude liver injection was prompt and dramatic. My hands cleared up completely.

I still require a liver extract injection once a month. If I skip it, I invariably develop a lesion near the nail on the fourth finger of my right hand. Equally invariably, it clears up again after the injection. When I take desiccated liver capsules by mouth, or eat another vitamin B-rich compound such as brewers' yeast, the dermatitis is not prevented. Hence, I conclude that not only do I need crude B-complex vitamins, but that these must be taken by injection to be effective in my case. Apparently the oral route does not result in sufficient absorption.

VITAMINS ARE VULNERABLE

In our modern environment, it's difficult to meet our vitamin needs. Not only is the vitamin content of food greatly reduced by the way it is handled before we eat it, but factors such as smog vastly increase our need for several vitamins—notably C and E. We end up with a reduced intake of vitamins and an increased need for them. Remember that smog is not limited to Los Angeles and New York. It is blight that covers almost all of the country and much of the world. Even in remote mountain regions of Appalachia the natives speak of the deterioration of visibility during their lifetime.

Freezing destroys vitamin K, and vitamin C is destroyed by cooking. What few vegetables we get in our modern diet are overcooked, so that much of the vitamin content is lost.

Drugs are another hazard. Many widely-used drugs (such as aspirin, birth control pills, and antibiotics) either destroy vitamins, keep them from being absorbed, or interfere with their utilization. Diuretics are frequently prescribed for women who suffer from edema (fluid accumulation). These eliminate the excess fluid along with vital sodium, potassium, magnesium, and B vitamins. Birth control pills interfere with vitamin B_{12}, folic acid, and vitamin B_6 metabolism.

Louis F. Wertalik of the Ohio State University College of Medicine, reported that in a group of healthy young women, birth control pills had greatly reduced serum B_{12} levels, and had somewhat diminished serum folic acid levels. He was unable to explain the mechanism by which the oral contraceptives produced this effect. Despite the low serum B_{12} levels, he had found the women's tissue levels to be adequate. It may therefore be that the serum levels were simply not reduced for a sufficiently long time to cause a reduction in the tissue levels, and that if oral contraceptives had been continued, the tissue levels would have shown a drop within a year or two.

Mineral oil blocks absorption of the fat-soluble vitamins A, D, and K. Iron, which is frequently prescribed for anemia and forms part of many over-the-counter tonics, interferes with the absorption of vitamin E.

The use of tobacco is very destructive to vitamin C and blocks vitamin B_{12} co-enzymes. Radiation therapy is destructive to many vitamins.

PEOPLE ARE IN TROUBLE

In recognition of these and many other detrimental circumstances, George M. Owen, M.D., of Ohio State University Children's Hospital, has stated a fact that cannot be sufficiently emphasized: The current nutritional status of the people of the United States is simply not known. But we have plenty of alarming clues: The U.S. Department of Agriculture, through then Assistant Secretary of Agriculture George L. Mehren, stated some time ago that at least 38 percent of the families in this country live on diets that do not even meet the minimal nutrition requirements set forth by the National Academy of Sciences. Even the Food and Nutritional Board of the FDA has stated that its guidelines concerning allowances for nutritional substances don't necessarily reflect the needs of any one person or group, since these can only be determined by clinical and biochemical examinations.

Nor is poor nutrition confined to "backward" rural areas in the poorer Southern states. A survey of 642 New York City children revealed that 73 percent subsisted on diets that did not measure up to the National Research Council's recommendation for daily allowances. According to the Bureau of Nutrition of the New York Department of Health, these children had low blood levels of many of the B vitamins, especially vitamin B_{12} and niacin, and suffered significant reading disabilities. Dr. George Christakis, director of the survey, urged that these children be given vitamin supplements.

A recent survey in England of 172 unselected psychiatric patients revealed that 47 percent of them had frank vitamins deficiencies.

Since excess amounts of the water-soluble vitamins are excreted by the body, it is my firm opinion that reasonably large amounts of these vitamins can and should be taken. (See precautions about vitamin B_6 in the section discussing that vitamin.) On the other hand, with the fat-soluble vitamins (A, D, and E), the possibility of toxicity does exist under certain circumstances, and much closer attention must therefore be paid to their dosage. The guidelines of the FDA are, however, too general and are useful only on the public health level. The optimal dosage for each person must be worked out on an individual basis.

EVERY CELL NEEDS EVERY VITAMIN

I dislike writing about one vitamin at a time, saying vitamin C helps wound-healing or that vitamin D is needed to absorb calcium. Each cell in the body needs every vitamin. Indeed, vitamins do not occur in the food we eat one at a time, isolated from each other.

Space makes it impossible for me to expand on the subject as I would like. This is a practical book in which I hope to teach you, with the help of your doctor, what vitamins to take and how to take them.

If you want to know about the separate vitamins intimately, you will find many books by experts without clinical experience who can enlighten you. But not many people who write about vitamins are physicians who sit across the desk from patients day after day, year after year, helping people work out their specific dietary supplements. This is the unique information I have. You bought the book to get that special knowledge.

With this preview in mind, let me give you a very brief introduction to vitamins to help you say hello to them.

TAKE VITAMINS AFTER MEALS?

When you first start taking vitamin, minerals and other nutritional supplements, I suggest that you take them directly after eating. If you wish, later you may test and learn whether you tolerate supplements on an empty stomach.

Iron is an exception. It should be taken on an empty stomach. It absorbs better in an acid medium. Iron and vitamin E should be taken at different ends of the day. If taken near the same time, selenium also interferes with absorption of vitamin E.

Vitamin A

Numerous studies have proved vitamin A is one of the vitamins most frequently low in the American diet. This deficiency has been noted many times in surveys of children in New York City. Remember, vitamin D and calcium cannot work properly without vitamin A, since vitamin A deficiency affects the skeleton and limits its growth.

The central nervous system of growing children can sustain severe mechanical damage because the brain and other parts of the central nervous system continue to grow without a corresponding increase in size of the bony structures.

In adults, this deficiency causes a number of symptoms, among them the well-known "night blindness," and the appearance of rough, scaly skin patches, especially on the upper arms. I well remember suffering from the latter condition myself during my teens, and have no doubt that it was brought on by vitamin A deficiency.

Although vitamin A deficiencies are frequently seen in this country, deficiencies of vitamin A are often devastating in poorer nations. Children by the tens of thousand are severely injured by a deficiency in this vitamin, often to the extent that they are blind.

Night blindness was first described in Egypt in 1500 B.C. Interestingly, fried liver was eaten to cure it. Liver is a rich source of vitamin A, of course.

The vitamin protects us against colds, pneumonia, and influenza, and a deficiency may result in inadequate protection of the mucous membranes against infection.

It also protects against cancer and bladder stones and has been used in the treatment of acne and psoriasis.

The vitamin occurs in large amounts in carrots, liver, and sweet potatoes, and in smaller amounts in many other vegetables. But I do not think it wise to depend upon food intake for an adequate supply. This applies especially to diabetics, who have difficulty in transforming the carotene of yellow vegetables to vitamin A.

Because synthetic forms of vitamins A and D are apparently more toxic than natural ones, I suggest that you confine yourself to supplements made from natural sources of these two vitamins.

SHERMAN AT COLUMBIA

Dr. Henry Sherman of Columbia University was able to increase the longevity of rats by giving them added amounts of Vitamin A.

In his experiments he used the Osborne-Mendel strain of rats, that had been doing quite well on a diet of whole wheat and milk for 67 generations, and whose lifespan was precisely known. If there had been any significant defects in this diet, they would of course have shown up long before 67 generations had come and gone. Nonetheless, by doubling the amount of vitamin A in their standard diet, Dr. Sherman caused the male rats to live 5 percent longer, and the females to live 10 percent longer than expected. When he redoubled the amount of vitamin A, the males lived 10 percent longer and the females 20 percent longer. A second doubling of the vitamin A dose did not result in further increase of lifespan.

In terms of humans, it might mean that our lifespans could be increased from about 70 to about 110 or 120 years.

No one as yet knows whether these or similar findings are applicable to humans. But since we are betting our health and our lives on our intake of nutrients, I, for one, am going to place one of my bets on supplements of vitamin A.

VITAMIN A HELPS THE HEART

F. C. Ross, M.D., and A. H. Campbell, M.D., reported on an interesting study in which they administered vitamins A and D for ten years to a group of patients. In the treated group, the incidence of coronary heart disease was 5.8 percent; in the untreated group it was 15.8 percent. This may tie in with the well-known fact that the cholesterol level has a tendency to drop when vitamin A is administered.

In laboratory animals many birth defects have occurred in the offspring of mothers deficient in vitamin A. Do you want to take the chance of having malformed children or do you want to take vitamin A?

To avoid toxicity, which can be serious, the FDA recommends that no more than 7.5 mg of retinol (about 25,000 units of vitamin

A) be consumed daily. If you eat liver, be sure to include the vitamin A from liver when calculating your daily total.

Relatively large doses of vitamin E seem to give some protection against vitamin A intoxication. Vitamin A intoxication is rare, and usually involves the artificially produced vitamin. (One of the signs of toxicity of vitamin A may be emotional instability.)

The forms of vitamin A used in large doses to treat acne and psoriasis must be taken only under the strictest supervision of a physician.

VITAMIN A FOR THE COMMON COLD

As a preventative and treatment for the common cold, vitamin A has not had the press coverage of vitamin C. In my experience, however, vitamin A is even more important than vitamin C for the prevention and treatment of the common cold.

I take about 12,000 units of natural vitamin A daily from cod liver oil. If I feel a cold starting, I increase it to 75,000 units daily (by adding capsules of vitamin A) but *never for more than 5 days*.

Twelve-thousand units daily is also the minimal dose level I recommend for all of my adult patients. Patients with cancer or a strong history of cancer may get more, but only under close supervision. Vitamin A is not a vitamin to be adventurous with.

I also take a Beta-Carotene capsule, 15 mg every third day. The body turns this precursor of vitamin A into vitamin A. There is some evidence that it is more helpful in preventing cancer than the regular vitamin A. I feel certain that it has a great ability to prevent infections, including upper respiratory infection.

Many people take too much carotene. If the palms of your hands are beginning to turn orange, you're getting too much.

Your Vitamin B_1 Needs

Thiamine (vitamin B_1, sometimes spelled "thiamin") is the granddaddy of the "nerve" vitamins. It's essential for the proper functioning of the central nervous system. Its lack can result in almost any nervous manifestation you can name: depression, loss of memory, difficulty in concentration, fatigue, tension, heart failure, hyperactivity, confusion, hallucinations, numbness in the arms or legs, and many more.

Although the brain makes up only 2 percent of the total body weight, 25 percent of total metabolic activity takes place within it. Therefore the brain is extremely sensitive to a lack of vitamins.

Thiamine also acts as a co-enzyme necessary for the oxidation of alpha-keto acids, including pyruvic acid, which is a step in the process of carbohydrate metabolism. Since carbohydrates are the central nervous system's prime source of energy, thiamine is particularly important to the proper functioning of that system. (Don't worry about not eating carbohydrates. The body can make carbohydrates from fats.)

Vitamin B_1 is also needed for one nerve ending to properly stimulate (and thus pass along impulses) to other nerves.

A person doing heavy physical labor needs extra thiamine to compensate for a stepped-up carbohydrate metabolism. (The average laborer is likely to get many calories from carbohydrates.) For this reason the amounts required for good health vary somewhat, but the FDA states that 1.5 mg of thiamine per day is your recommended daily allowance. I personally take 500 mg daily.

Thiamine can be destroyed by drinking tea or eating raw fish. Both contain a vitamin B_1 antagonist. Alcoholics seemed to have a special need for extra amounts of vitamin B_1.

WHERE TO GET IT

Vitamin B_1 is present in many foods but tends to be depleted by the consumption of sugar, alcohol, and tobacco.

Vitamin B_1 is lost in storing and preparing food, especially when an alkaline salt like sodium bicarbonate (baking soda) is added to foods during cooking. High temperatures destroy much of the thiamine in meat. When water is used for cooking vegetables, thiamine is leached out.

One of the greatest losses of thiamine is caused by the milling of grains. When the outer husk of the grain is removed, much of the vitamin and mineral content is removed with it. White bread and white rice are, therefore, relatively thiamine-deficient foods.

Even though thiamine may be added to enriched bread, it is partially destroyed again by toasting.

SYMPTOMS OF DEFICIENCY

The symptoms of thiamine deficiency were described by a Chinese physician in 2600 B.C.

In 1872 a young Japanese naval scientist, Kanehiro Takaki, became appalled at the amount of beri-beri (a deadly form of neuritis, an inflammation of the nerves) occurring among sailors on long voyages. It seemed logical to suspect a dietetic cause. A crew of 276 left Japan for a trip to New Zealand, South America, Hawaii, and back. Of this crew, 169 developed beri-beri and 25 died of it. Another ship was sent on the same voyage, but with increased rations of meat, fish, and vegetables, and decreased amounts of rice. Wheat and milk were also added to the sailors' diet.

On this second voyage no deaths from beri-beri occurred, though fourteen men developed the disease. These fourteen, it so happened, had not eaten the full diet as prescribed.

Takaki reported his findings in the British medical journal *Lancet* but the article was ignored by the medical profession, which at the time was convinced that beri-beri was an infectious disease.

The struggles proving beri-beri to be a nutritional deficiency were much like those undergone by James Lind in proving that vitamin C deficiency caused scurvy in the British Navy. Joseph Goldberger, early in this century, had great difficulty proving that pellagra was a nutritional disease rather than an infection. (A group of establishment doctors appointed by the Federal government studied pellagra and—incorrectly—concluded that it was an infectious disease!)

THIAMINE IS WATER-SOLUBLE

Since thiamine is water-soluble, it's rather quickly excreted by the body and cannot build up to toxic levels like vitamins A, D, and E. I therefore have no qualms about taking and prescribing it in substantial amounts.

Patients sometimes get such a lift from thiamine that they need a sedative to calm them down. I vividly remember one doubting physician to whom I once gave a 500 mg tablet. A few hours later he called to tell me that he felt as if he had taken a handful of speed tablets. A sodium amytal capsule was necessary to bring him "down" to working level. This memorable experience convinced him of the tremendous chemical changes which vitamins can evoke.

Oddly enough, thiamine in large amounts can have a lifting effect on tired or depressed people and a tranquilizing effect on excited people.

To some patients I administer as much as 1000 mg of thiamine three times a day, and find it to be the decisive nutritional supplement which makes the difference between their feeling ill or well.

Very rarely individuals do better on thiamine by injection. Physicians experienced in the treatment of alcoholics have often found that thiamine in massive doses helps provide relief from the emotional and physical symptoms of alcoholism.

CAREFUL!

If given by injection, the physician must give thiamine in very small doses and gradually build up. Patients have died from allergic reactions to this vitamin when given by injection. Since the vitamin is well absorbed, it's very rare that a patient needs it by injection.

Your Vitamin B₂ Needs

Although widely available in nature, riboflavin (vitamin B_2) is among the most common dietary deficiencies in our society. Unless baking soda is used, cooking does not destroy a great deal of it; light causes some destruction. Probably the most common cause of riboflavin deficiency is poor dietary habits.

The vitamin is available in relatively large amounts in liver and brewers' yeast, and there is a fair amount in many vegetables. But these items do not form a significant part of modern man's diet.

If you take a relatively large dose of riboflavin it's easy to prove whether or not you are absorbing it properly. If you are absorbing substantial amounts, your urine will turn a rich yellow color.

Riboflavin is active in several enzyme systems, and its lack may cause a wide spectrum of symptoms, including cracks in the corners of the mouth, scaly rashes on nose and forehead, burning and dryness of the eyes, inability to tolerate bright lights, burning of feet, depression, dizziness, and numbness in the arms and legs. Any or all of these deficiency symptoms may coexist, as well as night blindness similar to that caused by lack of vitamin A.

Riboflavin is necessary for proper growth. Evidence says that its lack may increase your susceptibility to infections.

Lack of riboflavin has produced nerve degeneration and malformed offspring in laboratory animals.

My usual riboflavin intake is 200 mg one or two times daily. Some authorities believe that riboflavin intake should equal B_6 intake. I'm not certain about this, but why not?

Your Vitamin B₃ Needs

Vitamin B_3 was one of the vitamins that interested me early in my exploration of the world of nutrition. It's also known as niacin, niacinamide, nicotinic acid, or nicotinamide.

Vitamin B_3 is widely used in the body chemistry as a coenzyme, especially in protein metabolism and oxygen-reduction reactions in tissues.

Niacin has been one of the vitamins neglected by mankind during the entire course of civilization. Its severe lack has resulted in pellagra, the consequences of which are dermatitis, diarrhea, dementia—and death.

I saw my first case of pellagra in 1928. My playmate's grandfather sat on the front porch for most of the day staring at nothing. He had red scaly skin where his hands and neck were exposed to daylight. He was diagnosed as having pellegra and recovered after his family doctor advised his daughter to feed him liver. (Even at that time, the local small town doctor knew that pellagra was a deficiency disease, though the Federal government in all its bureaucratic wisdom—and the professors who advised it—still thought pellagra was an infectious disease.)

Since Vitamin B_3 was added to flour in this country starting in 1939, pellagra is thought to be rare. As a medical student at Duke University in the early 1940's, I saw pellagra many times. The last time I visited the eastern parts of South Carolina (1969), I saw many cases of pellagra in the poorer farm families that grew and ate their own corn and potatoes and hence did not get the vitamin from "store-bought" foods. A local physician confirmed pellagra's prevalence.

Today in New York, mentally incompetent patients not kept in hospitals are allowed to wander the streets, eat garbage and sleep in doorways. Tragically, any summer day in New York, you can see dozens of cases of pellagra in these people lying about on the sidewalks. The evidence: their confused speech and acts, as well as the red scaly skin over their hands and ankles where they are exposed to daylight.

EVEN MORE TRAGIC . . .

But perhaps more tragic are the innumerable people who have missed out on optimal emotional and physical health because of their less-than-optimal niacin (and other vitamin) levels.

There is evidence that niacin may prolong life and put off the senility which too frequently mars our final years. See chapter 23.

Edwin Boyle, M.D., former director of research at the Miami Heart Institute, states that when he administers niacin to middle-aged people for the prevention of heart attacks, they almost invariably return to his office with dramatically increased vigor. Their faces are shining. They have an increased feeling of well-being. They are as full of hope and plans as they were twenty years earlier.

Niacin, along with other dietary supplements, has a wonderful ability to reduce cholesterol. People, however, should take niacin in megadoses only under the care of a doctor who is familiar with its use. If taking more than 250 mg of niacin daily, liver function tests need to be carried out at regular intervals.

STARTING DOSE

When giving a patient niacin, I usually prescribe a starting dose of 250 mg three times a day. I have gone up as high as 30,000 mg daily, but doubt if I ever would again.

Because niacin releases the histamine from the basal cells, most people develop a flush when they first begin taking it. This flush is harmless, and usually disappears within an hour, even though it may be severe at first, so severe that you even feel it in your eardrums. It can be reduced by taking two aspirin or an antihistamine an hour before the niacin, or by taking it with food and cold water.

Some people tend to be over-stimulated by niacin during the first month. This can be handled by reducing the dosage. Your life may simply take on a more active cast, involving more participation and less standing on the sidelines. Some people engaged in sedentary work like bookkeeping or mechanical drawing may find it somewhat difficult to carry on their occupation after going on niacin. But this is far from universal, and can only be tested through trial and error.

I've seen many people who have done much better at their occupations, including artists who had reached an impasse and inability to create but were able to resume work with new vigor and creativity after being placed on niacin.

NIACIN REDUCES BLOOD CLOTTING

Not only does niacin lower serum cholesterol, but it also tends to keep the blood from clotting too easily and increases the oxygen-carrying capacity of red blood cells. Another important property is its tendency to raise blood sugar. A good many depressed or tense people suffer from errors in carbohydrate metabolism resulting in hypoglycemia. For them niacin is sometimes useful.

If, on the other hand, you have diabetes, ulcers, high blood pressure, or porphyria, niacin must be taken strictly under the supervision of a physician with wide experience in vitamin therapy.

Niacinamide and nicotinamide (it has nothing to do with nicotine) have the vitamin effects of niacin but do not cause a flush, and they lack the cholesterol-lowering effects and some of the other beneficial properties of niacin.

Beware: Sometimes the niacinamide form of B_3 causes depression and/or fatigue.

Niacin and niacinamide may cause serious side effects such as liver damage. They should be taken only under the supervision of a physician.

Pantothenic Acid Needs

Pantothenic acid was discovered by Roger Williams, the distinquished professor of biochemistry at the University of Texas and, from 1941 to 1963, director of the Clayton Foundation Biochemical Institute, where more vitamins and their variants were discovered than at any other laboratory in the world.

This man, who knew more about pantothenic acid than anyone, believed that if pregnant women were given 50 mg of this B-complex vitamin per day, the incidence of miscarriages and malformed babies would be greatly reduced. He pointed out that people have taken 250 times this dose without adverse effect—that, indeed, they have been better able to withstand emotional stress with this added vitamin supplement.

There is good reason to believe that humans require larger amounts of pantothenic acid than other mammals. Muscle is the most abundant tissue in the body, and our muscles contain about twice as much pantothenic acid as those of other mammals.

Almost every food we eat contains pantothenic acid. As in all other nutritional problems, the question remains: what is the optimal daily amount?

Pantothenic acid (it is usually given in the form of calcium pantothenate) is essential for the formation of steroid hormones, which means that it is particularly important for individuals under stress, since such persons secrete more adrenal cortical hormones than others. But since the vitamin is used in many co-enzyme systems throughout the body, no cell can function properly without its proper supply of pantothenic acid.

As yet, we do not know the specific daily requirements of this vitamin. Relatively good sources of it are egg yolk, kidney, yeast, and liver. It is available to some extent in almost all unpurified foods, but 57 percent of it is lost when wheat is turned into white flour, and 33 percent is lost during the cooking of meat.

I take 218 mg of calcium pantothenate at bedtime. Most people, in my opinion, would do well on this, though I may give a tense patient up to 436 mg of calcium pantothenate four times a day.

This vitamin is thought to be almost nontoxic for man. Doses up to 10,000 mg daily have been given with only minor gastriontestinal upsets.

Folic Acid

All of the B vitamins interact with one another, but folic acid is especially needed in conjunction with vitamins B_{12} and B_6. Whenever large amounts of those vitamins are taken, extra amounts of folic acid should also be administered.

Since folate is essential for the formation of DNA, it's especially essential for every cell in the body. Quite possibly it becomes even more essential with advancing age.

Anyone who uses alcoholic beverages should take extra amounts of folic acid.

It has been reported that up to 60 percent of psychiatric patients have low serum folic acid levels.

I routinely test all new patients for folic acid. Quite often I find patients deficient in this essential vitamin.

Folic acid is necessary to help the body absorb pantothenic acid, which is the vitamin into which the body breaks down calcium pantothenate when taken by mouth.

In this country, folic acid is not sold over the counter, except in small quantities. If you're deficient in vitamin B_{12}, folic acid may mask that deficiency.

I have tried up to 15 mg daily of folic acid in patients with emotional disorders and find that some patients respond well to it. However, I must say that a fair number of people feel absolutely awful on even small additions of folic acid to their nutritional programs.

Depending upon the individual, megadoses of folic acid may either stimulate or sedate. Often people simply experience an increased feeling of well-being, which, after all, is the prize we all seek.

After taking large amounts of folic acid for several weeks, we may need to lower the intake. As with many other vitamin supplements, the dosage must be "played with," adjusted upward and downward to find the right level.

I take 1 mg of folic acid two times daily. Everyone should have his serum folic acid level tested.

Folic acid is especially important for pregnant women. It prevents birth defects, especially birth defects in the nervous system.

FOLIC ACID AND SEIZURES

Folic acid has been reported to counteract the antiepileptic effect of several drugs that are used to control convulsive seizures. Other studies, however, have not supported these findings. Until the matter is settled, folic acid should be taken with caution and only under the strict supervision of a physician whenever a patient is taking anticonvulsive medication. The nasty rumor that folic acid causes convulsions, however, is completely without foundation.

Your Vitamin B₆ Needs

I have a special interest in vitamin B_6 (also called pyridoxine) since I must take it in relatively large amounts to feel good on a high-protein, high-animal-fat diet.

Vitamin B_6 is one of the vitamins (along with B_{12}) that people would kill for. I once made that statement on a taped interview. The producer stopped the taping and asked if I meant to say that some people would kill for vitamin B_6. I assured him that indeed I did mean what I said.

Vitamin B_6 is known to assist more than 60 different enzyme systems. It's small wonder that many people feel much better when taking it.

Pyridoxine is involved in many stages of protein metabolism, and thus assumes special importance in the vitamin regimens I advocate for many patients who are on high-protein, high-fat diets.

In rats, we find that vitamin B_6 deficiency causes a puffy swelling in the body, restlessness, and convulsions. Many allergic, sniffling children are suffering from pyridoxine deficiency.

These children often exhibit stunted growth, high-arched palates, crooked lower teeth, and a pale, puffy complexion. Dr. Leon Rosenberg, Dean of Yale University School of Medicine, has done much work on pyridoxine-dependent children—youngsters who have convulsions and fail to thrive unless given massive doses of vitamin B_6.

Roger Williams has drawn attention to the pyridoxine-dependent state. He believes that persons on a high-fat diet need added amounts of vitamin B_6 in order to prevent arteriosclerosis and heart disease, as well as hardening of the cerebral arteries and premature senility.

Gruberg and Raymond, physiologists at the Massachusetts Institute of Technology, have written a convincing book which argues that lack of vitamin B_6, not an elevated serum cholesterol, is the most important key to preventing arteriosclerosis, the cause of the great majority of strokes and heart attacks.

Others have presented evidence that vitamin B_6 protects against arteriosclerosis, including patients with peripheral arterial disease.

It's been observed that smoking lowers the body's vitamin B_6 and thought by some that this lowering of B_6 levels may account for the increased incidence of cancer in smokers.

A form of vitamin B_6 has actually been injected into melanomas (a type of cancer that may develop from moles) in laboratory animals and shrunk the growth.

There is some evidence to indicate that B_6 deficiency is at least a contributory factor in the premenstrual edema of women, and may manifest itself in such diverse symptoms as abdominal upsets or stiffness of the neck.

Women on "the pill" have been found to have low B_6 levels. Patients taking medication for tuberculosis need extra amounts of B_6. Certain drugs used to treat Parkinson's syndrome are inactivated by B_6, so it must not be given even in small amounts to people on such medication.

Depression has been observed in people who are deficient in B_6. Nerve damage and/or skin lesions have commonly been observed in patients suffering from a B_6 deficiency. Anemia may also be caused by a lack of the vitamin. Vitamin B_6 is also important for the function of the adrenal cortex.

It is especially important to have relatively large doses of pyridoxine if you are under any kind of stress, whether emotional or physical. Good sources of pyridoxine are yeast, liver, and—to some extent—eggs and leafy vegetables.

I take 200 mg of pyridoxine three times a day by mouth. If you take more than 50 mg daily of pyridoxine you should be under the close supervision of a physician with wide experience in nutritional therapy.

POSSIBLE DANGER FROM VITAMIN B$_6$

Several years ago the *New England Journal of Medicine* reported severe nerve damage in several patients who took 2000 mg or more of vitamin B$_6$ daily.

I have been using large amounts of this vitamin for many years and have never seen this happen. It may be because I give multiple vitamins (including equal amounts of B$_2$) along with the vitamin B$_6$.

On several occasions I've had patients develop a slight tingling of the fingers shortly after taking as little as 200 mg a day of B$_6$. (I remember that once it happened to a pianist!) I've always thought this was due to an allergy. The tingling stopped as soon as the vitamin was discontinued.

Such tingling can happen with any vitamin, or with many different foods. I've even seen it happen in a patient with MS who visited a movie house soon after it was sprayed for cockroaches.

Patients should not take more than 50 mg a day of B$_6$ unless supervised by a physician.

L-Carnitine

L-carnitine is usually referred to as vitamin B$_T$. It's been known since 1905, but has had little attention.

The body can make its own carnitine, but will not be able to without adequate supplies of vitamins B$_3$, B$_6$, and C, plus iron, and the amino acids lysine and methionine. Lysine is well supplied by meats, but it's easily destroyed by heat.

The body cannot utilize carnitine unless it's also given a good supply of the B vitamin pantothenic acid.

In 1983, under contract with the FDA, the Federation of American Societies for Experimental Biology published their conclusions about carnitine. Low body levels of carnitine were found in patients suffering from heart disease, cirrhosis of the liver, kidney diseases, neurological disorders, high serum cholesterol and triglycerides, certain muscles diseases, malnutrition, and low thyroid function.

Most often L-carnitine has been used to lower serum cholesterol levels and raise the HDL (high density lipoprotein) levels. Cholesterol is the "bad" fat in the blood and HDL is the "good" fat. You don't want cholesterol, you do want HDL.

L-carnitine has been recommended in the treatment of many kinds of heart disease and in some quarters is thought to be helpful for the heart muscle tissue itself.

In several of my patients I have seen angina (heart pain brought on by physical activity) ameliorated after they went on L-carnitine.

There have been reports of increased energy in people taking carnitine supplements. Because it helps the utilization of fats, it's been used to help weight reduction.

L-Carnitine capsule (Brand: Twinlab or Solgar) 250 mg, one capsule 2 times a day.

NOTE: *Do not take D-carnitine or DL-carnitine. There have been reports of toxicity from those forms.*

Although I have tested many patients for carnitine deficiency, I've only found one patient frankly deficient in it. I have, however, had a number of people tell me that they had more energy and experienced a feeling of well being when carnitine was added to their supplements late in their treatment programs. L-carnitine tends to block and reduce allergic reactions.

Your Vitamin B₁₂ Needs

Because of its enormous importance in the treatment of many serious emotional illnesses, this member of the B-complex family will be treated more fully in a later chapter. Let me say here only that I feel very strongly that everyone should have his serum vitamin B_{12} level determined. This is vital because many people can't absorb B_{12} when it's taken orally, so even when they take vitamins in large quantities they may still be deficient in vitamin B_{12}.

The anemia that eventually develops from a vitamin B_{12} deficiency may be corrected by taking 2 to 3 mg daily of folic acid; however, folic acid will not prevent the nerve damage (brain degeneration, destruction of the nerves in the spinal cord, etc.) which results from a vitamin B_{12} deficiency.

Also, many people have difficulty transporting vitamin B_{12} from their blood streams into other parts of their bodies, to the muscles and brain, for example. For this reason, in my view everyone should have a few trial injections of vitamin B_{12} (in the hydroxocobalamin form). If people feel better with this injection, they learn to give their own injections and continue the injections indefinitely.

Extra B_{12} is especially important for vegetarians, doubly so for vegetarians who are pregnant.

Your Vitamin C (Ascorbic Acid) Needs

In a conversation I had with the late Dr. Albert Szent-György, he reiterated, among many other things, his conviction that we are a long way from uncovering all the elements required for ideal human nutrition.

For breakfast Dr. Szent-György ate a banana sprinkled with two tablespoonfuls of wheat germ. (Most of my patients do not tolerate wheat germ well at all. I never take it and never recommend it. There are exceptions to everything. Dr. Szent-György may have been such an exception. On the other hand, he's not knowledgeable about the clinical practice of medicine, or about food allergies.)

He thought there is a natural food supplement (probably a B or B-like vitamin) in wheat germ which is essential to the proper functioning of ascorbic acid, and that this unknown factor is also crucial to vitamin C's role in preventing the common cold.

He was convinced that requirements for vitamin C vary enormously from individual to individual, and that it is tragically naive of the medical profession to think of scurvy as being the only result of a deficiency of vitamin C. Scurvy merely presents the ultimate stage of a disease which manifests itself in many earlier symptoms routinely missed by physicians.

GROWTH AND VITAMIN C

An article by Man-Li S. Yew, entitled "A Plus for Pauling and Vitamin C," describes that author's studies regarding the effect of vitamin C on growth, wound healing, and resistance to surgical stress in guinea pigs.

Dr. Yew found that large amounts of vitamin C are required for optimal functioning within these areas. Small amounts safeguarded the guinea pigs against scurvy, but did not allow them to grow to their ideal size, to heal wounds quickly, or to recover promptly from stressful surgical situations. On the basis of his findings he recommended, among other things, that children should be given approximately 1500 mg of vitamin C daily.

Some years ago, I shared a speaker's platform with Irwin Stone, a researcher who spent much of his life studying vitamin C. Stone, in fact, introduced Linus Pauling to the virtues of vitamin C. Pauling in turn, dedicated his book *Vitamin C and the Common Cold* to Stone.

Stone addressed his audience as "fellow mutants," meaning that we are each the result of a chance mutation in our genetic code that prevents us from manufacturing vitamin C in our own body like most mammals.

During the last century we have discovered any number of ways to destroy the vitamin C content of food during processing and storage, and our diet has been altered in an extraordinary way, often substituting bare sugar for the vitamin C-rich fruits eaten by our ancestors. This perversion has led to a host of deficiency symptoms, including decreased ability to fight disease and infection, and to emotional illnesses. We know that schizophrenics require as much as one thousand times the vitamin C used by a "normal" person, but we don't know as yet if this is caused by further chance mutation (causing such people to be born with a wildly exaggerated need for certain vitamins) or whether the enormous stress of being emotionally disturbed creates the need for extra vitamins. Probably both factors are at work.

Vitamin C is a Powerful Detoxifying Agent

It is possible that vitamin C can fight a toxic condition in a schizophrenic because many people with serious emotional problems certainly act as if they were poisoned, even if we cannot always identify the toxin.

One physician reported that he gave ascorbic acid intravenously to a highway patrolman who was overcome and unconscious from carbon monoxide poisoning. Before the needle was removed from the man's arm he was conscious and talking in a rational manner.

Tests have also proven that large doses of ascorbic acid will detoxify the venom from snakes (including rattlesnakes) and keep dogs from developing symptoms after having been bitten by these snakes.

A number of my patients have hypersensitivities that are greatly reduced by ascorbic acid. For example, I have one patient who is so sensitive to tobacco smoke that she can go to a theater where smoking takes place and be so affected that she reels home. But if she takes about 5 g of ascorbic acid before going to the theater she can sit through the movie, survive the smoke in the atmosphere, and walk a straight line home.

Aside from its connection to emotional illness, vitamin C has been found helpful in combating an impressive array of conditions—from counteracting the effects of environmental pollutants like carbon monoxide to the prevention of bruises caused by capillary fragility. Additionally, it has been used in the treatment of toxic insect bites, burns, diabetes, high cholesterol, overdoses of barbiturates, colds and other respiratory ailments, and possibly even malignancies like cancer of the bladder. Evidence of more astounding qualities of this vitamin is constantly accumulating.

The optimum daily intake of vitamin C is not yet known. Probably it varies widely not only from person to person but also in the same person at different times and under different conditions.

The Food and Nutrition Board of the National Academy of Sciences suggests an intake of 60 mg daily for an adult male—and that, you may be sure, is not the optimum amount for many people. I would be fascinated to know the hard scientific facts they used to decide that 14-year-olds need 50 mg a day and 16 year olds need 60 mg a day.

Linus Pauling takes 10,000 mg of ascorbic acid per day. (He keeps edging up on his dosage. By now he's probably taking more.)

My own dose is 15,000 mg a day.

One need only consult the sales figures of the major manufacturer of vitamin C in this country to learn that the use of ascorbic acid has risen sharply each year over the past 15 years. This increase in vitamin C consumption coincides with the decrease in the number of strokes and heart attacks suffered by the population. The American Heart Association feels that the reduction has been brought about by the reduction in the amount of saturated fat eaten by the population.

Both Pauling and I believe that we can thank the increased consumption of ascorbic acid for reducing the number of strokes and heart attacks.

Many studies have illustrated the protection vitamin C gives against cancer. At MIT, both vitamin C and vitamin E have been found to give protection against cancer-causing nitrosamines. Especially interesting is a recent research report showing the dramatic reduction in gastric cancer associated with increased consumption of vitamin C.

Your Vitamin D Needs

Vitamin D is necessary for the formation of a protein in the intestine which helps absorb calcium and other minerals. In turn calcium is a mineral which exerts a strong influence on the stability of cell membranes, particularly those of the central nervous system. And, of course, it is present in large amounts in bones.

When vitamin D—and therefore calcium—is low, the central nervous system becomes irritable. This irritability can range all the way from simple tension to the ultimate in nervous-system hyperactivity: convulsions.

When I was an infant, vitamin D deficiencies were quite common, and I am certain that I myself suffered from rickets and the hyperirritability which accompanies lack of calcium. My mother tells me that I cried for most of my first six months, and sometimes the only way the family could quiet me was to take me for a ride over bumpy roads in an automobile. Such stimulation would tend to discharge tension in the central nervous system; it would also stimulate the production of adrenal cortical hormone, counteracting any effect of the hypoglycemia and food allergies that probably were produced by the sugar in my formula.

The adult in our society is likely to lack sufficient vitamin D not only because of dietary deficiency but also because he receives very little skin stimulation from sunshine (which produces natural vitamin D). The problem is compounded in the elderly, who lack not only the stimulation produced by adequate light and vitamin D but also live on a diet poor in calcium and magnesium. Older people also produce diminishing amounts of various hormones. Taken together, these factors lead to demineralization of the bones; bone tissue becomes brittle, fractures easily, and heals with difficulty.

In addition, depleted calcium reserves can certainly contribute to the emotional problems of old age.

I personally prefer not to depend upon dietary sources of vitamin D such as livers and viscera of fish and animals that feed on fish, and therefore take 600 units of natural vitamin D daily in the form of cod liver oil, much the best way to get it.

Since vitamin D—like vitamin A—is stored in the liver for long periods, it is possible to accumulate toxic amounts of it. The synthetic form of vitamin D is far more toxic than the natural form. Some people are "vitamin-D fast," and require massive amounts.

I strongly recommend that no one take this vitamin in large doses without very strict medical supervision.

Your Vitamin K Needs

Vitamin K is primarily involved in the clotting mechanism of the blood. Formed in the intestines of humans, it is of little clinical importance except for persons with specific diseases such as jaundice. For this reason I do not take any vitamin K, and do not generally recommend it.

Your Vitamin E Needs

Vitamin E is another fat-soluble vitamin important for emotional health. It exerts a powerful influence on the cell membrane and the cell's utilization of oxygen. The brain cells are particularly dependent on a ready supply of oxygen. Also, vitamin E is an aid in hydrogen ion transfers, and thus again affects every cell in the body. Studies continue to show the importance of vitamin E in the prevention of cancer.

Probably the world's greatest authorities on vitamin E were the Shute brothers in Canada. I corresponded with Wilfrid E. Shute, M.D. He informed me that in his opinion most vitamin E preparations in the United States are not reliably labeled, and that one cannot be certain how much vitamin E one is getting unless one uses a reliably labeled product. He recommended the Key-E products put out by the Carlson Laboratories in Chicago. The Shute brothers were primarily interested in vitamin E for its cardiovascular effect, especially in preventing coronary artery disease and ameliorating angina pectoris. Those of us interested in megavitamin therapy for emotional disorders have found it equally useful. It is particularly helpful for patients who are depressed and tired—two very common complaints among persons suffering from emotional illnesses.

Vitamin E has been used extensively for menopausal symptoms, and can often substitute for hormone therapy in women. It probably aids sexual function in the female. All my patients are treated with multiple vitamins, nutritional supplements, and specific dietary recommendations; so when an impotent male becomes potent, it is hard to say which of the elements of his regimen was responsible for his return to the sexual arena. I can only say that if I had a potency problem, I would certainly include vitamin E in my regimen.

Unfortunately, vitamin E is one vitamin that can cause difficulties. When I first started taking it, I was unable to take more than 150 units daily without raising my blood pressure. Ordinarily, my blood pressure runs around 110 over 70, but whenever I took more than 150 units of vitamin E, it quickly rose to 140 over 90, to the accompaniment of a sizeable headache. It took me at least two years to gradually raise my vitamin E intake to its present level.

Daily at breakfast, I take Key-E, 200 IU (the succinate form), plus 400 IU of mixed E's ("mixed tocopherols") that contain the D-Alpha as well as the Beta, Delta, and Gamma tocopherols as they occur in nature. I consider this mixture added insurance, just in case we do not yet have the final word on all its active principles. As more insurance I also take 800 IU of Alpha-tocopherol acetate at lunch. (Note: "tocopherol" is sometimes spelled "tocopheryl")

It is my feeling that everyone should take vitamin E supplements in amounts of at least 100 or 200 IU a day, and possibly much more—for instance, if menopausal symptoms are present, or if there is depression and lack of energy.

Vitamin E should not be taken more than twice daily, since it interferes with iron absorption. Take vitamin E with breakfast and lunch. This leaves you free to absorb iron later in the day. Also, vitamin E should not be taken at the same time the mineral selenium is taken.

Your family doctor should make certain your blood pressure does not go up too high as you increase your vitamin E.

If your blood pressure does increase, it often normalizes if you stay on the same dosage level of vitamin E for several weeks. Your elevated blood pressure will fall quickly if you interrupt your vitamin E intake for a few days and then go back to a reduced level.

I usually start patients on Key-E capsules, 200 IU daily after breakfast. Since vitamin E may cause bleeding during surgery, many surgeons here in New York advise that it be discontinued 10 days before surgery. (I am not sure whether it truly causes bleeding.) Since it helps protect against the type of blood clots that occur in the legs following surgery, I think it advisable to begin taking it again on the second day following surgery. Be sure to ask your surgeon's advice.

Why Use Crude Sources of Vitamins?

Since it is likely that we have not yet discovered all vitamins and vitamin-like substances, I feel it is desirable to include crude vitamins in a vitamin program. If a Nobel Prize-winning nutritional chemist such as Szent-György includes crude sources of vitamins in his diet, I think it wise for you and me to do so.

Szent-György, however, is not sophisticated about food allergies which explains (I feel) his incorrect choice of wheat germ.

LIVER POWDER

Desiccated liver powder (or capsules) is an excellent source of crude B vitamins. Unfortunately a number of people are allergic to it; therefore, it's not a source of vitamins that I prescribe for patients until we are well along in the treatment program. (But far fewer people are allergic to it than to wheat germ.)

I take ½ teaspoon of liver two or three times a day mixed in with my powdered ascorbic acid and dolomite. I don't give more than a teaspoon twice a day to my patients.

Most people should not take yeast.

Lecithin

While it is not strictly a vitamin, I believe that a regular intake of lecithin often promotes good health.

Problem: Lecithin contains soya products and *many people are allergic to it*. For that reason, I hold off and don't give my patients lecithin until later in their treatment.

A non-soya lecithin made from the brains of calves is available: however, I would not advise using it. There are some viruses that occur in brain tissue that are very difficult to kill—even by cooking.

Lecithin is an emulsifier, but also contains the two B vitamins, inositol and choline. It is used in making chocolate and margarine because it breaks down their gummy consistency and allows them to flow readily through the production process.

Similarly, it works like soap in the bloodstream to emulsify fats and reduce cholesterols to a form that can be readily burned, instead of coagulating in your arteries.

Lecithin is abundant in egg yolk, sunflower seeds, melons, safflower oil and seeds and cereal seeds. Lecithin not only helps to dispose of cholesterol, but it also aids in the absorption of the fat-soluble vitamins, and may act to prevent gallstones.

Your body can manufacture lecithin, but to do so it needs three substances: the B vitamins inositol and choline, both of which are present in lecithin itself and also in yeast; and a particular amino acid (a building block of protein) called methionine, which is also present in yeast.

But in addition to yeast, if tolerated, I feel you should take lecithin itself, particularly if you are on a high fat diet.

Lecithin comes in granules, capsules, and syrup. Granules are best, because it's difficult to take enough capsules to do much good. The syrup sticks to the spoon and to the roof of your mouth; also, it is not delicious.

Try the granules, two to four tablespoons a day, straight, as if it were a cereal. Keep the lecithin in the refrigerator after opening the bottle.

Lecithin is an excellent source of two of the less publicized B vitamins: choline and inositol. Studies of these two vitamins in man are very incomplete, but the evidence is quite clear that laboratory animals require these vitamins.

Choline protects the liver. When this vitamin is low, massive fatty infiltration of the liver occurs. When puppies are fed choline-deficient diets they die within three weeks. Rats show kidney damage after being fed choline-poor diets for only four or five days. Also, cancer, muscular dystrophy, anemia, and heart and vascular disorders have been reported in laboratory animals on a choline-deficient diet.

Personally, I want choline and think you do too. Lecithin gives me mine.

Inositol also remains much of a mystery as to exact human requirements, but we do know that it is part of the phosphatide present in large amounts in brain tissue. Beef heart, as well as lecithin, is a good source. Why is it present in such large amounts in this heart tissue? I don't know. But if it's there the heart must need it. I don't want my heart muscle to go hungry.

The growth rate of mice is influenced by inositol, as growth is influenced by so many other vitamins, minerals and nutritional substances.

Human tissue maintained under artificial conditions grows better with adequate inositol.

Growth in and of itself may not seem too important, but lack of growth means that the body cells are being blocked from reaching their full potential.

The Value of Unsaturated Oils

Every cell in the body is surrounded by a fatty membrane. This membrane—the cell wall—requires unsaturated fats to maintain it and to help it function normally.

Also, prostaglandins require unsaturated fats for their formation. Prostaglandins are required for contraction of smooth muscle (such as that found in the intestinal tract and in the uterus) and to aid the action of certain hormones. Also, prostaglandins help lower blood pressure.

Researchers have concluded that fish oils which contain the poly-unsaturated fatty acid eicosapentaenoic acid (EPA), decrease platelet aggregatory effect, increase bleeding time, and help explain the low incidence of heart disease in Greenland Eskimos.

Cod liver oil is, of course, a fish oil, and one that I strongly endorse.

Both kinds of fats, saturated and unsaturated, are necessary for good health. Saturated fats come mostly from milk fats or meats.

Since the human brain is made up largely of fats, it's especially important that growing children have an adequate supply of fats.

Unsaturated fats come mostly from fish and vegetable sources. They too are essential for good health; they help the body handle saturated fats and lower cholesterol levels. A deficiency can lead to dandruff, acne, eczema, dry lusterless hair, loss of energy, impaired sex drive, and other symptoms.

The active ingredients in unsaturated oils are three fatty acids. They are present in almost all vegetable oils (except olive oil) but the best sources are linseed oil (*not the one you buy at the hardware store to mix with paint!*) and safflower oil.

I recommend—and take—one teaspoon of each of these oils every other day. These may be taken directly by the teaspoon or used as a salad dressing.

As stated previously, I recommend and take a teaspoon of cod liver oil daily. This is an excellent source both of unsaturated fats and vitamins A and D.

Oil used in cooking should not be counted since heat destroys some of the beneficial properties. For the same reason, you should choose cold-pressed oils rather than the heat-processed variety (the label will tell you). Be sure the oil contains no preservatives, and keep it in the refrigerator after you open it.

Lecithin and essential fatty acids often occur together in nature. Both help to handle saturated fats in the bloodstream; but lecithin, like vitamin E, is also an antioxidant preventing the oils from oxidizing.

NOTE: Do not take more unsaturated oils than mentioned above unless under strict medical attention. You must take adequate amounts of vitamin E when taking unsaturated oils.

Biotin

Biotin is another of the little-publicized B vitamins. Your body manufactures this vitamin so you don't need to take a supplement. Just be certain you don't destroy your own biotin by eating raw egg whites—*never, never, never eat the whites of raw eggs.* They will block this vitamin. Humans have become very ill by producing biotin deficiencies in themselves. How would you like to be tired, have numbness and muscle pains in your limbs, suffer from eczema-like skin rashes, have nausea and loss of appetite?

If you take antibiotics for an extended period of time, you must have blood tests to make certain your biotin (and other vitamin) blood levels remain normal.

Your Paba Needs

Para-aminobenzoic acid is the scientific tongue twister that designates another little publicized vitamin, usually referred to as PABA.

S. Ansbacher demonstrated that laboratory animals require PABA as an indispensable nutrient. We still, however, don't know the human requirement for PABA.

It is widely believed that PABA is not required in the diet of humans although PABA would be difficult to avoid since it is present in most foods. Yeast is an especially rich source.

PABA has gained some fame as an "anti-gray hair" vitamin (along with calcium pantothenate). Laboratory animals deficient in this vitamin develop gray hair, which clears up after PABA is returned to their diet. Whether this happens in humans remains to be proven. I once appeared on a talk show with nutritionist Carlton Fredericks, Ph.D., and commented upon the lack of gray in his hair. He attributed it to the 500 mg of PABA he took each day.

I haven't been able to make up my mind about the anti-graying effect of PABA. As of now, I have no problem with graying of the hair on my head, although my beard is getting quite gray. A few jokesters have commented that I'm getting old from the bottom up.

Several times I have tried taking PABA for a number of weeks, then stopping, then starting it again. I have never been able to decide whether or not the PABA has any effect on grayness. But I have frequently seen gray hair on my patients' heads turn dark after the patients have been placed on a proper diet along with adequate nutritional supplements. These supplements do not ordinarily include PABA.

Is the prevention of gray hair really important in the overall scheme of existence? Who can say for certain? We do know that graying of hair represents a failure of enzyme systems, and generally takes place as we grow older. More people die with gray hair than with the original color of their hair. A hundred years from now we may have the answer, but that won't do you and me much good. So again we must decide which horse to bet on.

I take PABA 500 mg daily and sometimes give it to patients.

Only last evening I saw a patient who visits me every six months to review his nutritional status. He is the most avid PABA advocate I know. Apparently he has a PABA dependency. If he leaves the vitamin off for more than a day or two, the inside of his mouth becomes covered with canker sores. When he starts the vitamin again, they disappear.

Ordinarily, food or other allergies are the cause for canker sores. Usually if patients eat the diet that's free of foods to which they're allergic, they have no trouble.

This patient is quite sophisticated about testing himself for food allergies and seems to have ruled them out as a cause of his trouble. Interestingly, as a self experiment he recently went up to two 500 mg PABA tablets three times a day. On that dosage, for a short time he developed a patch of gray in his hair. Then—after several weeks—the patch turned dark. Though he's in his fifties, his hair is now quite dark. As with me, his whiskers remain gray.

(In a later chapter we'll discuss other uses of a form of PABA; Ana Aslan, M.D. has developed what is called H-3 or Gerovital.)

A Few Practical Points

First, you should take in as little binder and artificial coloring as possible with your vitamins. Choose straight powder or clear capsules, or sugar-and-starch-free tablets that are clearly labeled as such. Regular tablets often upset the stomach or cause other undesirable side effects. For instance, diarrhea is often cause by ordinary vitamin C tablets. Sweetened chewable tablets are least desirable of all.

You should be aware that you may be allergic to one line (or brand) of vitamins, but you may well be able to tolerate another brand without difficulty.

And remember: you might conceivably feel worse when you take a particular vitamin. Several times I have found a particular vitamin disagrees with a particular patient, even when the patient is not allergic to the vitamin. Your particular enzyme system may function less well with mega-doses of a particular vitamin. This is not common, but it is possible. Only trial and error will answer this question for you.

TABLE 1.
My Usual Nutritional Supplements

cod liver oil	1 teaspoon daily (A, D, Unsaturated fats)
beta carotene cap. 15 mg	1 cap every 3rd day
Hy B Complex-50	1 cap 1 or 2 times a day
B_1 500 mg cap	1 cap 1 or 2 times a day
B_2 200 mg cap	1 cap 1 or 2 times a day
B_6 200 mg cap	1 cap 1 or 2 times a day
calcium pantothenate 218 mg cap.	1 cap at bedtime
folic acid 1 mg tablet	1 tablet 3 times a day
B_{12} (Hydroxocobalamin) (by injection)	3 to 6 cc in AM and 1½ cc in afternoon
L-carnitine 250 mg cap	1 cap 2 times a day
vitamin C (powder)	1½ teaspoons 2 times a day
vitamin C cap (Super C) 500 mg	3 at bedtime
vitamin C cap (Time release) 500 mg	1 at bedtime
Key E cap (Succinate form)	200n units 1 every 3rd day after breakfast
acetate E cap 400 units	1 every 3rd day after breakfast
mixed tocopherols 400 units	1 every 3rd day after breakfast
linseed oil capsule	1 every day
dolomite powder	½ teaspoon 2 times a day (checked to make sure it con-

	tains no toxic amounts of lead or other heavy metals)
zinc gluconate 60 mg cap	1 cap 3 times a day
manganese gluconate 133 mg cap	1 cap at bedtime
selenium 200 mcg tab	1 tab after supper
kelp tablet	1 every 3 days
liver injection	1 cc 1 time per week

CHAPTER SEVENTEEN

MINERALS FOR YOUR NERVES

A few years ago the 23-year-old wife of a law student was brought to my office by her husband and her mother, each holding one arm to prevent her from running away.

At first glance, Mary looked like the happiest soul alive. She babbled about amusing people she had just seen on the street, made fun of her mother-in-law's derriere, and skipped blithely from subject to subject. Her body was as active as her mind; she kept pacing back and forth in the office ignoring me when I invited her to sit down and talk. Her husband leaned against the door, to keep her from bolting.

Her effervescence—like that of all people suffering from mania—was contagious. I found myself smiling at her jokes and listening in fascination to the flow of witty words, that leaped forth like pirouetting dancers.

Mary, the family told me, had been trying to finish college for the past six years, but intermittent periods of depression and elation had repeatedly interfered with her studies. She had earned credit for only a year and a half of work. Although she was intelligent and efficient during her normal periods, she was too depressed and slow-moving during her down swings to study effectively.

But the worst times were the upswings, like the one she was experiencing at the moment. She could not even sit still long enough to attend classes, let alone absorb anything from a lecture.

LITHIUM IS A MINERAL

For the past few years, psychiatrists have been using the mineral lithium carbonate with great success in the treatment of manic states. I don't know why Mary wasn't given lithium. Perhaps her previous doctors had seen her only during her depressive states, and had not realized that she suffered from the dramatic mood swings that characterize the true manic-depressive illness.

I prescribed lithium at once, and saw her again three days later.

On her second visit she was accompanied only by her mother. This time she appeared neither unduly elated nor depressed. She talked about her difficulties in a thoroughly rational manner. She realized that her life passed through abnormally steep up and down cycles. She stated that for no obvious reason she would grow more and more restless, take on too many extracurricular activities at school, lose sleep, and finally become so disorganized that she could no longer function.

Weeks later she would descend to a comfortable level for a short while and then pass on down into the black caves of depression.

LITHUM SHOWS THE POWERFUL EFFECT MINERALS HAVE ON BRAIN CHEMISTRY

The transformation that a mineral, lithium carbonate, can bring about in manic-depressive illness such as Mary's is one of the most spectacularly satisfying experiences a psychiatrist can have. This simple mineral can literally transform broken lives into useful ones.

Typically, lithium was ignored for a generation after J.F. Cade, M.D., discovered a medical use for it. In 1949, this general practitioner in the Australian hinterlands learned that lithium carbonate could work what seemed like a miracle in the treatment of manic-depressive illnesses. He wrote a convincing scientific paper describing his findings, but the paper was studiously ignored by the medical establishment. Perhaps if Cade had been a professor of medicine at some prestigious university, his findings would have been taken more seriously. His story is typical of the neglect the medical establishment often heaps upon men who make new discoveries.

At least Cade was luckier than Joseph Goldberger, who discovered that pellagra was caused by a vitamin B deficiency, not by germs, as everyone believed. Goldberger died believing his findings had been rejected. Cade lived to see lithium widely used in the United States a mere twenty years after he developed a new use for it.

P.S. After we got Mary calmed down, we tested her and discovered she had marked allergies to tobacco, wheat and sugar. These were removed from her diet. We were then able to gradually take her off her lithium.

She did well for about six months, then started smoking again and cheating frequently on her diet. She returned to see me in another manic state. Again lithium brought her down. She stopped smoking and went back on her diet and once more we were able to take her off lithium.

I happened to run into her on the street a few months ago. She told me she had been doing very well. She had stayed off cigarettes and food, cheating only on her birthday and New Year's Eve.

WHY NOT STAY ON LITHIUM AND SMOKE AND EAT PIZZA?

We live in a society of people brought up to believe they can have their cake and eat it too. I only wish such were true. Mother Nature, unfortunately will not bargain with us. It would be possible for Mary to continue taking lithium for the rest of her life and get away with smoking and eating the foods to which she had cerebral allergies, *but* she could do so only by paying a price. Lithium, in the high amounts it would be necessary for her to take, eventually interferes with thyroid function. Also, in my view, it has a subtle blocking effect on some parts of the central nervous system.

The late Joshua Logan went on television now and then and told of how he was maniac and how lithium controlled his difficulty. He added that patients must stay on it for the rest of their lives.

I don't know for certain whether it's true, but if Josh Logan was anything like the manic patients I've seen, he too had cerebral allergies to such things as tobacco and certain foods. In all probability he could have gone off lithium if he eliminated the things to which he was allergic.

"But he did well on lithium" you say.

True, but he probably paid a price for it. The physiological and psychological effects on long-term usage of lithium are still being explored. His creativity died.

Lithium treats a symptom. That's always a poor third or fourth best way to treat a patient.

I like to get to the cause of the symptom and treat that.

I find less than the usual therapeutic dose (300 to 600 mg daily) helpful for some patients with food and environmental allergies regardless of the symptoms they feel.

YOUR BODY MUST HAVE MINERALS

When most of us think of minerals we have visions of quaint novelty shops with spears of gleaming quartz or bookends made of petrified wood. Such minerals seem to have little to do with human emotions. Our bodies could not function without minerals. You'll recall that all of the body's chemistry takes place with the help of enzymes, and that enzymes are made up of a protein, a vitamin and a mineral. Minerals are especially important for the normal functioning of the nervous system.

Physicians are aware that iron, sodium, potassium, and calcium are needed in the proper amounts for good health. However, their knowledge quickly fades away when it comes to copper, manganese, chromium, magnesium, zinc, and others.

TESTING FOR MINERALS

I suspect lack of good tests for body mineral levels is one of the reasons physicians generally aren't very interested in minerals.

Other than checking for extremely high or low levels of minerals, blood tests are of little use. For example, it's possible to do a blood test for zinc, then have the patient walk up and down a few flights of stairs and test again. The second test will often be quite different from the first.

You see, the blood is only a medium for the transportation of minerals—and many other things.

WHAT IF YOU TESTED THE UNITED STATES FOR MONEY?

Think of the United States as the body of a person and think of money as a mineral for which you want to test.

If you test the U.S. for its total money supply, you could carry out the test by taking a sample of all the money that was being transported. You could stop every tenth armored truck and count how much money it was carrying.

But what about all the money that's flowing into and out of the country? What about all the money locked up in safes and bank vaults? What about the new money that was being printed in Washington and the old money that was being burned?

Estimating the amount of a mineral in the body is even more complicated. If you test the blood for calcium you don't know whether the calcium in the blood came from drinking a glass of milk, or whether the body is drawing calcium out of the bones and leaving them calcium-poor.

THE ONE ACCURATE TEST FOR MINERALS

There's only one really good test for body minerals: burn away all the organic material in the body and measure the calcium, zinc, and other minerals left in the ashes.

Very few people want that test. It's not covered by Blue Cross/Blue Shield!

MORE TESTS FOR MINERALS

Excretion tests give a fairly good—but far from perfect—idea of the body's supply of minerals.

For example, it's possible to collect urine for 24 hours and measure how much magnesium the body puts out by way of the kidneys in one day.

Then it's possible to give an injection of a known amount of magnesium and collect another 24 hour urine.

The amount of the magnesium "saved" (not excreted) gives some idea about how starved the body was for magnesium.

Clearly, testing for every mineral in this manner is a great deal of work . . . and even when you get the answer it's far from a perfect one.

OTHER TESTS FOR MINERALS

Rather than test the blood for minerals (where the minerals are always in transit), it's generally better to test body tissue. For example, if the doctor does a biopsy and takes out a sliver of bone, the bone can be analyzed for its calcium and other minerals.

Most people don't want major surgery to learn their mineral status.

It's possible to remove a bit of muscle from the body and get some idea of the body's mineral levels. Not everyone wants this, and again the answer it gives is far less than perfect.

WHAT SHALL WE DO!

Last year the *New York Times* and the country's press services ran news items condemning the testing of hair for body mineral levels.

Here's the real problem:

1. There is no practical, perfect test for body mineral levels.

2. Hair tests for minerals—as generally performed—have become something of a racket.

(Many things in the field of nutrition are more or less a racket. Ads that recommend sugar for "quick energy" are more or less a racket. Saying that the use of corn oil for cooking "may reduce your cholesterol" is more or less a racket; and taking two additional percentage points of caffeine out of coffee and selling it as "decaffeinated coffee" is more or less a racket.

So it's not surprising that resourceful entrepreneurs have tried to turn hair tests for minerals into a racket. Here's how they've done it. You send certain mail order laboratories a sample of hair. They'll have it analyzed for minerals, then put the information in a computer and the computer will give a long complicated printout telling what each mineral does for the body and the symptoms that can come from a deficiency in the mineral.

So far so good.

But the computer doesn't know when to stop. It then turns out a long, complicated diet telling you what to eat at each meal to help furnish the missing minerals. (This the computer is willing to do even though it doesn't know whether you get hives from strawberries or have diabetes or suffer from PKU.)

Of course choosing a diet on the basis of a hair test is nonsense, but good theater—and profitable.

Rightfully such use of hair tests for minerals should be stopped—along with ads for "decaffeinated" coffee.

My Experience with Hair Tests

For nearly twenty years I tested every new patient's hair for minerals. I've probably had more clinical experience with hair tests than anyone else. I don't have to read about other people's studies on the tests. (I would like to add that the cost of my first office visit covered both a psychological test and a hair test for minerals. When a rare patient does not want the tests, the charge is the same. No one can say I profit from hair tests. I seldom get more than one repeat hair test.)

Hair tests are of value.

How do I know?

1. Repeatedly I've seen a pattern of overall mineral deficiency in alcoholics and others who give a history of following a mineral-poor diet.

2. I've given these patients supplementary minerals and tested their hair again and found that their mineral levels became normal.

3. By using hair tests for minerals, I've discovered high lead levels in patients several times. These high lead levels were confirmed by blood and urine tests.

4. When I find a patient with a high mercury level, I always ask him if he frequently eats canned fish. Almost all of them do.

5. In general I do not consider the sodium and potassium hair levels accurate, but routinely the most emotionally disturbed patients I see have high potassium hair levels.

Note

Hair tests can be very misleading if patients use certain shampoos—anti-dandruff shampoos that constrain selenium, for example.

Dyes—especially the dyes used to darken gray hair—may leave lead in the hair (and in the body—be careful!).

Under such conditions it's sometimes useful to test pubic hair rather than hair from the head.

Sometimes fingernail clippings are tested in place of hair.

HISTORY OF HAIR TESTS

Hair tests were originally developed by veterinary nutritionists to plan optimal diets for beef herds. It happens that much of our hard evidence about nutrition comes from intensive studies in animal husbandry.

There's money to be made raising healthy cattle.

Unhappily, the big money in human health care is made by diagnosing and drugging people after they're sick.

I've stopped testing hair for minerals. People who know little about the test have damned it so often in print that it's seen by insurance companies and medical controllers as a racket procedure.

Like everything else, it can be a racket.

If used properly, it can be useful.

As Edward T. Hall has said, "We are tyrannized by our culture."

And, as Tolstoy said, "What men consider sacred and important are their own devices for wielding power over their fellow men."

YOUR CORRECT MINERAL LEVELS

As with vitamins, there is probably no such thing as a "normal" requirement for any mineral.

Some people feel better on what appears—by our present standards—to be an abnormal level of a mineral. For example, a "normal" intake of magnesium will induce drowsiness in some patients while other patients function best on doses of magnesium clearly higher than "normal."

Furthermore, a person's need for a certain mineral may change with age or during times of physical and emotional stress.

Before menopause, women need more iron than men; women also need different levels of certain minerals at different times in their menstrual cycle. Premenstrual cramps can often be controlled with temporary large doses of dolomite—a mixture of magnesium and calcium.

Older people are more likely than younger ones to have mineral deficiencies—because of poor diets, or because they absorb food poorly, or both.

Pregnant or lactating women need more minerals than they would otherwise.

OFTEN MINERALS WORK TOGETHER

Not only is the total amount of a mineral in your body important, but mineral levels should be maintained in certain ratios to each other. Sodium and potassium work together. You need both calcium and magnesium, but to function properly you should have about twice as much calcium as magnesium.

CAUTION: You can overdose with minerals. Some excess minerals may not be quickly eliminated in the urine. Toxic levels may be reached. Follow your physician's advice.

UNDERSTANDING BETTER HOW MINERALS WORK

To illustrate how minerals affect the way you feel, let me explain how two minerals act in nerve stimulation.

Whenever a nerve is stimulated, there is an exchange between sodium and potassium across the nerve membrane. In the resting state most of the sodium remains outside the cell membrane and most of the potassium inside. But when the nerve is stimulated, sodium moves into the cell and potassium moves out of it. This causes an electrical charge in the cell which is passed down the cell body, releasing "catecholamines."

The chemical released—the catecholamines—pass through the "neural clef" and stimulate the next nerve. (Nerves are not like the copper electrical wiring in your house. A space exists between one nerve and the next. This space is called the "neural clef.")

After the movement of the sodium and potassium through the

cell membrane, the sodium must be pumped out of the nerve before it's ready to react to another stimulation.

A magnesium-activated enzyme system known as ATP (adenosine triphosphate) pumps the sodium back out of the cell and allows the potassium to flow inside.

If you have a deficiency or a marked excess of the minerals sodium or potassium, your nerves cannot respond normally to stimulations.

If the nerve membrane cannot allow the sodium and potassium to pass easily in and out, your nerves cannot function properly.

If you lack magnesium, the sodium pump will not work correctly.

During convulsions, sodium and potassium have a massive interchange through cell membranes.

One of the theories about why electroshock therapy is helpful for some patients with emotional symptoms: nerve cell membranes are altered by the electrical shock so that sodium and potassium can pass through the membrane in a more normal manner.

How Calcium Works as a Nerve Relaxer

Calcium salts are present in the body in the largest amounts of all the minerals. We all know how important calcium is in developing bones and teeth, but there are also sizeable amounts of calcium in the body fluids and cells.

Furthermore, calcium has a marked effect on the excitability of the nervous system.

Many years ago, I witnessed a demonstration of calcium's dramatic effect on the central nervous system.

While I was a resident in internal medicine, a 34-year-old clerk came to the hospital's emergency room one Saturday night. He hated to bother the doctors at that late hour, but he had a severe headache and couldn't find a drug store that was open. Could he please have a couple of aspirins?

He was given a check-up by the intern on duty, who discovered papilledema—a condition in which the nerve endings at the back of the eyes bulge out. This is a common finding associated with increased pressure in the skull due to a brain tumor.

The patient was told that he might have a tumor and was urged to admit himself to the hospital for a complete work-up. He wouldn't hear of it, and continued to demand aspirin, which had always helped his headaches before. The intern continued to insist on hospitalization and eventually called the man's family. They pressured him into entering the hospital.

During the next four days, the patient was subjected to extensive neurological tests, including skull X-rays, brain scans, and all the other special tests performed when brain tumor is suspected.

Much to everyone's surprise, the tests showed nothing abnormal. The team of doctors was unable to decide on a likely location for a brain tumor, but after a conference they decided to open the patient's skull for an exploratory operation.

On the night before surgery, the patient began complaining of severe cramps in both legs. At first, the nurse thought he was simply nervous about the surgery, and paid little attention to him.

During midnight rounds, however, they found the patient lying rigid, with the muscles of his arms and legs contracted. His throat was so tight that he made a crowing sound with every breath. They called the resident on neurosurgery who examined the patient and then asked for a medical consultation. I was an assistant resident in internal medicine at the time, and on call.

Just before I arrived on the floor, the patient suffered a convulsion, and was only semiconscious when I saw him.

I suppose it's only natural for surgeons to think in terms of surgical disorders, and for internists to give priority to medical problems. I was immediately struck by the similarity between his condition and that of people suffering from an extremely low calcium level, and began to test my hunch by tapping with two fingers along his facial nerve. This brought on a twitching of the muscles of his mouth, nose, and eyelids.

I asked for a syringe and an ampule of calcium gluconate. Before we had finished injecting the solution into the patient's vein, his body relaxed, the crowing sound stopped. Soon he was fully conscious and able to talk rationally.

This therapeutic test with calcium gluconate clinched the diagnosis of "hypocalcemia" and saved the man from unnecessary and possibly dangerous, surgery.

It happened that this patient was suffering from a deficiency of the parathyroid gland, which reduced his calcium to very low levels.

Minerals are greatly affected by body hormones, and such a dramatic calcium deficiency rarely occurs unless there is some accompanying defect like lack of vitamin D or low parathyroid hormone. Nonetheless, this case is a good illustration of the inability of the central nervous system to function properly without an adequate supply of a particular mineral: calcium.

Obviously, we don't often see people collapsing in the street, jerking with muscle spasms and making crowing sounds while breathing. But I wonder how many people might be suffering from milder forms of calcium deficiency, and how much emotional suffering is caused by a calcium deficiency.

The same is likely to be true of much of the non-patient population suffering from nervous tension "due to stress."

An ordinary diet supplies calcium in fairly generous amounts through milk, cheese, egg yolk, beans, lentils, nuts, figs, cabbage, turnip greens, cauliflower, and asparagus. (I have already discussed in chapter 13 why milk and milk products, nevertheless, should be avoided by most people.)

Supplementary calcium can be taken in several forms. I usually recommend one half of a teaspoon of dolomite powder 2 times daily, since this provides much-needed magnesium as well as calcium.

Magnesium deficiency is very common in our society—much more so than calcium deficiency.

WARNING: Some sources of dolomite have been found to contain lead and other heavy metals in toxic amounts.

PROBLEMS WITH CALCIUM ABSORPTION

On a high-protein diet, approximately 15% of the calcium taken in by mouth is absorbed. On a low-protein diet only 5% of calcium is absorbed.

The phytic acid in grains forms an insoluble compound called calcium phytilate. In this form, calcium is bound in such a manner that it cannot be absorbed. Oxalates (organic chemicals) in certain foods (especially spinach) also combine with calcium to form calcium oxalate, an insoluble chemical which the body cannot use.

Magnesium: The Neglected Mineral

Magnesium salts are the most neglected minerals in the Western world, though they are amply available in nuts, soybeans, seafoods, beans, and peas, and in the supplement dolomite. The human body contains about 21 grams of magnesium. Something like 70 percent is combined with calcium and phosphorous to make bone; the rest is in the body's soft tissues and fluids. About one part magnesium for two parts calcium should be taken into the body.

Magnesium, like calcium, affects the permeability of the cell membrane. A defect in the cell membrane may result in distortion of perceptions and mood alterations, all the way from euphoria to stupor. Studies show that alcoholics tend to be quite deficient in magnesium. This deficiency helps lead to the psychosis brought on by alcoholism: the DT's, the infamous "pink elephant" stage of alcoholism.

As mentioned earlier, some people need higher than "normal" amounts of magnesium. Some people have more energy with added magnesium. Other people feel sedated by it and take it only at bedtime.

Symptoms of Magnesium Deficiency

Suspect a magnesium deficiency if you have any of the following symptoms: irregular heart beat, excitability, muscle spasms, twitching, tremors, confusion, disorientation, weakness, depression, easily fractured bones, a wish to die.

Indeed, if you drink milk or eat cheese or live in the Western World and eat a "modern" diet, the chances are very great that you have a magnesium deficiency.

Certain foods are high in magnesium, but you shouldn't chose foods because of their mineral or vitamin contents. The figures are unreliable. Also, you should chose your foods on the basis of whether or not you are allergic to them.

Get your vitamins and minerals separate from your food. Buy them at a health food store.

CAUTION: If you drink milk or eat cheese you will be getting calcium without getting magnesium. Since calcium and magnesium must have each other in certain ratios for the body to work correctly, you are increasing your magnesium deficiency when you drink milk and eat cheese. Instead of helping your biochemistry, you are giving it more difficulties.

You cannot absorb calcium and magnesium without vitamin D.

Pregnancy, of course, increases the body's need for both calcium and magnesium. Doctors give pregnant women extra calcium, but they do women (and their babies) a great disservice when they neglect to also give them magnesium and trace minerals.

And please don't forget, bone must have a matrix (a protein network) to hold the calcium and magnesium. Without vitamin C, the bone matrix will not form properly.

If you use alcohol, cortisone, the male hormone testosterone, or digitalis, you may need extra magnesium. Consult your physician under these—and all—circumstances.

A Case of Acute Magnesium Deficiency

In a letter published in the medical journal *Lancet*, Dr. Joan Caddle of the George Washington School of Medicine discussed the importance of adding magnesium when thiamine (vitamin B_1), or other B vitamins are given.

In order to use the B vitamins, the body needs a compound called thiamine pyrophosphate, which cannot be formed without magnesium.

In Nigeria, Dr. Caddle observed extremely malnourished children who had been treated with vitamin-B-enriched milk with added protein. She discovered that the addition of these B vitamins actually increased the children's physical and emotional symptoms.

Some children became immobilized and simply sat and stared, while other developed nervous tics of the eyelids, and still others showed tremors of the hands and feet and became unable to walk with a steady gait. A few even developed convulsions, which constitute the ultimate irritability of the central nervous system.

Dr. Caddle uncovered a magnesium deficiency in these children. When magnesium was added to their other nutritional supplements, all their symptoms promptly disappeared.

These children represent an extreme case, but magnesium deficiency on a lower level is extremely common among Westerners. Since magnesium is so critically important to your physical and emotional health, you have little to lose and much to gain by adding a magnesium supplement—dolomite powder—to your diet.

If you take vitamins and don't get a lift, or if you get a lift from vitamins that later fades, chances are great that you need more magnesium. Half a teaspoon of dolomite in water two or three times daily may do the trick.

You Must Have Every Nutrient

Now do you see why I keep saying that everyone must have every nutrient? Chemically speaking, our bodies are orchestrated. Toot the horn too much or roll the drums at the wrong places and you have noise rather than music. In the body, you have biochemical confusion and you become nervous, or depressed, or tired—or have any one of a hundred other unpleasant symptoms.

Why Sodium Is Important

We're all familiar with the mineral sodium through our use of table salt (sodium chloride).

In the earlier chapter section entitled "Understanding Better How Minerals Work," I have talked about the critical importance of the body's "sodium pump," how sodium and potassium work as a team and move in and out of the nerve cell as the nerve fires. It might be a good idea to review that section.

Since sodium is used in the ATP energy transfers that take place in every cell, it's essential to life.

There can be no question that sodium imbalance produces a profound effect on the nervous system. In Addison's disease, for example, adrenal cortical hormones are too low. Adrenal cortical hormones help us retain sodium in our bodies. When these hormones are low, the body loses sodium.

When sodium levels become low, patients become profoundly weak, tired, and depressed. Fortunately, full-blown Addison's disease is rather rare. The real question is: how many people who are only somewhat tired and depressed suffer from a sodium deficiency?

WE USE TOO MUCH SALT

We are constantly told that we use too much salt. Why do people use too much salt? Possibly because their bodies need it. Some people feel a great deal better if they use liberal amounts of salt.

HERE'S THE POINT THAT'S MISSED

People use a great deal of salt—they "like the taste of it"—because they need it. They need it because they're eating high carbohydrate diets.

CHECK THESE IMPORTANT FACTS

Cows, and other animals that live on carbohydrates, must have a source of salt outside their diet.

Lions, on the other hand, who live off proteins and fat, need no outside source of salt.

Back in my carbohydrate eating days, I too enjoyed salt—I probably needed it.

Now that most of my calories come from fish-fowl-meat, I dislike the taste of salt. I haven't used any salt on food for at least 20 years.

My Conclusion

If people crave salt, if they feel better when consuming extra salt, they are probably eating a diet that's wrong for them.

Of course with certain medical diseases (high blood pressure or congestive heart failure, for example) patients do not tolerate salt well.

Let me add that almost all high blood pressure is the result of one or more food allergies. The most common offenders are grains and sugar. I have, however, seen high blood pressure caused by tea and many other foods.

People with Addison's disease must have added salt.

Heat Exhaustion ("Sunstroke") is a Sodium Deficiency

Profound changes in the central nervous system take place during heat exhaustion, in which the body is depleted of sodium. Patients with such a syndrome often suffer from headache, weakness, confusion, and drowsiness which can lead to coma. You might not think of coma as a manifestation of a central nervous system disorder but the contrasting states of coma and convulsion represent the two extremes of excitation in the nervous system.

Coma is the ultimate in nervous tissue depression; convulsions represent the height of nervous overactivity—of nervous tension.

REMEMBER: Hair tests for sodium and potassium levels are rather inaccurate.

Potassium—A Sea Story

Some years ago an elderly lady came to see me who insisted that she felt well only when she took kelp tablets. She was in her seventies, a stubborn little woman, determined to discover the reason for this oddity.

I was quite unable to shake her conviction that kelp was of great benefit to her. She had read up on the subject and believed that the iodine in kelp made her feel better by helping her thyroid function more effectively. At the time I was still rather naive about nutrition, and I suspected that she was simply a foolish old woman with a fixed idea. But as I worked with her I gradually realized that her faith in kelp might not be unwarranted.

To see what differences it would make in her condition, I began giving her kelp one week and taking her off of it the next week.

While taking kelp she was bright-eyed, alert, and energetic.

During the weeks without it she dragged into my office depressed, tired, tense and argumentive.

I then tried giving her a placebo (a bland tablet) one week and kelp the next. I could still see that she was much better with kelp than with the placebo. Next, I gave her a placebo which I said had a very high iodine content—higher than that of kelp—to test again whether her relief of symptoms was a product of auto-suggestion.

But even on this supposedly high-iodine placebo she did not feel at all well.

I began asking myself whether the high potassium content of kelp could be making her feel better. When I substituted another form of potassium for the kelp, she maintained her feeling of well-being.

At last we had the answer. Indeed the sea kelp was helping her and her self-therapy had been sound.

Too Much Potassium Means Trouble

Never take potassium on your own. Only take it under the close supervision of a physician.

Excessively high blood levels of potassium usually occur in patients with kidney failure, in those patients who are in shock, in people who are acutely dehydrated, or in people with Addison's disease. Sometimes patients who are taking oral potassium while under medical care get too much and have symptoms from it.

The symptoms of elevated potassium are confined mainly to the central nervous system and to the heart. The heart may be slow and emit poor sounds. Ultimately there may be cardiac arrest. Central nervous system symptoms include mental confusion, tingling in the arms and legs, and numbness, sometimes progressing to the point of paralysis.

TOO LITTLE POTASSIUM ALSO MEANS TROUBLE

People with low potassium levels are frequently tired. Most cases of potassium deficiency are brought on by medications classified as "diuretics." These are usually taken for a common form of swelling often complained about by women (almost always it's due to an undiagnosed food allergy). Diuretics are also often given for high blood pressure and to control the swelling or breathing difficulty experienced by patients with certain types of heart trouble.

Sulfur-Protein Equation

Sulfur is used not only to make the proteins that form part of the body's enzymes, but also to make the actual cells of the body . . . and the protein complexes that help hold the body's cells together.

Man's sulfur needs are met by the protein he eats. Two amino acids—systeine and methionine—are rich in sulfur.

Sulfur in its plain mineral form is poorly metabolized. Grandma meant well, but I'm afraid her sulfur and molasses spring tonic didn't do much good. Give your grandchildren a good fish, fowl, or meat meal and you'll be giving them a good supply of sulfur.

Your Iron Needs

Although iron is present in the body in much smaller amounts than magnesium, sodium, sulfur, potassium, phosphorous, and calcium, iron salts are known to everyone because of their widely advertised role in preventing anemia.

People's needs for iron change greatly at different times of life. You need extra iron while you are growing, during pregnancy or breastfeeding, or whenever you have lost blood (from accident, surgery, heavy menstrual flow, etc.). During these stressful periods, iron supplements may be necessary.

But in general, only small traces of iron are needed for healthy adult men and for women past menopause. Even young women need only about 18 mg a day during periods of stress such as childbearing and lactation.

The best food sources of iron are liver, kidney, heart, and spleen; next best are egg yolk, fish, clams, oysters, nuts, figs, dates, asparagus, beans, molasses, and oatmeal.

As you've heard me say before, however, choose your food according to your allergies, not according to what it has in it. If I ate molasses, I'd get more iron, but the sugar in the molasses would make me too tired to write this book.

For the body to use iron properly, some traces of copper must be present. Also, iron is better absorbed when there is hydrochloric acid in the stomach. This means: if you take an iron pill, take it an hour before meals.

Vitamin C also helps iron absorption by reducing it to a more soluble ferrous state. Some iron pills have added vitamin C, which makes sense.

Phytic acid, which is found in many cereals and oxalates (such as occur in spinach) bind iron into insoluble compounds and thus prevent its absorption. As mentioned, vitamin E and iron interfere with each other. Take E in the morning and, if needed, take iron at night.

Because anemia tends to cause exhaustion and depression, proper iron levels are certainly important to the adequate functioning of the nervous system. However, iron is one of the nutritional supplements that you can overdo. Excessive amounts cause harmful iron deposits throughout the body.

Consult Your Physician Before Taking Any Iron Supplement.

Most physicians, I am happy to say, are more knowledgeable about iron than any other aspect of nutrition, and certainly more so than about any other phase of mineral metabolism.

Your Copper Needs

Copper, essential for cellular metabolism, works in many enzyme systems. Together with iron, it is necessary for the formation of hemoglobin. Copper is also needed to maintain the myelin sheath around the nerves. The sheaths act as insulators, like insulation around wires, so that impulses traveling along them are not passed haphazardly to other nerves.

Copper deficiency is rare in "normal" human adults, but occasionally my hair test reveals low copper deposits in a patient. The exact clinical significance of this has not yet been determined, because usually a patient low in copper is also deficient in other minerals. In private practice it is impossible to do control studies by administering only one mineral at a time; patients are not expected to lend themselves to experiments.

Whatever deficiences exist must be treated immediately. But definite copper deficiencies are sometimes found in children on a high milk diet, and in some adults who suffer from severe diarrhea and lack of absorption from the gastrointestinal tract.

One result can be copper-deficiency anemia.

For copper, eat shellfish, other seafood, liver, kidney, lamb, and brewers' or primary yeast.

The most significant disorder associated with copper metabolism is Wilson's disease. This involves profound changes in the brain and liver, due to abnormal copper deposits caused by metabolic defects. The disease causes marked tremors, difficulty in speech, drooling, poor coordination and muscle rigidity due to improper nerve stimulation. Accompanying emotional symptoms include changes in behavior and neurotic and psychotic reactions.

It is felt by some that mildly elevated copper levels are often associated with schizophrenia, and attempts have been made to lower the copper levels of patients suffering from schizophrenia by using penicillamine. Most psychiatrists reject this drug because it frequently causes severe toxic reactions; giving zinc (zinc gluconate capsules 60 mg, three times a day) will often lower high copper levels.

Avoid copper cooking utensils, copper water pipes, and copper beer cooling coils.

Hair tests of people with red hair often show high copper levels although these levels must be very high before it is likely to be clinically significant.

Your Iodine Needs

A few generations ago iodine received much publicity after it was discovered that an iodine deficiency could cause a goiter, a swelling of the thyroid gland. The deficiency was found in places distant from the oceans, such as Switzerland or America's Midwest, where vegetables are grown in iodine-poor soil.

Iodine deficiency can cause hypothyroidism, a low functioning thyroid. But more about this disorder in the chapter on hormones.

The average adult iodine requirement is only 100 to 150 mcg daily, which you can easily get from iodized salt. Since iodized salt often contains impurities, including sugar, I consider kelp a much more desirable source. The body stores what iodine it needs and discards the rest, so there is virtually no chance of getting too much. A kelp tablet once or twice a day is your best source of iodine.

Iodine in kelp or iodized salt rather frequently causes skin eruptions similar to acne.

Your Manganese Needs

Manganese is required in amounts of only about 4 mg a day, and clear deficiences in man have not been adequately studied. In my hair tests I rather frequently find patients deficient in manganese but these people usually have multiple deficiencies. It is difficult to know just what symptoms come from a lack of manganese.

The enzymes arginase and phosphotransferases require manganese as a cofactor. Arginase aids in protein metabolism and phosphotransferases aid energy systems.

Copper, iron, and manganese act as catalysts in the formation of hemoglobin.

In tests on male laboratory animals, manganese deficiency has caused a loss of interest in sex and eventual sterility. I've had several male patients with low manganese hair tests who had low sexual interests and performance. Several have improved after being placed on manganese. One of them commented, "I've heard of putting lead in your pencil, but manganese in your pencil, that's ridiculous. But it worked!"

Female test animals low in manganese refused to suckle their young.

What else do you need to know about manganese? It's found in nuts, but unfortunately most people in our world react to nuts. I suspect it's often due to the mold or the preservatives used on nuts. Leafy vegetables and brewers' yeast or primary yeast are good sources of manganese.

I often give patients managanese gluconate capsules. I've never had a patient get into any trouble from one 133 mg capsule at night.

Your Cobalt Needs

To date there is not much definite information about cobalt deficiencies in adult humans, though some reports indicate that cobalt therapy has helped anemic children. Typically, we know more about the effects of the deficiency on livestock than on humans.

It's well known that cattle and sheep grazing on cobalt-deficient land may develop pernicious anemias and severe disorders of the central nervous system. Their symptoms are relieved by adding cobalt to the diet.

Cobalt is incorporated into the vitamin B_{12} complex.

I've already mentioned that I believe everyone should have a serum test for vitamin B_{12}, and that everyone should try a few injections of vitamin B_{12b}. While cobalt deficiency per se has not been proven in humans, vitamin B_{12} deficiencies definitely have. Do some people feel better with extra vitamin B_{12} because of the cobalt it contains? I don't know but I do know that seafood is rich in cobalt.

Your Zinc Needs

During the past few years physicians have begun to show an interest in zinc. I was surprised when I interviewed Robert A. Goode, Ph.D., M.D., for my book *Vitamin C Against Cancer*. At the time he was president of and research director for the Memorial Sloan-Kettering

Cancer Institute. One of the first things he told me was that he had been having a love affair with zinc for years.

Zinc is a common deficiency in our society. It's important for the support of the immunological system, and thus, it's especially needed to prevent both infections and cancer.

Surgeons find that zinc helps wound healing. Pediatricians have prescribed it as a popular ingredient of diaper rash ointment.

Some researchers have concluded that persons suffering from schizophrenia require extra amounts of zinc.

Zinc has become one of the "name" minerals because of its widespread use in important enzyme systems throughout the body, including one that works with insulin and the one required for the metabolism of brain cells.

People suffering from alcoholism have a special need for zinc. Once they develop cirrhosis of the liver, their average serum concentration of zinc is only 66 mcg per 100 ml, about half the amount found in well people. Apparently, persons suffering from alcoholic cirrhosis are unable to store zinc and lose large amounts in their urine. Since zinc is required in the metabolism of alcohol itself, it's prudent for heavy drinkers to add a zinc supplement to their diet.

I routinely give my patients zinc gluconate capsules, 60 mg. three times a day. I have never observed zinc toxicity from this dosage.

Zinc supplements are said to be especially important for the treatment and prevention of benign prostatic hypertrophy. I'm not so sure about that.

Men lose a great deal of zinc in their ejaculations. Men who are heavily into sex should be especially careful about their supply of zinc.

Your Chromium Needs

Chromium acts in concert with insulin in the metabolism of sugar. In studies on animals maintained on low chromium diets the animals developed a diminished sugar tolerance, which could be reversed by the addition of chromium. Rats maintained on severely chromium-restricted diets showed impaired growth, and did not live out their normal life span.

Recent research indicates that chromium deficiency in humans is extremely widespread. Chromium is useful in preventing and lowering high blood pressure. It also helps reduce cholesterol and hardening of the arteries. This means chromium might help fight the mental changes accompanying senility.

Meat, shellfish, and chicken are good sources of chromium.

Selenium Too Is Becoming a "Big Name" Mineral

Briefly, here's what you need to know about selenium.

Like vitamin E, selenium is an antioxidant. That means it's likely to postpone aging and prolong life. Evidence is accumulating that it prevents cancer. In tissue cultures, it inhibits cancer growth.

A deficiency in animals is associated with heart disease. Is the same true for humans? Probably.

In areas of low selenium, there are more strokes and there's more cancer.

Like water, too little selenium is deadly and too much is deadly. The right amount is about 200 mcg daily. Go higher than that and you're on your own. Toxic symptoms have been reported from 1000 mcg daily.

I have had several older men who found selenium did wonders for their in-bed life.

CHAPTER EIGHTEEN

FINDING YOUR IDEAL VITAMIN AND MINERAL PROGRAM

Vitamin Deficiencies And Vitamin Dependency Disorders

Physicians understand simple vitamin deficiencies. A patient is deficient in vitamin B_{12}, for example, and becomes anemic. The physician gives injections of vitamin B_{12} and corrects the deficiency.

Many physicians, however, do not understand biochemical individuality and vitamin dependency disorders.

Biochemical Individuality

The late Roger J. Williams, professor emeritus of chemistry at the University of Texas and a past president of the American Chemical Society, and others, have stressed that each person has a different need for every nutrient, especially for every vitamin. Recently Dr. M. Levine of the National Institutes of Health, published a paper in the *New England Journal of Medicine* admitting that we have little knowledge about the ideal amount of vitamin C people should take. The paper used the term "new concept" in its title. Perhaps

205

the idea was new to the government and to the editor of the *New England Journal of Medicine*, but was not new to the readers of *Lancet*, which published a paper on the subject nearly forty years ago. The implication of Levine's paper is that we do not know the optimal level for any vitamin.

When we learn more about individual needs, we will probably find that each person's ideal vitamin level falls on a bell-shaped curve. Many people who fail to thrive in our society probably fall at the neglected far end of the bell curve.

Vitamin Dependency Disorders

A vitamin dependency disorder is a biochemical defect. Because of the defect, the person with the disorder needs more than the usual amounts of one or more vitamins. Rosenberg at Yale reported on children whose convulsions he could control only by giving vitamin B-6 in amounts several hundred times the accepted norms. These children suffered not from vitamin deficiencies but from vitamin dependency disorders.

Popular medical textbooks neglect the subject.

The Heinz Handbook of Nutrition, not widely read by physicians, but with a distinguished editorial board, states: "The typical individual is more likely to be one who has average needs with respect to many essential nutrients but who also exhibits some nutritional requirements for a few essential nutrients which are far from average.

The more widely available and equally distinguished *Merck Manual* states: "Vitamin dependency usually relates to those vitamins with coenzyme function and results from an apoenzyme abnormality that can be overcome by administration of doses of the appropriate vitamin that is many times the RDA. The medical literature describes many vitamin dependencies."

How to Diagnose Vitamin Needs as Well as Vitamin Dependency Disorders

The only practical way to find your ideal vitamin needs is to increase and decrease the amounts of vitamins—one at a time—and discover whether you feel better when taking a large amount.

Some people feel worse on a large amount. I've seen patients who felt great on 7 mg. a day of folic acid (a B vitamin) and terrible on 12 mg. a day.

Directions for testing follow.

BUT REMEMBER

As I have emphasized, establishing your best nutritional levels can be complicated and is an ongoing process. You can't just "set it and forget it." I've been fine-tuning my own nutrition program for years.

It's a physiological reality that from time to time our body chemistry and/or our general health shifts. That requires us to raise or lower our levels of nutrients. Inevitably, too, we experience times of unusual physical or mental stress. We develop allergies. Our hormone levels change with age, pregnancy, or menopause.

Try not to be discouraged by the thought that you'll probably never hit on one particular combination of nutrients that will suit you for the rest of your life. Look at it this way: Almost nothing important in life remains constant. Just when we think we've got everything nailed down, we change jobs or get a promotion; or our children grow up; or our marriage cracks; or the market drops. Our lives must be changed to accommodate the new situation. Life is indeed a process, and no process is a static thing.

Before continuing, I must say once more that the information I give is valid in general. It works for most people, but it's possible that it won't be suitable for you. Since nutrition affects your body profoundly, it follows that altering your nutrition can have a significant—and (rarely) even harmful—effect on your body chemistry. Again I urge you to consult your physician before embarking on a nutritional voyage of discovery.

I'm aware that this advice raises problems. If every doctor knew what he should about proper nutrition, you wouldn't need this book. Instead, your doctor may be less well-informed on the subject than you. He may be discouraging or even scornful of your interest in nutrition partly because he knows too little about it and doesn't want to expose his lack of knowledge. Nevertheless, I recommend that you go over your plans with him so you can be sure you know if there is any *solid* reason to expect trouble.

Have you ever had rheumatic fever? Do you have high blood pressure? Do you have diabetes—or low blood sugar? Do you have a tendency toward depression? Do you have an ulcer, or any digestive problem that could be aggravated by large doses of vitamins? Are you taking any drugs (such as antidepressants or anticoagulants) that might be affected by your vitamin intake?

As you know, I cannot prescribe specifically for you without examining you. If you were my patient, I would test you for those conditions. I would design a specific vitamin and mineral program for you based on your special chemistry. And then I would follow you throughout your treatment.

Even if you decide to design your own nutritional program, you still should arrange to have medical guidance, especially in the beginning. If you can persuade your doctor to read up on nutrition and vitamin therapy, so much the better. If not, at least have him do a physical examination on you and perform the laboratory studies mentioned in the next section.

If he tries to talk you out of taking vitamin supplements, make sure he explains his objections in detail. Ask him for medical references, for the names and dates of publication of scientific papers and textbooks that you can read. That will help you separate lack of knowledge and prejudice from sound medical judgment.

Chances are he won't have any references to give you. Probably he will be passing a negative judgment without proper information.

The Minimum Tests You Need

Have your doctor order a complete blood count, a routine urine, a VDRL, SMA 24, HDL, T-3, T-4, IgE, and, if a man, a serum testosterone. Everyone should also have serum vitamin levels. They should be done a certain way. Have your local laboratory telephone

Vitamin Diagnostics, Route 35 and Industrial Road, Cliffwood Beach, New Jersey 07735 (Tel: 1-201-583-7773).

This laboratory will give your laboratory directions for preparing and mailing the blood samples to them for testing. This laboratory is the only laboratory I know of that uses a biological method for testing vitamin levels. Not only is it more accurate than other methods, but it's also less expensive.

All tests should be done first thing in the morning. Have nothing to eat, drink, or smoke after 10 P.M. the night before.

IF YOUR DOCTOR WON'T COOPERATE . . .

If your family doctor refuses to cooperate with you than you have two choices. First, you can try arm twisting. Your doctor, after all, is providing a service. He can give you advice based on his best scientific judgment, but he shouldn't refuse you a treatment that you want if he does so on the grounds of simple prejudice.

If your lawyer refused to handle your divorce case on the grounds that your wife is a wonderful woman and you shouldn't want to divorce her, you would be perfectly justified in seeking legal service elsewhere. You can point this out to your doctors although I'm sure you're aware that it is not likely to improve relations between you. Perhaps the preferable alternative is to locate a second doctor for this treatment alone. When you call for an appointment, make it clear to him or his secretary that you are coming specifically for certain tests.

WHY YOU NEED A NUTRITIONAL BASE

Megavitamins are doses of vitamins that are higher than needed to prevent clinical symptoms of malnutrition. Each vitamin has different properties, and may be of special benefit to one person or another. You can determine the amounts that will help you.

But before we begin let me say that, like the FDA, I believe that there is a base level of vitamins that should be taken by virtually everyone.

Unlike the FDA, however, I think that if you live in the "modern" world and eat "modern" food, there is almost no chance that you are getting your ideal levels of vitamins and other nutrients from diet alone. Therefore, the first thing you should do is bring your nutritional level up to an acceptable line.

START BY GOING BACK AND READING CHAPTER 16 ON VITAMINS

After checking with your physician and after reading chapter 16 on vitamins, set up a daily, unsaturated oil-mineral-vitamin program for yourself. This will be the base we'll work from.

NOW STEP UP TO MEGAVITAMIN LEVELS

When you have lived with your base level of vitamins for about two weeks, you may begin experimenting (tailoring would be a better term) to determine whether you feel better with mega levels of certain vitamins.

Increase only one vitamin at a time, so that if you experience a reaction (good or bad) you will know which one did it.

One more tip before you begin. The most common difficulty people experience with megavitamins is indigestion, "gas," or a burning feeling in the stomach. Most people can avoid those discomforts if they will take their vitamins directly after eating.

If you take tablets be sure they are labeled "free of starch, sugar, and artificial dyes."

Better to use capsules when available. It's better still to use the straight powders when you can get them. That way you avoid all the binders and fillers that may cause upset stomach in some people.

In any case, never take vitamins that are colored and coated. Don't even take those labeled "protein coated." Many people do not tolerate them well. We're trying to solve problems, not cause them.

If in spite of following the above directions you still have trouble from your vitamins, change forms. If you've had an upset stomach from tablets, change to capsules—or vice versa.

If you still have trouble, change brands. Some people will tolerate one brand of vitamins (and other supplements) better than another.

WHAT'S YOUR TYPE?

Some people must change types of vitamins. For example, one may be unable to take straight ascorbic acid powder but may tolerate the delayed action type, or calcium ascorbate—possibly sodium ascorbate.

CAUTION: Sodium ascorbate contains sodium so should be taken only with the strictest supervision of your physician.

Some people cannot tolerate the ordinary B-complex vitamins, but can tolerate B vitamins *from* rice bran sources. Schiff makes such a vitamin capsule. Careful: companies try to fool you. Some "rice bran"-labeled B vitamins only have a rice bran filler. Schiff even has such a line—in addition to B-complex *from* rice bran.

If the label says a B-complex vitamin has 50 mg of thiamine (B_1) in it, you may be certain it's not *from* rice bran but rather *with* rice bran. The tablet with B-complex *from* rice bran will have only 5 or 10 mg of thiamine.

If you change forms of the vitamin and change brands and still have trouble, I would try reducing the dose of the vitamin to see if you can tolerate it at a lower dosage.

If still unable to tolerate the vitamin, try taking it only once every four days.

If still unable to take the vitamin, then it's quite possible you will not be able to take it. I have several patients who cannot take any vitamins at all. Now and then I see a patient who—strange as this may sound—can take vitamins only by injection.

Rarely a patient can tolerate the injectable form of the vitamin by mouth; they buy the injectable vitamin, withdraw it into a syringe, then squirt it in a inch or two of water in a glass and drink it.

Why can they tolerate this? Who knows? The human body can measure things in quantities that are too small for machines to measure.

Vitamins A and D

Vitamins A and D aren't do-it-yourself vitamins for experimenting with high levels. Do not increase these above the levels given in chapter 16.

Beta-Carotene

Beta-Carotene is a pre-vitamin A that the body can change into vitamin A. Like E and selenium, it's an antioxident and may retard aging. Reliable reports indicate that it is important in the prevention of cancer. There is no question in my mind about its being important in the prevention of infections, such as colds.

Usually I have patients take Beta-Carotene capsules (Solgar) 15 mg (25,000 IU) every third day. You may increase and decrease your dose by a capsule or two to see if you notice any difference in how you feel.

CAUTION: Check the palms of your hands. If they begin getting an orange tint, reduce your dosage. Most people can take only 15 mg of beta-carotene every third day.

How to Establish Your Vitamin E Level

As you learned in chapter 16, vitamin E is important for treating emotional symptoms. If you are tired, listless or depressed, experiencing menopausal symptoms, under emotional stress or stress from a polluted environment, increased doses of vitamin E may help you.

Research indicates that vitamin E may well prolong your life and some men swear it increases their sexual vigor.

The Drs. Shute in Canada spent their lives studying vitamin E. They threw the vitamin E advocates into a turmoil since one of these physicians now believes that Alpha-tocopherol (sometimes spelled tochopheryl) *acetate* is the most important form of vitamin

E, and the other brother came to believe that Alpha-tocopherol *succinate* was better. As a result, many nutritionists now suggest that patients take each type of vitamin E to make certain they are covered. I think it might be a good idea also to throw in a capsule of natural mixed tocopherols (E complex), about 400 units daily.

It is particularly important that anyone with heart disease receive close supervision while taking vitamin E. I am one of the very many physicians who believe that the use of vitamin E is essential for the proper treatment of many kinds of heart diseases, but the proper dosage differs for different kinds of heart trouble.

CAUTION: People with rheumatic heart disease (valvular heart disease) must have especially close supervision by a physician when taking vitamin E's. Generally, people with rheumatic heart disease do not tolerate E's in large doses.

CAUTION: Some people's blood pressure rises if more than 200 units of vitamin E are taken per day. The blood pressure promptly drops to normal after the dose is reduced. Some of these patients can take higher levels of vitamin E if the dose is increased very slowly.

For almost two years I couldn't go above 350 units daily. Then, gradually, I could step this up without having my blood pressure rise. Now I seem to be able to take almost any amount without difficulty.

Since vitamin E may be stimulating, I advise that it be taken early in the day. Because E interferes with the metabolism of iron, it should never be spread out over the day. The gastrointestinal tract should be left to absorb iron at night. The E should be taken at breakfast and lunch.

Always read labels on vitamin-mineral tablets. Since iron and vitamin E aren't compatible, you know the company is selling you a very questionable product if the tablets contain both iron and vitamin E.

I suggest that people start on 100 to 200 units of mixed tocopherols daily after breakfast. Almost everyone can take this amount without worrying about increasing blood pressure. If you wish, this amount can gradually be increased over the course of about two weeks to 400 units.

Have your physician follow your blood pressure.

If you want to increase your level of vitamin E, add 100 to 200 units of Alpha-tocopherol succinate at lunch. (I like the brand Key-E, made by Carlson Laboratories.)

If all goes well, try adding 200 units of Alpha-tocopherol acetate, also at lunch.

After a few weeks, some people double the above dose.

If using vitamin E to increase sexual vigor, take it an hour or two before having intercourse.

How to Establish Your Vitamin C Level

I'm convinced that there are large variations in the amount of vitamin C that people require to feel their best. Linus Pauling says that about 4,000 mg a day is the minimum amount of vitamin C most people require. From my clinical experience, I'm inclined to go along with him.

Both of us have observed, however, that many people feel better on much higher doses of vitamin C. Here again, the only way to discover at what level of vitamin C you feel best is to increase it gradually to larger doses.

You can start with your base dose of one-quarter teaspoon four times a day (4,000 mg), then build up by adding about 2,000 mg every four days. Remember to take it well diluted in room temperature water. Ascorbic acid flavors hot tea as if it were lemon, but unfortunately heat destroys the vitamin.

If you have an ulcer or have a tendency toward ulcers, your stomach may not be able to tolerate the acidity. (Most people with ulcers can tolerate ascorbic acid.) The acidity can be eliminated by mixing your dolomite with the vitamin C.

If that doesn't do the trick you might try switching to one of the other forms of C, such as the time-released.

KIDNEY STONES AND VITAMIN C

A few years ago there was a great storm in the press about the possibility of vitamin C causing kidney stones. There are some theoretical reasons why a high intake of vitamin C might increase the formation of calcium oxalate stones.

The threat, however, has remained theoretical. These of us who have been giving—and taking—daily vitamin C doses of 20,000 mg and higher simply haven't had patients develop kidney stones.

There is some factor which we don't as yet understand that makes one person develop stones and the next person with the same diet and biochemistry fail to develop stones.

It may be that infection in the kidney causes the stone formation. We know that kidney infections are unlikely to happen when the urine is acid. Ascorbic acid (vitamin C) tends to acidify the urine. Perhaps that's why patients don't develop kidney stones on large doses of vitamin C.

Another possible reason why patients don't get in trouble with large doses of vitamin C: pyridoxine (vitamin B_6) tends to inhibit kidney stone formation. Almost all of us giving large doses of vitamin C also give vitamin B_6 along with it.

It's probable that magnesium also protects patients from kidney stones.

FINE POINTS ABOUT VITAMIN C

As mentioned, the ordinary vitamin C tablet you buy at the corner drugstore is not dye-, sugar-, or starch-free unless it says so on the label. This common ascorbic acid tablet gives many people gas, abdominal pains, and diarrhea if taken in reasonably large amounts.

A better source of vitamin C is the dye-, sugar-, starch-free tablet so labeled. Better still is the clear capsule containing vitamin C.

The straight powder is the best, although even it may produce diarrhea when taken in very large amounts. Again, start slowly and build up the dosage gradually.

Two warnings! First, use the ascorbic acid powder only if it looks like talcum powder. A granular substance (granular like table sugar) is also often labeled "ascorbic acid powder." Avoid the granular form. It frequently causes all sorts of difficulties: diarrhea, upset stomach, rashes, emotional difficulties, etc. How do I know? Not long ago there was a shortage of ascorbic acid powder and many of my patients (along with me) switched to the granular type. Almost all of us had many reactions from it.

Secondly, some companies have started to cut (dilute) their ascorbic acid powder with inert ingredients. This means you get short-changed and you will be taking the wrong dose. The proper strength: one teaspoon equals about 4,000 mg of ascorbic acid.

These may seem like small points but they are very important. They can make the difference between success and failure in your vitamin program.

A FEW PEOPLE NEED GIANT AMOUNTS

Do not take large doses of C—or any other vitamin or mineral or unsaturated fats (oils)—unless under a physician's care. By large doses of C, I mean 1000 mg or more.

A few of my patients feel best on 30,000 mg of vitamin C a day. I have one patient with an extremely unusual biochemistry who functions well only on the heroic dosage of 60,000 mg daily.

This gifted woman has marked food allergies and was for a number of years an alcoholic. When she stopped drinking she became very obese because of allergic addictions to certain foods.

Tests revealed that the patient was sensitive to almost every food, but especially to all red meats. Only when we took her off all meats and gradually increased her ascorbic acid to 60,000 mg daily was she able to control her weight and feel good. By "good" I mean that she lost her chronic depression and tiredness.

She had been suicidal when I first saw her, but she has now attained significant heights in her profession, takes pride in her slender figure, and finds that life is worthwhile again.

We have repeatedly tried reducing her ascorbic acid intake but she simply does not feel good at lower levels.

If your uric acid is elevated, it may go higher with more C, though I have seen it fall with large doses of vitamin C. Usually your cholesterol will drop while you take large amounts of vitamin C.

If you're pregnant, inform both your obstetrician and your pediatrician-to-be about the vitamins you're taking and ask their advice. Generally, I lower vitamin C levels for pregnant women to about 1000 mg three times a day.

(A physician—now deceased—with wide experience in the use of vitamin C stated that he had given 10 grams or more a day to very many pregnant women without difficulty. I have caught him in several untruths, however, and would be afraid to take his word for it.)

One of the problems in giving large doses of any vitamin to pregnant women is that the baby also gets large amounts of vitamins while in the uterus. Once the baby is born, the vitamin supply is suddenly reduced—though this is less of a problem when the baby nurses. Still, no one knows whether she will be able to nurse until it's tried.

Having a sudden reduction in vitamin levels leaves the newborn infant with a *relative* vitamin deficiency. This makes the infant more susceptible to infections.

The whole matter can be solved if the pediatrician will immediately place the newborn on generous amounts of vitamins. Seldom, however, does one find a pediatrician with the knowledge needed to do this.

CAUTION: The birth of a baby to a non-nursing mother who has been on large amounts of vitamins is an emergency situation that must be dealt with at once!

HOW TO TEST YOUR VITAMIN C LEVEL

If you're curious, you can test your own urine to get a general idea about your body levels of vitamin C. At a drugstore, buy a 5% aqueous solution of silver nitrate. Using an eye dropper, place ten drops of this solution in a clean cup. Add ten drops of your urine. Wait two minutes. The solution will become white-beige, smoky gray, or charcoal in color. The darker it is, the more vitamin C you are spilling. If you excrete little or no vitamin C, your system is using all it can get, and probably needs more.

How to Establish Your B Vitamin Levels

In order to be sure your basic B vitamin needs are met, I suggest that patients start by taking a multiple B_6 vitamin, one that contains nothing but B vitamins. Generally I give my patients Hy-B Complex 50, which is the brand name for a multiple B vitamin. If the patient has a history of allergies, I have him start by taking ¼ to ½ a capsule for a few days to make certain it's tolerated.

The next question is always, "How do you take half of a capsule?"

A reasonable question.

Pull the capsule apart, shake out the unneeded vitamin, push the capsule back together again, wipe it off, and swallow it.

How to Test for Levels

Finding your own best level of B vitamins is a two-part process. After you have found your level for C and E, you begin with the B vitamins, one at a time. Take one until you discover what amount makes you feel best, then stop that vitamin temporarily while you test the next B vitamin. You should keep a written record of both your mental and physical reactions. When you have tested each B vitamin and arrived at a complete schedule of B vitamins for yourself, you may find that taking them in combination produces different effects.

You may need to test all over again using different combinations at different levels.

Water-Soluble

Because B and C vitamins are water-soluble and easily excreted in the urine, there's little danger that extra amounts will accumulate in your body. In order for them to be readily excreted, however, it's advisable to drink at least a quart and a half of water a day.

CAUTION: As mentioned many times, you must have your doctor's supervision while following any directions given in this book. It's especially important that you have your physician's supervision if you take pyridoxine (vitamin B_6) in amounts larger than 50 mg a day. Nerve damage has been reported from taking B_6 in large amounts over a long period of time.

In all fairness, others have found vitamin B_6 safe to take in doses up to 1000 mg daily. However, I think it unwise to depend upon this figure.

You should also keep in mind that the B vitamins are an interlocking complex. You need all of them.

VEGETARIANS PLEASE NOTE!

If I were following a vegetarian diet, I would either have an injection of vitamin B_{12b} once a month or have my serum vitamin B_{12} level checked every three to six months. Vegetarians are especially prone to develop low levels of vitamin B_{12} when subjected to unusual stress. Most types of stress use up vitamin B_{12} in massive amounts.

For example: Bill Hawkins was a psychologist referred to me by his therapist for a nutritional workup. The man had been locked up on the psychiatric floor of one of New York's major hospitals. They had diagnosed him as suffering from schizophrenia, paranoid type.

My tests showed that the patient had a low serum vitamin B_{12} level. His paranoid symptoms cleared quickly after he was given vitamin B_{12b} by injection. Through trial and error, we discovered that he needed an injection of 1 cc once a week to remain symptom free.

Trial and error also told us that if the patient drank an alcoholic beverage, he needed the B_{12b} injection every three days.

The chemical stress by the alcohol was enough to more than double his need for vitamin B_{12}. I've seen the same thing happen with a strep infection or following surgery.

PREGNANCY IS A STRESS

One of the greatest stresses is pregnancy. The baby gets its nourishment both from what the mother eats and from her body reserves.

Again, let me remind you that pregnant vegetarians are likely to be deficient in vitamin B_{12}.

How to Establish Your Thiamine (B_1) Level

Many people feel better after they start taking vitamin B_1 in megadoses, particularly people who eat many sweets and other carbohydrates, and those who frequently drink alcoholic beverages. Especially are they likely to be helped by large amounts of vitamin B_1 if they suffer from symptoms such as tiredness or depression.

To discover your best dose of vitamin B_1, with your physician's approval, I suggest that you begin with 100 mg. Less is rarely worthwhile. I suggest that you start after breakfast on a Saturday because it's possible that you'll experience a high and need time to come down.

If you discover you tolerate 100 mg without difficulty, gradually move up to a 500 mg capsule. After you have adjusted to one such capsule a day, try three a day, one with each meal. If your sense of well-being has not increased at this point, you should drop back to a more modest dose.

You may want to try raising the levels again when you are taking megadoses of each of the B vitamins to see whether your reactions change.

How to Establish Your Riboflavin (B_2) Level

I've seen only a few people with emotional difficulties improve by taking riboflavin (B_2) alone. Still, vitamin B_2 has a marked effect on certain physical symptoms such as red, burning tongues, painful cracks at the corners of the mouth, and eyes that are sensitive to light.

Many people who wear dark glasses all the time because bright light hurts their eyes, are suffering from a riboflavin deficiency.

Wearing dark glasses much of the time is harmful because the natural light entering your eyes is an important source of stimulation to your nervous system. (You'll read all about it in the chapter on light.)

Riboflavin deficiency can also cause myelin (nerve sheath) degeneration. A lack of vitamin B_2 has been found to cause atrophy of male sex glands in rats.

I often recommend that patients try a 200 mg capsule of riboflavin three times a day for a week. After completing this trial, record any change in your physical or emotional state.

Then put riboflavin aside until you have completed testing the other B vitamins.

How to Establish Your Niacin or Niacinamide (B_3) Level

Niacin and niacinamide (different forms of vitamin B_3) are important today mostly from a historical standpoint. At one time I relied heavily on them, but as I've learned more about food and environmental allergies, I seldom use niacin or niacinamide.

Vitamin B_3 has proved to be useful in the fight against severe emotional disorders. Sometimes it benefits other people who are nervous, tired, depressed, or mildly overwrought.

As you know, niacin can also have significant physical effects, reducing blood cholesterol and the danger of blood clots, and raising blood sugar levels, which can mean difficulty for diabetics.

Because vitamin B_3 can have such important physiological effects, I especially recommend that you take this supplement only with the supervision of your doctor. If he hasn't already done so, get him to read the medical literature on niacin.

THE TWO TYPES OF VITAMIN B_3

There are two commonly used types of vitamin B_3: niacin and niacinamide.

Usually I find that people who are slowed down and depressed do better on niacin. Those who are tense and hyperactive often react more favorably to niacinamide.

CAUTION: Niacinamide can make some people tired and depressed.

When using niacin, I commonly start my patients on a 250 mg capsule three times a day. After three days, I have them go up to a 500 mg capsule, then double the dose every four days until they're taking 1,000 mg three times a day. Vitamin B_3, especially, should be taken as a straight powder or in the clear capsule form.

Niacin may cause flushing, and occasionally, nausea. Megadoses of niacin may give a lift and a feeling of buoyancy to older people in general, and to depressed people in particular. After a few days, the flush from the initial dose should decrease and disappear.

The standard minimum dose for people with emotional difficulties is 100 mg three times a day, though some schizophrenics must sometimes go higher. I have given as much as 30,000 mg a day.

CAUTION: I cannot stress enough how important it is for you to have medical supervision by a physician well trained in the field of nutrition and especially knowledgeable about the use of large amounts of niacin.

Many people feel great on as little niacin as 250 mg once or twice a week.

Keep in mind that while most people feel better within days of beginning a niacin regimen, some require longer to feel its benefits.

If it's discovered that you do better on niacinamide than on niacin, I do not recommend pushing the dosage beyond 4000 to 8000 mg daily.

CAUTION: As with niacin, niacinamide treatment is not a do-it-yourself project. Take it only under the advice of a physician.

When you reach higher levels of niacinamide or, especially, niacin, you might be plagued by nausea. This nausea is often more marked in the morning and may come on before you take your after-breakfast dose of the vitamin. For this reason, you may not suspect the vitamin as the cause of your difficulty. Skip your vitamin B₃ for a day. If it's causing your nausea, the nausea should disappear.

Nausea is very common with the garden variety of niacin tablet you pick up at the corner drugstore. It is less common when taking the starch-free, sugar-free tablets and much less common when taking the colorless, sugar-free, starch-free straight powder or capsule.

Don't let anyone tell you a product is sugar-free and starch-free unless it is so labeled by the manufacturer.

WHEN TREATING SCHIZOPHRENIA . . .

When niacin is given to patients suffering from schizophrenia, the dose should generally be built up gradually over a period of several weeks.

When the patient experiences nausea, as most people do at some level, they should skip the vitamin for twenty-four hours and go back to a slightly lower dosage, say about 1500 mg per day lower than the level that produced the nausea.

If a patient doesn't experience nausea at 30,000 mg a day, there's no point in pushing higher. People who do not improve on that level do not improve on higher levels.

Niacin and niacinamide in mega (large) amounts may give positive liver function tests. Tell your physician about it. If you take more than 250 mg daily of niacin or niacinamide be sure that your physician monitors your liver function tests and uric acid levels.

Niacin is sometimes useful for people with severe food allergies. It seems to act as a nonspecific detoxifier. I once had a patient who could scarcely function on less than 30,000 mg of niacin per day. But after we discovered that she was allergic to beef and eliminated it from her diet, she needed no niacin at all. Indeed, only small amounts of it would make her feel ill.

Many psychiatrists find that using vitamin B₃ decreases a patient's need for tranquilizers. Often the amount of tranquilizer can be cut in half soon after the patient starts megavitmin doses of B₃.

NB: Nowadays, I seldom prescribe more than 50 mg a day of vitamin B_3.

In the treatment of most emotional illnesses, unsaturated oils, minerals and vitamins (with the exception of Vitamin B_{12b}) are about 25% in importance, cleaning up the environment is 15% in importance, and diet is about 60% in importance.

Because the above facts are not observed, many people fail in an attempt to get help from nutrition for their emotional troubles. Physicians in the field of nutrition—and patients—are not aware of the above facts.

Very few nutritionists understand the complexities of food allergies.

How to Establish Your Pyridoxine (B_6) Level

Insofar as I know, there are only two vitamins that people would kill for. One of them is vitamin B_{12} and the other is vitamin B_6.

If vitamin B_6 is going to help you, you know it right away. It's especially important for anyone on a high-protein diet. It's needed for protein metabolism and can help to keep blood cholesterol levels low.

It also plays a part in carbohydrate metabolism, which makes it particularly valuable for people with hypoglycemia or diabetes. B_6 is essential to prevent certain types of anemia. It reduces tooth decay and some important studies indicate that it may reduce the incidence of certain types of cancer. It reduces heart disease and the formation of kidney stones. Allergic states are often improved by large amounts of pyridoxine.

A deficiency of vitamin B_6 can make you irritable, tired, or restless; an acute deficiency can even lead to convulsions.

When you begin taking pyridoxine, you may find that you have more energy, feel less tense, lose the bloated feeling in your body; that the bags under your eyes disappear; that your arthritis improves. You may find that it relaxes you to the point of sleepiness. If this happens, take your B_6 at bedtime.

Begin with 50 mg of B_6 once a day.

CAUTION: If you go higher than 50 mg daily, it's especially important that you have a physician supervising your voyage of discovery. There have been reports of severe damage with the use of high doses of vitamin B$_6$.

If your physician agrees, increase your B$_6$ level to one 200 mg capsule three times a day.

I have several patients who function well only if they take as much as 600 mg of vitamin B$_6$ three times a day. Needless to say, you must have the strictest of medical supervision if you take that amount.

A few people cannot tolerate high doses of pyridoxine. If it makes you nervous, irritable or slightly nauseated, take it in clear capsule form, with no coloring or binder. If it still bothers you, ask your doctor for a prescription for injectable B$_6$. Take the liquid out of the bottle with a needle and syringe, squirt it into water, and drink it. Some people can tolerate this form and no other.

A NEW FORM OF VITAMIN B$_6$

In order for pyridoxine (vitamin B$_6$) to be utilized by the body, the body chemistry must turn it into its active form: pyridoxal 5 phosphate. Some people have a defect in their chemistry that will not effectively carry out this conversion. For that reason pyridoxal 5 phosphate has been placed on the market so the active form can be taken.

Off hand, that seems to be the ideal solution to the problem. Actually, it's a mixed blessing.

Many people have digestive systems that do not assimilate pyridoxal 5 phosphate well. As a result you are never quite sure how much they're getting.

While some people feel better on the pyridoxal 5 phosphate than on the straight pyridoxine (B$_6$), others do best when taking a mixture of pyridoxine and pyridoxal 5 phosphate. Only trial and error will give your answer.

NOTE: Pyridoxal 5 phosphate comes in 50 mg capsules. I've used the one put out by Klaire Laboratories. It's said to be five times as strong as straight vitamin B_6, but of course that depends upon how well a person absorbs it.

I have seen a number of people do better on pyridoxal 5 phosphate than on the straight B_6. On the other hand I've seen a few people who feel terrible on it.

I have the impression that pyridoxal 5 phosphate is more toxic for some people than the straight B_6.

Do not take pyridoxal 5 phosphate without close supervision by your physician.

Generally I've had negative results with the riboflavin 5 phosphate form of riboflavin (vitamin B_2).

Taking vitamin B_6 is said to sometimes cause a deficiency of vitamin B_2. With large doses of viatmin B_6, I usually give 200 mg of B_2 three times a day.

How to Establish Your Vitamin B_{12} Level

The lower limit of "normal" is given as 150 by some textbooks, and as 200 by others. Every textbook will inform you that 226 is a perfectly normal B_{12} level. Yet several years ago I learned that the "normal" B_{12} level is not necessarily normal for every individual.

I had tried many things to get a patient with a B_{12} level of 230 feeling better. Once, on nothing more than a hunch, I gave the patient an injection of vitamin B_{12}.

Immediately she felt like a new person. She stopped complaining about back pain and depression, got out of bed and began caring for her family again. Vitamin B_{12} completely changed her life—and later the lives of many of my other patients.

Since that experience, I've made it a policy to give all of my patients a therapeutic trial on B_{12b} by injection. As a result, I have learned a great deal about the vitamin and made a number of discoveries concerning it.

As time passes, I find less and less use for massive amounts of most vitamins, but more and more use for vitamin B_{12}. Clinical experience has been my teacher. I am not one of those smart alecks who thinks he knows more than anyone else about everything. I think I'm being honest, however, when I say that I probably know more about the clinical use of vitamin B_{12} than anyone else in the world. Way back in 1972 I published a paper in which I reported on 221 cases of vitamin B_{12} deficiency from my practice. Since then, I've seen many more.

And that doesn't include the many cases of vitamin B_{12} dependency disorders that I've diagnosed and treated.

Every New Year's Eve I used to think, "Well, I won't learn anything new about vitamin B_{12} this coming year."

By February, I always learned something new.

Now on New Year's Eve, I say, "I wonder what fascinating new things I'll learn about vitamin B_{12} during the coming year."

VITAMIN B_{12} IS A COMMON PROBLEM

As you know by reading this far, vitamin B_{12} deficiencies and/or vitamin B_{12} dependency disorders are very often a significant cause of emotional illness.

Unfortunately, people with vitamin B_{12} deficiencies are often unable to absorb vitamin B_{12} when taken by mouth. That means they must have it by injection.

Experience has taught me several things about vitamin B_{12}:

1. Every person should have blood tests for vitamin B_{12}.

2. Every person should be given several injections of vitamin B_{12b} (regardless of what the blood tests show) as a test for a vitamin B_{12} dependency disorder.

VITAMIN B_{12} AND VITAMIN B_{12b}

Vitamin B_{12} comes in several forms, the most important of which are cyanocobalamin (vitamin B_{12}) and hydroxocobalamin (vitamin B_{12b}).

Cyanocobalamin (B_{12}) is the one most commonly found in physician's offices. Many physicians do not know of the existence of hydroxocobalamin (B_{12b}). Because they know nothing about it, they say all sorts of things to patients to hide their lack of information.

I've had patients tell me that their doctors told them that hydroxocobalamin was "a rare and expensive form of B_{12}," that it's "only used in research centers," that it's "unavailable in this community," and on and on.

Nonsense. Hydroxocobalamin is a standard, widely used, inexpensive form of vitamin B_{12}.

True, most drug stores don't stock it—and that explains why druggists try to tell patients that there's "no difference between cyanocobalamin and hydroxocobalamin." Hydroxocobalamin can easily be ordered from a drug wholesaler.

Advantages of Using the Hydroxocobalamin (B_{12b}) Form

In order to utilize vitamin B_{12}, the body must convert it from cyanocobalamin into hydroxocobalamin. Why not start out using the hydroxocobalamin form and save the body a biochemical step? Also, why risk coming across someone who lacks the biochemical machinery needed to change B_{12} to B_{12b}?

Cyanocobalamin has been reported to be toxic for some people suffering from amblyopia (dimness of vision without a demonstrable cause). Indeed because of this toxicity, there has been a movement afoot in Great Britian to remove the cyanocobalamin form of B_{12} from the market.

Another advantage of hydroxocobalamin: it keeps blood levels of the vitamin at high levels approximately three times longer than cyanocobalamin.

One more problem with cyanocobalamin: it contains the "cyanide" radical. It's well known that cyanide is toxic for people. Why introduce cyanide into the body when it can so easily be avoided?

All of the information I'm about to give about vitamin B_{12} applies to hydroxocobalamin (vitamin B_{12b}) rather than to cyanocobalamin (vitamin B_{12}).

I have not had wide clinical experience with cyanocobalamin and do not first-hand know what it will not do. However, I would be very hesitant to use the cyanide form of vitamin B_{12} in large amounts over a long period of time. I have personally used hydroxocobalamin and have given it to very many people over many years.

I've seen only minor complications from it:

1. An overstimulation that's included insomnia. (Very rare.)

2. An allergy to the vitamin that produces a mild flushing for a few minutes. (Rare.)

3. An allergy to the vitamin that leaves a mild swelling and redness at the site of injection. (Very rare.)

4. A hemoglobin pushed to the upper limit of normal when taken along with testosterone enanthate over a number of months.

The books warn that hydroxocobalamin can:

1. Give some people an allergic reaction.

2. Uncover a hidden case of polycythemia vera. This means if you already have polycythemia vera—a condition in which your hemoglobin rises too high—and your hemoglobin has not yet actually gone up, the use of hydroxocobalamin (or cyanocobalamin) may cause your hemoglobin to rise to the levels it was about to rise to anyway. I have checked for this repeatedly, but never seen it.

3. Cause eye damage if given to persons suffering from hereditary optic nerve atrophy (Leber's disease). This occurs only in males and I have never seen it.

CAUTION: Do not use the cyanocobalamin form of vitamin B_{12}. Do not let a druggist or a physician tell you that there's no difference between cyanocobalamin (vitamin B_{12}) and hydroxocobalamin (vitamin B_{12b}).

To Discover Your Best Level of Vitamin B_{12b}

Since the injectable form of vitamin B_{12} is a prescription item, you will have to have the cooperation of a physician to try it.

It's not easy to educate a physician, but if he's open-minded, give him a copy of this book and ask him to at least read this section on vitamin B_{12}. Just as a lawyer charges for the time he spends researching a case, it's only fair that a doctor do the same. Tell your physician that you will pay him for the time he spends reading the section on vitamin B_{12}.

Here We Go!

Ask your physician to give you an intramuscular injection of 0.2 cc (200 mcg) of hydroxocobalamin. (If you are quite allergic, start with 0.05 cc, and build up more slowly. I have had a rare, extremely allergic patient develop a mild allergic reaction to this dose—a slight flush that lasted 5 or 10 minutes.)

If the first dose was well tolerated, a few minutes to a few days later (but not longer than a month) give a second injection of 0.4 cc, followed at the same interval by 0.5 cc, 0.75 cc and 1 cc.

If by this point you have had no increase in energy or feeling of well being, it's likely you do not have a vitamin B_{12} dependency disorder; however, the matter is not yet wholly settled.

I have had patients—especially depressed patients—who do not respond until they are given as much as 5 or 6 cc of B_{12b} at one time. (Do not give more than 3 cc at one spot. See Appendix 4 at the end of this book for detailed instructions for giving injections of B_{12b}. The details are important.)

I think of one patient particularly, a spectacularly successful designer who had made so many millions so quickly that he began enjoying the "finer things of life" too much and had overdosed his nose to the point that he fell into a horrendous depression.

Later, I'm sad to say, he abandoned B_{12b}, got off his diet, started freebasing and ended up a penniless bum. (Earlier he had been a rich bum.)

In any case, if you feel no better with a 5 cc injection of vitamin B_{12b}, you can forget about it—unless your blood test showed that you were low in it.

CAUTION: If your blood test showed you were low in vitamin B_{12}, you must have injections of vitamin B_{12b} all of your life whether or not you feel any better with it.

I would suggest 1 cc a month as a minimum amount. Better too much than too little. This is no small matter. You can have brain damage, and spinal cord damage from lack of vitamin B_{12}. I have had low B_{12} patients diagnosed as suffering from Alzheimer's disease. Another patient with a B_{12} deficiency arrived in my office in a wheelchair. Since vitamin B_{12} deficiencies and dependency reactions tend to be hereditary, everyone who is blood-related to you should also be tested.

> **CAUTION, CAUTION! If you get more energy or a feel-
> ing of well being after an injection of vitamin B$_{12b}$, the
> effect may last only half an hour and then wear off. (More
> commonly the effect lasts 2 or 3 days before wearing off.)**

When the effect wears off, you may feel profoundly weak and depressed. The weakness may be so bad that you feel someone has pulled the plug out of your body and all of your life has drained away. You may feel deeply depressed, suicidal in rare cases.

This letdown will gradually wear off in anywhere from a hour or two, to two or three days. Also, the letdown will be cured by another injection of vitamin B$_{12b}$.

Be thankful for the letdown. It probably means you have found the vitamin that will change your life. Jack Kennedy has been quoted as having said he would never have become president without injections of vitamin B$_{12b}$! Many an actor would not have an Oscar without vitamin B$_{12}$ injections and a number of athletes would not have moved into the million-dollar ranks without B^{12}— those ruddy drops that cheer sad hearts—and strengthen faint hearts.

WHAT TO DO

If you have the letdown mentioned above, it's best to get another injection of vitamin B$_{12b}$ as soon as possible. If this happens a time or two, then it will be clear that you have a biochemistry that will function best only if it's supplied by a higher than normal amount of vitamin B$_{12}$.

HOW MUCH, HOW OFTEN?

There's no test that will tell you or your physician how much B$_{12b}$ you need or how often you need it.

Your body knows, however, and will tell you if you will listen to it.

You don't want to spend the rest of your life on a roller coaster— sailing up in the air, and then crashing down to the ground. You want to feel neither high nor low. You want a good, steady feeling of well being.

Here's How to Get What You Want

Start out by giving yourself (after having been taught how to do so by your physician) an injection of hydroxocobalamin (vitamin B_{12b}) in the amount that experience so far has proved to be neither too much nor too little. Many people start by giving themselves ½ to 1 cc every other day. (In the beginning, it's best to give it first thing in the morning.)

If you get a lift from your injection, then you have waited too long to get it. Inject the same amount of vitamin B_{12b}, but try giving it every morning—or even morning and afternoon.

When you do not get a lift, that's the right interval. Your interval might (very rarely, and then only temporarily) be every 3 hours. Your interval might be once every week or two. Your body is the boss.

After you find your right interval, then you need to find the right dose. Try going up ½ cc each time until you reach 3 cc. At this point, with more B_{12b} given at each injection, you might find that it lasts longer.

If you feel no better on a higher dose and if it lasts no longer, then go back down on your dosage until you find the amount that does not allow you to feel your best, then go up again to find the right amount for you.

Very rarely patients require more than 3 cc. I had one history professor who for years could not go to work unless he took 26 cc (yes, twenty-six cc!) every morning.

Gradually he has come to need less and now takes 26 cc only every four or five days. Often people need less as time goes by.

As mentioned earlier, if under stress, such as menstruation or surgery you may need more.

Sound Strange? Let Me Explain.

If you get a lift after your injection of B_{12b}, it means that your chemistry has less than the ideal amount of vitamin B_{12} that it needs to run at peak efficiency.

Think of it this way: If you have an eight-cylinder car that has two spark plugs that won't fire, then you will be driving the car using only six cylinders. The car will still go on six cylinders. It will take you to the shopping center and get you to the golf course. But the car won't be very lively. It will struggle to get up hills, will lack pick up and the engine might knock a bit.

You want your biochemistry to purr along all the time on eight cylinders—not to sputter and falter.

If the doubting Thomases of the medical profession could only take a vitamin B_{12b}-dependent patient home to live with them a few weeks, they would be absolutely convinced about what I advocate regarding vitamin B_{12} therapy.

WHAT NOT TO DO

Now and then I see patients who have felt "run down" at some time in the past and visited a physician who gave them a "course" of vitamin B_{12} injections. The patient felt much better after the "course" but then gradually settled down into his or her old "run down" rut. For some reason it seldom seems to occur to either the patient or the doctor that the injections must be continued indefinitely.

The other week I saw a patient from the midwest who felt a great deal better when her doctor gave her an injection of vitamin B_{12}. The effect, however, lasted only a few hours. In spite of pleading on the patient's part, the physician would give her no more than 0.3 cc of B_{12} once a month.

He arrived at this figure because 0.3 cc of B_{12} by injection is all that is needed to keep the blood picture normal when a patient is suffering from a B_{12} deficiency. However, he was not dealing with pernicious anemia. His patient had a vitamin B_{12} dependency disorder, quite another matter.

Everyone needs all the vitamins, but it's especially important to have an adequate supply of the B vitamin known as folic acid when taking large amounts of vitamin B_{12}.

How to Establish Your Folic Acid Needs

NOTE: Folic acid is unable to enter the body cells properly without an adequate supply of vitamin B_{12}.

As you know, you should have a serum folic acid test when you have the test for vitamin B_{12}. If you have a borderline or deficiency level, you must take folic acid all your life.

This B vitamin is available both in tablet and injectable forms. With a prescription you can buy a 1 mg tablet. Without a prescription you can buy a 0.8 mg tablet. (In Canada one can buy 5 mg tablets without prescription.) All tablets should be labeled "sugar-free, starch-free." If the tablets are yellow, don't worry about artificial dyes. Folic acid itself has a yellow color.

Textbooks of medicine say that people absorb folic acid if taken by mouth—unless the person is ill with some rare, serious intestinal disorder such as sprue. Much to my surprise I have discovered that some people without demonstrable gastrointestinal disorders do not absorb folic acid properly. I have checked this finding with Kurt A. Oster, M.D., of Bridgeport, Connecticut, who is especially interested in folic acid. His clinical experience agrees with mine.

People who cannot absorb folic acid must have it by injection, a rare situation. Since vitamin C causes a loss of folic acid through the urine, it's particularly important that people on ascorbic acid pay attention to their folic acid levels. Injections of vitamin B_{12b} help the gastrointestinal tract absorb folic acid.

Deficiency in folic acid has been associated so prominently with anemia that physicians seem to pay little attention to other possible symptoms.

It's known that guinea pigs have convulsions and become very lazy if they have a folic acid deficiency. At least one study at Yale University reveals brain damage caused by folic acid deficiency. I believe that many nervous disorders are caused by folic acid deficiencies and that its deficiency causes much depression and indeed may, like vitamin B_{12} deficiency, produce almost any emotional disorder. I strongly recommend that patients who are deficient in folic acid take at least 1 mg three times a day and that they have a repeat blood test after a month to see if they are absorbing it properly. If not, the dose should be increased to 5 mg three times a day. If the serum level still doesn't go up, folic acid should be given by injection.

Up and Down the Folic Acid Scale

Folic acid deficiency is rather common in our society. I see perhaps one new case a month. Some people have a folic acid dependency disorder, just as a vitamin dependency disorder can occur with any other vitamin.

I have an engineer as a patient who's a very careful observer. The last time I saw him, he told me he had recently been experimenting with levels of folic acid.

"If I take 7 mg a day, I feel fine and have no trouble," he told me, "but if I lower the dosage to 4 mg, after about a week I begin getting suspicious of all of my fellow workers and feel very uncomfortable around them."

To show how much variation there is in people, another patient telephoned me from Maryland the other day to tell me that she took ½ of a 1 mg tablet of folic acid and felt terrible. We find that she can only tolerate ¼ of a tablet every 4 days. (She's quite allergic to most foods, including vitamins. The only vitamins we've been able to find that she can tolerate come from Canada. I had to get a special research permit from the FDA to import them and give them to her.)

In testing yourself for your particular folic acid level it would be reasonable to start with 1 mg three times a day and work up to perhaps 5 mg three times a day.

After leaving it at this level for a week or more, you might try going down to lower levels.

Very rapidly patients feel the effects of folic acid. Either they feel a great deal better or a great deal worse.

Some patients feel stimulated by large amounts of folic acid and others feel sedated. Still others just feel rotten.

Only trial and error will help you and your physician find your correct level.

Folic acid is a very neglected vitamin. Since it helps niacin accept methyl groups, there is much theoretical reason why folic acid might be helpful to persons suffering from schizophrenia.

A nasty rumor has been circulating that high doses of folic acid might cause convulsions. This rumor is based on a misinterpretation of work done on an epileptic.

CAUTION: If you're taking anticonvulsant medication, however, you should tell the doctor who gives it to you that some anticonvulsants are neutralized by folic acid. In that case, folic acid might cause a convulsion.

Folic acid also cancelled the effects of some forms of cancer chemotherapy. If you're getting this type of treatment, be doubly sure to clear the vitamin with your physician.

If I had a demonstrated folic acid deficiency, I would take folic acid all my life and I would check my blood serum level every three months to make certain I was absorbing it. Otherwise, I would give myself a trial on it to see whether it seemed to benefit me.

An adequate supply of all vitamins and minerals is important for everyone all the time, but adequate amounts of B_{12b} and folic acid are especially important during pregnancy and lactation.

How to Establish Your Pantothenic Acid Level

Pantothenic acid, certainly a neglected vitamin, is important in the production of the adrenal cortical hormones and in carbohydrate metabolism. A deficiency can cause degeneration of nerve tissue, physical weakness, and depression. A generous supply has resulted in longer lives for laboratory animals. Will it do the same for you? We don't know, but I want to be certain that I have more than enough.

The exact amount of pantothenic acid needed by humans has not been determined, though it is probably in the order of 10 to 15 mg a day. Perhaps ten or twenty times this figure would be a good idea for many people; some people feel better when taking up to a hundred times the basic amount.

Since many people are relaxed by this vitamin, I usually suggest that it be taken at bedtime. If you are tense, hyperactive, and irritable, you might try it during the day. Start with about 200 mg at bedtime and increase it every night to 600 mg, or you can take 200 to 400 mg three or four times a day to learn what level is best for you.

L-Carnitine (Vitamin B$_T$)

In 1948, G. Fraenkel, while working out the folic acid requirements for insects, found that meal worms needed a nutritional factor which had not yet been identified. This substance was found to be carnitine, a chemical substance that had been identified by Gulewitsch and Krimberg in 1905.

If meal worms went more than 4 or 5 weeks without this vitamin, they died. Fraenkel dubbed the new vitamin B$_T$.

Carnitine hasn't turned out to be one of the glamor vitamins. In truth, not a great deal of work has been done on it.

Vitamin B$_T$ is especially important for fat metabolism. It might be important for people who are trying to control their weight and their cholesterol. People with heart disease should take extra amounts of carnitine.

The vitamin is widely available in such things as brewers yeast and red meats. It's available in 250 mg capsules, L-Carnitine (Solgar). You might try a capsule one to three times a day to check it out.

CAUTION: Do not take the DL-carnitine or D-carnitine forms. There have been reports of toxicity from the DL form.

How to Establish Your Paba Level

Para-aminobenzoic acid (PABA) is another one of the "minor" vitamins that appears to be more promising than the two just mentioned.

During the late 1940's an obscure physician, Ana Aslan M.D., practicing in Transylvania, heard that procaine (Novocaine, a common local anesthesia that used to be injected into your gums by the dentist) broke down in the body and formed the vitamin para-aminobenzoic acid. She also learned of occasional unpleasant reactions from the alkaline form of procaine, the form used as a local anesthesia.

Aslan made a buffered, acidified form of the procaine which she began injecting into patients and which carries the trade name of Gerovital (or H-3).

Dr. Aslan was particularly interested in preventing aging, and claimed to have increased the lifespan of her patients by 30 percent. A 30 percent increase in lifespan impresses me. If you are going to pass on at age 70, and you can add 30 percent more time to your life, you would be over 90 when you died.

Dr. Aslan also found PABA useful for many psychological complaints such as depression and fatigue. She reported success in treating Parkinson's disease and claims an 80 percent cure for schizoid patients, meaning people who are not frankly schizophrenic but who are severely disturbed emotionally. She also reported that her injections helped greatly in cases of impotence.

Incidentally, Dr. Aslan avoided sweets, alcohol, and tobacco, and advised all of her patients to do the same, since she felt these things accelerate aging.

In this country procaine injections have only been approved for use as a local anesthetic.

Not much work has been done on Aslan's use of procaine. Here in New York, Nathan Kline, M.D., found it a rather effective but briefly acting antidepressant.

Some time ago, several United States congressmen visited Dr. Aslan. They were impressed by the good results they saw and encouraged several American physicians to begin research on the subject but not much has come from this work.

I suspect that much of Aslan's good results came from taking her patients off sugar, alcohol, and tobacco, and giving them vitamins.

You can buy PABA tablets (sugar-free, starch-free, colorless, 500 mg) across the counter and give them a try. Some people are said to have more energy when taking PABA.

Do You Need Vitamins By Injection?

For some people, injection is the only effective way to get water-soluble vitamins.

I have already mentioned the need for giving vitamin B_{12b} by intramuscular injection because of unreliable absorption by mouth.

If repeat blood serum tests show folic acid is not being absorbed, then it should certainly be given by injection.

Occasionally I see a patient who is unable to take any form of B or C vitamins by mouth. Strangely, a number of them can tolerate injectable vitamins.

I think you should be suspicious of physicians who routinely give vitamins by injection—other than vitamin B_{12b}.

CAUTION, CAUTION, CAUTION: The injection of thiamine, vitamin B_1, (either by itself or in combination with other vitamins, either intramuscularly or intravenously) has caused death. If this vitamin is given by injection, it must be started in very small amounts and slowly built up to therapeutic levels. This rule is commonly ignored, especially in institutions where large amounts of B vitamins are given by injection to recovering alcoholics.

How to Fine-Tune Your Vitamin Regimen

As I said earlier, finding (and staying on) your best vitamin level is an on-going process. Once you have been through the one-by-one vitamin check I have described, you have an outline to work with. But the process is not finished by any means. You are now taking yeast, vitamins A and D, and your own levels of C and E. You are taking whatever additional doses of B vitamins you have found to be helpful to you. At this point, you should begin again to test higher levels of vitamins in combination. For example, vitamin C and vitamin B_6 are interconnected; when B_6 is low, blood levels of C tend to be low and when B_6 goes up so does the vitamin C. Therefore, you may be able to lower your level of vitamin C if you are taking extra B_6, and still maintain a feeling of well-being; on the other hand, you may find that pushing the doses of both vitamins still higher produces even better results.

CAUTION: See earlier warning about taking more than 50 mg a day of B_6.

Similarly, you may find you can reduce your vitamin E. Vitamin E compensates for stress in the body as do several B vitamins. When you take them together, you may feel best with a higher or lower level of both.

Over a period of time, you should continue to test your reactions to various combinations of vitamins. Go back to the beginning dosages of the B vitamins; take two together; push the doses of each to the top limits; observe the way you feel. When you hit on a combination that works for you, add the rest of the B vitamins, one by one.

As a rule, people feel best with a certain combination of vitamins, although the proportions and combinations change over time. Throughout, continue to take yeast; this will minimize the possibility of creating a deficiency of one B vitamin while experimenting with another.

Finding a Mineral Supplement

Finding your correct mineral supplement is more complicated than working out the vitamin levels that are right for you.

There are many ins and outs. For example, if you have a history of kidney stones, your doctor might want to do calcium excretion studies on you to learn exactly how much calcium you spill while taking various amounts of calcium. If you're taking medication, your mineral requirements may change. Sometimes it's a good idea to increase a certain mineral for a set period of time, then reduce it.

Earlier I gave information about minerals that are usually needed; however, taking minerals is a complicated subject that should only be approached with the help of a physician knowledgeable about the subject.

CHAPTER NINETEEN

DIET FOR ALCOHOLISM

It's possible to make some strains of mice drink more heavily if you bang bells and make them generally uncomfortable in their cages. You "drive them to drink."

But mark this: other strains of mice bombarded with the same banging of bells cannot be driven to drink.

We can only conclude that ultimately the individual's chemistry, not his stress decides whether or not he will become an alcoholic.

THE ALCOHOLIC BLAMES HIS PROBLEMS

It is not the alcoholic's problems that drive him to drink. It's his chemistry.

We tend to blame our unhappiness on our problems, but problems are a perfectly normal part of life. Since the world is not set up according to anyone's wishes, we all have problems. We never finish with our problems. As soon as we satisfy one need, we develop another need that we want to satisfy . . . and we're sure we'll be happy if only. . . .

We think we don't have enough love, enough money, enough respect. Real happiness, complete contentment seem always to be just over the next hill, at the end of the rainbow.

I have a secret to tell you, dear reader: problems are always a part of life and will be with us until the day we die.

As pointed out previously, problems become large and unmanageable only if our biochemistry is not working right. Then prob-

242

lems (the ones that are mountain-high) are only symptoms, not causes.

HOW TO SHRINK PROBLEMS WITHOUT GOING TO A SHRINK

If you think your problems are too large, check out your nutritional supplements and your food allergies. Once these are in ideal balance, your problems will be down around your knees instead of up above your head. You will be able to cope with your remaining problems with a little finger, even if it previously required both arms and shoulders just to keep your problems from crushing you.

Although this is a book on nutrition, I would like to commend the work of AA and encourage anyone with alcohol problems to seek AA's help. In general, AA has been hostile toward psychiatrists, mainly because of the unpleasant experiences AA members had during the '40s and '50s when psychiatrists routinely gave alcoholic patients barbiturates, merely changing them from addictions to alcohol to addictions to barbiturates.

But one of AA's co-founders, Bill Wilson, was a very strong advocate of nutritional approaches (including megavitamins) as an aid to anyone who wanted to give up alcohol.

The Special Nutritional Needs of Alcoholics

ANYONE SUFFERING FROM ALCOHOLISM MUST GIVE SPECIAL ATTENTION TO HIS NUTRITIONAL NEEDS.

The above sentence should be written in flashing red neon letters a yard high and placed in every room of the alcoholic's home.

First, the alcoholic should be on the basic nutritional program as detailed in chapter 15.

Second, it's most important for the alcoholic to check out his food allergies. Alcoholism is mostly a manifestation of food allergy. Allergies to foods other than alcohol are always present. If the alcoholic is not taken off foods to which he is allergic, his chances for recovery are greatly reduced. Some aspects of nutrition are especially important in treating alcoholism. Although these will be discussed in the next few pages, I want to remind the reader that every aspect of nutrition is important for the alcoholic.

Each person suffering from alcoholism should be given special tests for food allergies (as detailed in chapter 10). Skin tests are of no help. If tests are not done, then the alcoholic should assume he is allergic to table sugar, to grains, to milk products (other than butter), and to nuts and seeds. Non-sweet fruits can usually be tolerated in limited amounts.

THE DOLOMITE NEEDS OF ALCOHOLICS

Generally, it's particularly important for a person with alcoholism to get extra amounts of magnesium, taken in the form of ½ tea-spoon of dolomite in water 3 or 4 times a day. Be sure to check the package of your dolomite to make certain it does not contain excess lead and other heavy metals.

THE GLUTAMINE NEEDS OF ALCOHOLICS

Glutamine, an amino acid, constitutes, along with glucose, the bulk of nourishment used by the nervous system. Glutamine can give an enormous lift, especially to people who are tired or depressed. Glutamine can be very simulating—even overstimulating—to some people. When I take a couple of capsules I feel as if I have been pumped full of speed.

Glutamine often offers special relief to the alcoholic. An alcoholic, like a sugar addict, gets more and more hooked as he becomes more and more malnourished and has more vitamin and mineral deficiencies. Once this damaged metabolism extends to the appetite control in the hypothalamus, he is even more likely to spree drink.

A Plant Extract

A research scientist at the University of Texas, William Shive, became interested in an unknown substance present in extracts of many plants and animals able to protect living cells from alcohol poisoning. The unknown substance proved to be glutamine, an amino acid present in many protein foods but frequently destroyed, i.e., turned into glutamic acid. In laboratory tests, bacteria were poisoned by adding alcohol to the medium in which they grew.

When glutamine was added to the medium, the bacteria could tolerate much higher doses of alcohol without suffering damage.

When glutamine is given to alcoholic rats and hamsters, they lose their desire for alcohol, or greatly diminish their intake. Although long-range experiments on humans have not yet been conducted, some spectacular results have been documented.

J. B. Trunell reported one case of an alcoholic who was given glutamine without his knowledge (glutamine is tasteless). Abruptly and for no apparent reason, the man gave up drinking, got a job, and in a follow-up two years later reported that he no longer had any desire to drink.

Although glutamine is not a miracle cure by itself, and does not necessarily help every alcoholic, I recommend that it be given a trial by anyone with a drinking problem.

Dosage

If you wish to try glutamine, begin with one 200-mg capsule three times a day, for a week, increasing to two capsules, three times a day the second week, as part of your experimental nutrition regimen. You might later try 500 mg, three times a day. Some people get better results if they take it on an empty stomach.

If you're trying to control a drinking problem, take 500 mg, 1 to 3 capsules, three times a day. If it speeds you up too much, take it one hour before meals but not at bedtime. If necessary, decrease the dose and build back up more slowly.

There have never been any reports of unfavorable side-effects from glutamine (other than overstimulation) so you can take as much as you feel you need, though I see little point in exceeding 3000 or 4000 mg three or four times a day. Remember that the deleterious effects of alcohol may be more acute than the effects of simple malnutrition, so be sure you give glutamine time to help you recoup the losses that your nervous system may have suffered already.

As with other recommendations in this book you should follow your doctor's advice. Be sure you are taking *glutamine, not glutamic acid,* which does not protect against alcohol poisoning. Many doctors and druggists confuse the two.

THE THIAMINE NEEDS OF ALCOHOLICS

Special attention should be given to thiamine since some patients with alcoholism have long experienced a thiamine deficiency and often require massive amounts over an indefinite period. I recommend 500 mg three times a day. Again, some people find thiamine quite stimulating. It should be taken in doses that are not overstimulating and, of course, thiamine should be taken in conjunction with the other B vitamins since all the B vitamins work together.

Although thiamine has a stimulating effect on many people, some people find it has a marked calming effect.

THE VITAMIN B_{12} NEEDS OF ALCOHOLICS

The next emphasis should be placed on vitamin B_{12}. Remember vitamin B_{12} comes in two forms: cyanocobalamin (vitamin B_{12}) and hydroxocobalamin (vitamin B_{12b}). Most alcoholics do better with large injections of vitamin B_{12b}.

Once after I gave a speech in L.A., a woman came up to me and said that she had been an alcoholic for many years. Then she began taking vitamin B_{12} injections, 1 cc daily. After starting the B_{12} injections, she gave up alcohol, she said, and became schizophrenic. She increased the B_{12} injections to 3 cc daily and became an "ordinary neurotic." Soon she went up to 5 cc daily of vitamin B_{12} and became normal. Only with this large amount of B_{12} could she maintain her feeling of well-being. After learning about (vitamin B_{12b}) from one of my papers, she switched to that form of vitamin B_{12} and discovered she could cut her dose in half.

I had been especially interested in vitamin B_{12} long before I heard her story, but never before had I considered giving more than 1 cc at a time. I began trying various doses of vitamin B_{12b} on my patients and found a few people who did a great deal better on massive amounts of B_{12b}.

People suffering from alcoholism would be well-advised to have therapeutic trials of vitamin B_{12b} injections, regardless of what their blood levels show.

Most drug stores carry the *cyanocobalamin* form. That *is not* the form you want. Don't let a druggist or a physician tell you it's the same thing as *hydroxocobalamin*. (See chapter 16 on vitamins to learn where your physician may order hydroxocobalamin. It's readily available and inexpensive.)

Special attention should also be paid to the folic acid needs of patients suffering from alcoholism. Almost everyone with this problem needs 1 to 3 mg of folic acid three times a day.

How Drugs and Chemicals Destroy Vitamin B_{12}

Vitamin B_{12} absorption is reduced by a number of common chemicals routinely taken by many people. One of my patients came to me in a quite depressed state and was found to be low in serum B_{12}. He responded very well to injections of vitamin B_{12b}, but required it about every five days to maintain his sense of well-being. Whenever he drinks even a modest amount of alcohol he finds that he begins to build up steam and requires B_{12b} injections at approximately three-day intervals to calm down.

The alcohol destroys his vitamin B_{12}.

As I pointed out in my paper on vitamin B_{12b}, a drug called Dilantin, commonly taken by individuals suffering from epilepsy, may also cause a marked depletion in the body's B_{12} stores.

Birth control pills lower vitamin B_{12} levels. Without doubt, many other medications also lower serum B_{12} levels. It is my strong feeling that all people—especially as they get older—should have periodic tests of their serum B_{12} levels and serum folate levels, since their reduction has profound effects on the central nervous system.

A vitamin B_{12} deficiency can even cause brain damage and paralysis. I once had a patient with vitamin B_{12} deficiency arrive in my office in a wheel chair.

If low levels of vitamin B_{12} continue long enough, pernicious anemia develops and the patient dies.

Most physicians mistakenly believe that low serum B_{12} levels and low folic acid levels produce anemia prior to causing damage to the central nervous system and producing emotional symptoms. *This is absolutely incorrect. I urge you not to let a physician tell you that tests of serum B_{12} levels and serum folic acid levels are unnecessary and only experimental. This may be his way of trying to dismiss a subject on which he has not read up.*

I have talked with physicians from all over the world who report that patients, particularly those in advancing years, ask them for

B_{12} injections because they make them feel better. Almost invariably, these physicians think that the patients are asking for what amounts to a placebo. Often the doctors give in against their inclination just to pacify the patients. These physicians very rarely check the serum B_{12} levels of such patients to find out whether a deficiency does, in fact, exist. Nor do they consider the distinct possibility that the patient may be suffering from a hereditary vitamin dependency disorder and needs the vitamin in amounts vastly in excess of the average.

THE ESSENTIAL FATTY ACID NEEDS OF ALCOHOLICS

As explained in the chapter on vitamins, free fatty acids are essential for good health. They can be absorbed in small amounts from various vegetable oils. The best and safest sources are cold-pressed safflower and linseed oil, and, of course, cod liver oil. Everyone not allergic to it should have at least one teaspoon a day of safflower oil, in salad dressing or by spoon. Also, please take one teaspoon daily of cod liver oil. Laboratory experiments have shown that alcoholic rats reduce their alcohol intake when they consume fats, especially unsaturated fatty acids.

THE CALCIUM PANTOTHENATE NEEDS OF ALCOHOLICS

This substance may be of special help to alcoholics. I suggest from one to five 218 mg capsules at bedtime, or dispersed throughout the day if you do not find them too relaxing.

FOLIC ACID

Since alcohol interferes with the metabolism of folic acid, it's also especially important that anyone using alcohol have extra amounts of the B vitamin called folic acid.

SEX AND ALCOHOLISM

The Freudian cliches of several generations ago about alcoholics being orally fixated or having subconscious homosexual tendencies are largely nonsense, psychiatric fairy tales that are being dismissed by the younger generation of scientists.

It's true that the use of alcohol can cause liver damage which will make the ratio of female to male sex hormones higher than it should be in men. Always, a person suffering from alcoholism should have his hormone levels studied. If found deficient in testosterone, men should consider getting injections of testosterone at one- or two-week intervals. I might add that thyroid hormone in the form of desiccated thyroid tablets is also sometimes indicated.

PROPER NUTRITION FOR ALCOHOLICS

Alcoholism is, among other things, a nutritional deficiency disease. Every alcoholic is malnourished. Most people believe that this is a symptom of the disease, but Dr. Roger Williams, among others, believed that malnutrition may be the cause of alcoholism. It may be that nutritional and metabolic imbalances are precisely the factors that make one person susceptible to alcohol addiction while another is not. At any rate, he believes that it is impossible to become an alcoholic if you are properly nourished.

Obviously, correcting nutritional deficiencies is one of the first steps an alcoholic must take in recovering from his disease. (Proper nutrition can also help to prevent the potential alcoholic from becoming addicted in the first place.)

A deranged appetite mechanism is one of the most dangerous symptoms of alcoholism. This usually becomes apparent when the alcoholic no longer desires food at all, and craves only the empty calories of alcohol. But along the way to alcoholism (and the disease usually takes many years to develop), other signals may appear. For instance, alcohol sometimes seems to stimulate the appetite. Alcoholism is often—perhaps always–associated with hypoglycemia (low blood sugar). Therefore an alcoholic may become addicted to both forms of empty calories, alcohol and sugar. He may binge on both alcohol and sweets. The result is an overweight alcoholic who is nevertheless starving to death—and all the while he assures you that he must not be alcoholic because everyone knows alcoholics don't eat.

To break this cycle, either to prevent true alcohol addiction or to recover from it, a high-protein, high-fat, low-carbohydrate, no-table-sugar diet is essential. Of course, any true alcoholic must give up drinking entirely if he is to recover. But at any stage of the disease, a high-protein, high-fat diet that acts to keep the blood sugar stable will also act to inhibit the craving for alcohol by preventing the wild swings in blood sugar levels that contribute to the rush he gets from drinking and the drop that makes him need another.

ALCOHOLICS AND PSYCHIATRISTS

Psychiatrists and alcoholics have not had much use for each other in the past. The psychiatrist was frustrated because he discovered that psychotherapy ("talk treatment") simply did not work, and the alcoholic was frustrated for the same reason. While addiction to alcohol may certainly have emotional consequences for the patient, both he and the psychiatrist must recognize that they are dealing with a basically physical, organic condition, not an "emotional" disease.

Anyone dealing with alcoholics—and this goes for the patient's family as well as his doctor—should be prepared for some early frustrations. We must remember that addictions, whether they be to alcohol, drugs, or chocolate cake, are among the strongest forces motivating humans. The behavioral strivings to satisfy addictions can be stronger than the sexual drive, stronger than the drive for food and water, and may even become stronger than the drive for life itself. If those without addictions will remember this, they can be more patient with alcoholics.

NOTE WELL

Allergic reactions give many people a strong urge to eat carbohydrates (especially sweets) and make them want an alcoholic drink. If a person suffering from alcoholism has been on the wagon for a time, then feels an urge to drink, the reason is usually an allergic reaction. Possibilities: a food to which you're allergic (a candy bar, for example), a cat, perfume, tobacco smoke, bug spray, hair spray, a new carpet—almost anything you can name.

The trick is to think about such triggers and try to spot and avoid them. Often a mate can see connections missed by the patient.

An allergic reaction to something in a drink is often one reason alcoholics cannot control their drinking. Commonly they are allergic to one of the grains in hard liquors. They have a cerebral allergic reaction and lose all reason and perspective. They won't allow you to make them stop drinking. They would let you kill them, but not stop them!

If a man loses his girlfriend, he may start drinking. Our society teaches that alcohol is a tranquilizer. He thinks the alcohol will put his pain to sleep.

In fact, alcohol is a poor tranquilizer. Even more than most tranquilizers and sedatives, alcohol leaves a person depressed and disorganized.

WHY RICHARD NIXON LOST THE WHITE HOUSE

I doubt whether Nixon was any more devious than many other politicians. We know from published accounts that Nixon greatly increased his alcohol intake as the Watergate problems nipped ever closer to his heels.

I suspect that Nixon reasoned—falsely!—that a few good drinks would allow him to escape the problem for a time, would leave him refreshed and better able to handle the stress and the maneuvering needed to escape his pursuers.

Instead of leaving him refreshed, the alcohol left him more depressed and interfered with his brain's integrative ability. He became disorganized, panicked and ran.

Nixon was basically a tough, bright, resourceful man. If Nixon had had no alcoholic drinks during the Watergate trouble, I suspect he would have solved his problem and survived intact.

CHAPTER TWENTY

LIGHT IS FOOD!

Since 1970 I've been writing about the importance of full-spectrum light for good health. I have been using it in my office and in my home, and have asked my patients to use it.

In 1985-1986 I was glad to see reports about the importance of full-spectrum light issued by the National Institutes of Health. Their study showed many people were much less depressed if they were exposed to full-spectrum light. It's unfortunate that the NIH was 15 years behind the times on this important facet of health. Hopefully they will continue to make more "new discoveries."

WHY LIGHT?

You're probably wondering why a chapter on light is included in a book on nutrition and health. The answer's very simple: Light, like food, comes to us from the outside—from the environment. Light, like food, is taken in by our bodies and utilized in a large variety of metabolic ways. Light, therefore, is a nutrient every bit as vital as the vitamins and minerals we take by mouth.

The sun gives us full-spectrum light, light waves that go all the way from infrared to ultraviolet. This is the type of light our bodies need.

The full-spectrum light provided by the sun (you also get reflected full-spectrum light on hazy days and in the shade) extends from

290 to 3500 nanometers. All of this spectrum is necessary for optimum health.

Architects designing homes and offices usually work only with the narrow band of light waves between 380 and 770 nanometers. Clearly, this is far from full-spectrum level, and contains no ultraviolet light at all.

The poor light that most of us get is just as inferior as the food we eat. Poor light injures both our bodies and our nerves just as much as a poor diet.

Before we began civilizing ourselves into semi-invalidism, we got much full-spectrum light: the kind of light that nature gives us in the form of sunlight.

Most people now spend their time indoors and are exposed to a small fraction of the spectrum. If your company is really "up-to-date" you're probably working under fluorescent light, which may be an industrial engineer's dream of perfection—but happens to be the most nutrient-deficient light of all. Even ordinary light bulbs are preferable to the total artificiality of the fluorescent environment.

LIGHT AND VITAMIN D

Probably the one function of light that most people are familiar with is its power to provide our vitamin D needs. This vitamin—also popularly known as the "sunshine vitamin"—regulates the use of calcium, magnesium, and phosphorus in our bodies. Because of its role in the proper formation and functioning of teeth and bones, it is especially important in infancy, childhood and old age. Lack of vitamin D during childhood can cause rickets, retarded growth, and tooth decay; among the elderly, vitamin D deficiency is partly responsible for a condition called osteoporosis (brittle bones), which causes major fractures, such as broken hips, as a result of relatively minor falls.

But what about vitamin D deficiency during the middle years?

Obviously, adequate vitamin D intake is one way of helping to forestall osteoporosis—an affliction that besets a large percentage of post-menopausal women, and causes no symptoms until it has progressed to a near-irreversible state.

Helping to form strong, healthy bones, is only one small benefit from full-spectrum light.

THE CASE OF SYBIL

Not long ago a patient visited me who had been to see 40 different doctors over a period of several years. Sybil told me that she was sure something was wrong with her chemistry, but that no one had been able to discover any defect during dozens of physical examinations and extensive laboratory workups. These had revealed only that she suffered from low blood sugar. The proper diet for this condition had ended her fainting spells, but had done nothing for her other complaints: muscle cramps, burning sensations throughout her body, fatigue, headaches, and the simple feeling of being sick.

After exhausting their diagnostic means, the other physicians had always come up with the same diagnosis: Her troubles were due to "tension."

This wastebasket (variously labeled "tension syndrome," "hypochondriasis," or "constitutional inferiority") is a favorite wastebasket into which many doctors dump illnesses they can't diagnose. Having read this far, you probably know that my favorite patients are those who have visited 40 doctors without getting relief.

The additional tests I performed on Sybil revealed a borderline vitamin B_{12} level and very low vitamin B_3 level. Once these deficiencies were corrected, she improved somewhat, but not enough.

I also found she had an allergy to peanuts, hydrocarbons, cats, dust, pasteurized (but not raw) milk, wool, and mold. Also, she sometimes reacted to beef.

As far as possible, we removed all the offending foods and environmental substances. Nonetheless, she continued to be tired and suffered from muscle cramps.

She was sent to one more internist, who hospitalized her, biopsied her muscle tissue, and performed a battery of special tests on it, all of which turned out negative. Once more she was given a diagnosis of "tension," and turned back over to me.

Psychiatric training gives a physician several advantages over other physicians. One of these advantages is that they spend more time with their patients, and they listen to what the patients tell them—at least the good ones do. When I see a patient for half an hour week after week, little bits and pieces of seemingly unrelated information tend to gradually form into a meaningful pattern. Luckily, that's what happened with Sybil.

One day she said, "You know, it's a funny thing: I can eat all the beef I want without any allergic reaction at home; but every time I eat it for lunch at work I get a reaction."

There was a time when I would have dismissed such a comment as nonsense coming from a self-absorbed neurotic. But I long ago decided that there is no such thing as a hypochrondriac. There are only patients whose ailments resist diagnosis by traditional techniques. Once a doctor comes to this conviction, that doctor is forced to consider every possible lead that patients supply.

We had already checked Sybil's place of employment—a very large international corporation. She dealt with computers which, when they were warm, gave off volatile particles of plastic. Amazingly, this very allergy-prone patient was not sensitive to plastics. We had also checked the carpeting and air filters in the room where she worked. (Some fiberglass air filters are charged with oil or contaminated with fungus. Also, some air purifiers use electrostatic screens which put ozone in the air.)

Sybil apparently had no allergies to anything at work.

What happened next is a good example of how an intelligent patient can help a doctor—if the doctor will only permit it. (Too many of us in the medical profession feel too insecure to accept information tendered by our patients, fearing that our prestige might suffer if we don't appear omniscient. This is a great mistake. An intelligent and observant patient can often be of tremendous help to the doctor, sometimes even when it comes to making a relatively simple diagnosis.)

Sybil happened to mention that she only reacted to beef when she ate it under fluorescent lights!

We tested her and found her observation to be valid. Investigation into the subject revealed that John Ott, a private citizen interested in light, and R. J. Wurtman, a professor at MIT, had written papers on the importance of full-spectrum light.

The fact that throughout our evolution our ancestors lived under full-spectrum light meant to me that there was every reason to believe man's biology still required it.

Investigation revealed it to be true. Many of my patients felt much better if they used full-spectrum light.

The more I read about the research done on photo stimulation, the more clearly I realized that the most common pollution in the civilized world is light pollution.

THE CASE AGAINST LIGHT POLLUTION

From the time life first began on this planet, our primitive ancestors spent their daylight hours in the open, searching for food. Is it surprising that human chemistry came to incorporate light stimulation, and that our body's chemistry evolved with the assumption that full-spectrum light stimulation would always be available? True, certain species have adapted to life without light—for instance, the blind white fish found in the waters of places like Mammoth Cave. Their ancestors have lived in a dark environment for so many generations that they lost their ability to see, since nature tends to eliminate useless organs and chemical reactions and to conserve tissue for utilization in a more productive way.

But we humans have neither retained our old habits nor adapted to our new ones. As recently as a hundred years ago, 75% of the people in this country still lived off the soil and spent most of their time outdoors, where they received full-spectrum light stimulation. Now, with the overwhelming population shift from rural areas to cities, most people spend very little time outdoors. They commonly receive from 95% to 100% of their light stimulation from artificial sources, which are almost always lacking in some part of the spectrum.

Suppose you went to some foreign country, found a very rare and valuable animal, and brought it back to live in captivity; would you not try to provide it with an environment as similar as possible to its indigenous one? If the animal had been living in a hot, dry desert under perpetual sunshine, would you choose a dark, swampy area as its new habitat and expect it to thrive?

Obviously not. You would provide surroundings as similar as possible to its native ones.

Through a process of selective breeding supervised by Mother Nature, animals become uniquely adapted to life in their particular environment—and we tamper with this adaptation at great peril.

Eventually, those species that cannot thrive in a given environment simply die off, do not leave offspring, and their genes and genotypes are eliminated from the stream of life. Yet we blindly take man—a mammal who (yes, I need to emphasize this again) evolved as a hunter of meat—and chain him to an office by day and an apartment at night, and expect him to thrive in these two little environmental cells, neither of which provides the full-spectrum light stimulation under which he evolved.

Ancient civilizations were well aware of the vital importance of full-spectrum light. This is documented by their preoccupation with the sun. The Aryans worshipped the sun. They called it "Dyas," a word from which the Latin "Deus" evolved. In Egypt, during the fifth dynasty (2750 B.C.), a sun-oriented theology became the state religion, and sun worship became a central facet of Egyptian life. Ancient Persia's most important god was Ormusza, the god of light; and very close to him in importance stood Mithras, the sun god. The Phoenicians worshipped the sun god Baal, as did the ancient Hebrews, for whom he was also the god of health. Babylon worshipped Marduk, another sun god, whose father was Ea, the supreme healer. In ancient Greece, many healing powers were attributed to Helius, the god of light and sun. Sol, another sun god, was one of the twelve deities of the ancient Romans' religion. In Pompeii, we find many frescoes depicting people stretched out on rooftops, sunbathing. Most Roman houses also had solaria for that purpose.

While these examples might make it appear that glorification of the sun was a characteristic of mediterranean peoples, the practice actually extended far into the chillier climes—through Central, Eastern, and Northern Europe, all the way to Britain's sun-worshipping Druids.

With the advent of Christianity, Western man's attitude toward the sun changed. Worship of the sun was condemned, its healing powers ignored, and sunlight itself became associated with paganism. It was to take more than fifteen hundred years before opinion began to change again. The French court physician Theodore Tronchin led the way with his advocacy of walks in the fresh air and sunlight. The impact of Rousseau's back-to-nature philosophy completed the job of restoring sunlight to the lives of the people.

In 1796, the University of Göttingen awarded a prize to J. C.

Ebermaier for his paper on the effects of sunlight on the human body. He was one of the first scientists to recognize that rickets was much more common in low-lying, dark, and damp places than in dry, light-exposed ones.

Sunlight became a popular therapeutic measure and remained so through the first thirty or forty years of this century.

Since then physicians have become more preoccupied with chemotherapy at the expense of full-spectrum light. Despite all chemical advances, in the depth of winter most people will feel an instinctive longing for the warm, sunlit spots of the world. Those who are unable to indulge their inner promptings begin to look for substitutes.

Sunlamps have become a popular item. Lately the industry has begun to manufacture full-spectrum lights as well, which makes this important source of stimulation available to all people all day long.

Further research is also underway. Two scientific societies have recently been established to further the study of light: the American Society for Photobiology and the Environmental Health and Light Research Institute. Both these organizations are actively attracting attention to the subject of full-spectrum light, and encouraging research in the field.

WHAT CORRECT LIGHTING CAN DO

Interestingly enough, much current research is being done by a nutritionist, Professor Richard J. Wurtman of the Massachusetts Institute of Technology. One of his experiments was conducted at a home for retired people, and it provides an especially noteworthy illustration of the importance of the subject.

The home's elderly residents were divided into two groups. One group was exposed to full-spectrum light in their day-to-day activities; the other group was not. At the end of the experimental period, the patients in the group exposed to a full-spectrum light stimulation showed a marked increase in the absorption of calcium from their food intake.

Calcium metabolism is an especially important problem in the elderly, because of their tendency to osteoporosis, causing loss of calcium in the bones making them brittle and highly susceptible to fracture. Osteoporosis is really a two-fold problem. Most of the elderly persons so afflicted tend to have endocrine deficiencies as well. Hormones needed to build strong bones are lacking, which compounds the adverse effect of their defective calcium metabolism, Also, physical activity—especially walking—is needed for bones to retain their calcium.

In another study, Wurtman placed male and female rats under two types of light for 20 days. One group was born and raised under the standard "cool-white" fluorescent light tubes. These widely used tubes are very deficient in ultraviolet radiation, and have abnormal ratios of red and yellow—an imbalance which causes a great deal of difficulty in people exposed to it.

The second group of animals grew up under "Vita-Lite," a full-spectrum fluorescent light made to mimic the rays of the sun as closely as possible.

Spending a forty-hour week under the Vita-Lite bulbs is roughly equivalent to staying outdoors at noon for thirty minutes once a week in the summer sunshine.

At the end of the experiment, the animals were sacrificed. Those raised under full-spectrum light uniformly had smaller spleens, larger hearts, and larger sexual glands than those raised under standard fluorescent light.

It is no accident that this particular study was sponsored by the National Aeronautics and Space Administration, an agency with great interest in light research. Proper light stimulation is obviously of paramount importance for living in the totally artificial environment of space travel, and it will become more important as we penetrate farther into space and stay away from our home planet for longer periods. For similar reasons, the navy already utilizes ultraviolet stimulation for its personnel on submarine duty. This stimulation has not only been found helpful in preventing infections, but also in maintaining the men's emotional health under the stressful, confined conditions of their tours of duty.

Full-spectrum light stimulation is also routinely used in many hospital nurseries for the prevention and treatment of hyperbilirubinemia, especially prevalent in premature infants. Hyperbilirubinemia is a metabolic disorder in which certain bile pigments in the body increase so that a baby's skin turns yellow (jaundiced).

ONLY FOOD IS MORE IMPORTANT THAN LIGHT

Dr. Wurtman declares flatly that light is the most important environmental input, after food, in controlling bodily functions. To substantiate this finding he points to the importance of a chemical substance called melatonin, which is regulated by the pineal gland—one of the glands directly stimulated by light. Melatonin circulates in the bloodstream after it is released from the pineal gland. Because it is especially soluble in lipid (fat) solvents, it can pass through the blood-brain barrier without any difficulty. This blood-brain barrier is a very selective gateway; only compounds useful to the brain are allowed to pass through it.

Once inside the brain, melatonin apparently causes an increase of serotonin—one of a group of substances known as neurotransmitters. A neurotransmitter is a chemical that allows one nerve cell to stimulate another nerve cell. Unlike the continuous electrical wiring in a house, the nerve cells of the brain and body are not directly connected with one another. They stimulate each other by releasing minute amounts of chemicals that travel from one nerve fiber to another and thereby activate it.

It is hardly possible to overemphasize the role played by these neurotransmissions in influencing mood and behavior.

In the February 12, 1970, issue of the *New England Journal of Medicine*, Drs. R. J. Wurtman and Robert M. Neer discussed the effects of light stimulation and its two main avenues of influence on the body. The first is the direct effect due to photochemical stimulation of the molecules in the skin, or the tissues immediately beneath the skin; the second is the indirect effect obtained via the light-sensitive cells in the eyes.

The most important known effects of direct light stimulation of the skin are the increase of calcium absorption from the intestines, the decrease in circulating bile pigments, and the well-known tanning effect of ultraviolet light. In all probability, many more biological effects are brought about by such skin stimulation; we just are not yet aware of them. More germane, perhaps, is the effect of light stimulation through the eyes, which seems to be primarily endocrine in nature. Full-spectrum light strikes the retina of the eye and stimulates the optic nerve, which in turn sends out impulses to the hypothalamus—a part of the brain that exercises a profound effect on our emotions. From there, stimulation travels down to the pituitary gland, also called the "master gland," because it regulates the secretions of all other endocrine glands. Such stimulation of the pituitary causes an increase in the size of the sexual and other glands in mammals.

A City Without Sun

The influence light has on emotions was illustrated in an article entitled "The Murky Time," published in the January 1, 1973, issue of *Time* Magazine.

The article tells about the 10,000 people who live in the town of Tromsø, 650 miles north of Oslo, Norway, and 200 miles into the Arctic Circle. The people in Tromsø spend two months of the year—from November 25 to January 21—without any sunlight. During this period, which they call Morketiden (Time of Darkness), the mentally unstable people in the population become acutely disturbed. Even normally well-adjusted people grow tense, restless, vaguely fearful, and tend to be preoccupied with thoughts of death and suicide.

Even though everything is done to minimize the sense of darkness—lamps on the streets and in gardens burn twenty-four hours a day—the county sheriff of Tromsø, Knut Kruse, admits that the townspeople behave very differently during the sunless winter months.

They spend their time moodily philosophizing about life and tend to become too lackadaisical to pull themselves together for constructive pursuits.

Psychiatrist Harold Reppesgaard of Asgard Mental Hospital agrees. The entire town changes to a slower pace, he says. People are constantly tired; their powers of concentration are poor; their work efficiency is reduced.

Some of the citizenry blame lack of proper sleep for their symptoms. But an Oslo physiologist who has researched the emotional problems associated with the annual Tromsø blackout has concluded that it's the prolonged absence of light that brings out the people's worst behavior and accounts for the sudden increase in depression, envy, jealousy, suspicion, egotism, and just plain irritability.

Personally, I think most scientists knowledgeable about the subject would agree that the emotional upheavals are more likely to be caused by a lack of full-spectrum light, not by a lack of sleep.

Insomnia is merely another symptom caused by lack of full-spectrum light.

During the period of Morketiden the citizens of Tromsø spend much more money on sleeping pills, pep pills, and tranquilizers than at any other time of the year. Their use of hard drugs also increases sharply. People have more accidents and more psychosomatic illnesses. Despite their heightened irritability, they desperately need to be with each other. Restaurants, dance halls, and concerts are especially crowded during this time.

What these people want most of all is to escape their sunless world, if only for the briefest vacation in some sunny southern spot. Business firms encourage such vacations as a way of maintaining their workers' stability and efficiency.

The sun's return to Tromsø is marked by a special holiday called Soidag (Sun Day). On that day, schools and offices are closed. People stream out in the streets to watch the sun rise, shouting and clapping each other on the back ecstatically happy in the knowledge that life will at last return to normal.

What more graphic picture could be drawn to document the effects of proper light stimulation?

Explorers at the end of long polar expeditions—during which they have little full-spectrum light—return to civilization suffering from depression, lower sexual drive, lower blood sugar levels, and lower blood pressure.

It would seem that man, despite his almost infinite capacity for adjustment to his environment, has pretty much failed to adjust to a life without full-spectrum light.

Many other observations confirm this. In one radio station, for example, ordinary fluorescent lights were installed as part of a modernization program. Despite the scientifically engineered surroundings, people who worked there soon turned grumpy, began complaining of minor aches and pains, and expressed increasing dissatisfaction with their companions and their working conditions. They did not specifically mention lighting as one of their complaints, and almost certainly they were not aware of its bad effect.

As interpersonal relationships continued to deteriorate, and work efficiency declined, experts were consulted. As a result, full-spectrum light was installed.

Almost at once the former spirit of camaraderie returned and employees settled down to working efficiently together once more.

Such anecdotal evidence is interesting and, in the aggregate, highly meaningful. But to date, most of our hard knowledge concerning full-spectrum light stimulation still comes from research on laboratory animals, just as our knowledge of cancer and cardiovascular disorders continues to expand through laboratory experimentation.

I think it is of great interest that varying light sources can significantly affect the very lifespan of mice. A research strain of mice known as C3H routinely develops tumors at a certain age.

The emergence of these tumors has been greatly postponed by exposing these animals to full-spectrum light.

Dr. John Ott has discovered that rats kept under ordinary fluorescent lights develop myocarditis, an inflammation of the heart muscle; whereas rats kept under full-spectrum light do not develop this disease.

Not all animal research is necessarily directly applicable to humans; but it would seem reasonable to conclude from these experiments that light simulation has profound biological effects on living creatures, whether they be plants or animals.

We have every reason to believe that mankind's biology is similarly affected.

What Happens When Children are Deprived of Sunlight?

W. O. Loomis, M.D., professor of biochemistry at Brandeis University, is convinced that humans lack adequate vitamin D because they do not receive full-spectrum light stimulation. Thus, he says, the deficiency disease known as rickets is in effect the first air pollution disease, because air pollution in the cities cuts down sunlight. He also points out that the disease is far more prevalent in the northern regions of the world than in the southern ones. In New Haven, Connecticut, for example, 80% of the children between the ages of two and three years show clinical evidence of rickets; in Puerto Rico, only 12% of children in this age group show such signs.

Another interesting study was conducted by Harry S. Hutchinson of Bombay, India, who reports marked differences in the incidence of rickets among Mohammedans, upper-class Hindus, and lower-class Hindus.

Among the rich, well-fed Mohammedans, the incidence of rickets in those under twenty was 70%—a fact which Hutchinson attributes to the well-to-do Muslims' custom of remaining indoors and keeping their children constantly indoors. Among upper-class Hindus, the children are allowed outside more often; in this group, the incidence of rickets among people under the age of twenty was only 20%.

Among the lower-class Hindus almost no evidence of rickets was found, despite their very poor diet; presumably, both children and adults spend a great deal of time outdoors.

In 1973 I attended a meeting in Florida devoted to scholarly papers on light stimulation and its relation to the biological system.

Eighty-seven universities were represented at the meeting, in addition to scientists from the research departments of major corporations such as General Electric.

During a film presentation, we saw a series on hyperactive children. In the first part, the children were filmed during a routine hour in their classroom. Accustomed as I am to the vagaries of unstable people, I felt that these children were enough to make a saint hit them over the head with a Bible. They were totally incapable of paying any attention to the work at hand; they twisted about in their seats like contortionists, kicked each other and the furniture, climbed on top of the desks and crawled under them, raced around the classroom, and in general, behaved in the manner typical of the hyperactive-child syndrome. Their short attention span and absolute inability to remain in one position long enough to carry out even the simplest task demonstrates this.

At the time the movie was shot, the classroom was lighted with standard fluorescent tubes.

These fluorescents tubes were then replaced by full-spectrum tubes.

After the same children were exposed to the full-spectrum lights for several months, their activities were again filmed. The differences were startling. No longer were they climbing all over the furniture and making grotesque bodily contortions. Instead of charging about like wild animals, they now moved like normal children. They were markedly less self-centered, more willing and able to interact with each other in a meaningful way. They were also able to sit still in their chairs and attend to the work before them.

It might be interesting to see what would happen to a class full of normal children after a few months' exposure to full-spectrum light. I suspect that their behavior as well as their grades would improve. In fact, a recent study of students, sponsored by the Center for Improvement of Undergraduate Education of Cornell University, seems to confirm it. The study was conducted by James B. Maas, Jill K. Jason, and Douglas A. Kleiber, who report that objective measurements revealed less fatigue and better visual acuity in students studying under full-spectrum rather than the traditional cool-white fluorescent lights.

Soviet Research Shows . . .

The Soviet Union had great interest in preventive medicine, especially in pediatrics. In one study, M. A. Zamkov, E. I. Krivitskaya and A. I. Hertsen of the Pediological Institute in Leningrad reported on the favorable effects of ultraviolet radiation on children. In an experiment lasting from October, 1963, through March, 1964, two groups of children were housed in their school under similar conditions; the difference was that one group worked under weak overhead ultraviolet radiation and the other group under standard fluorescent lights.

The students who had received ultraviolet radiation showed a shorter reaction time to light and sound, which meant that their nervous systems were working more efficiently than those children who had not received ultraviolet stimulation. They showed less eyestrain and a generally increased working capacity, resulting in significant improvement in their academic standing as compared to the group exposed to standard fluorescent light.

On the basis of these results, the authors advocated ultraviolet radiation for all schoolchildren—a conclusion that certainly sounds reasonable to me, except that I would extend it to the entire population.

There have also been a number of reports from the Soviet Union concerning the beneficial effects of ultraviolet light on arteriosclerosis and arthritis. Ultraviolet's effect of reducing cholesterol levels has been known for some time. In this way it offers protection for people prone to high blood pressure, coronary disease, and hardening of the arteries of the brain—sometimes the cause of emotional disorders associated with senility.

In another Soviet study, N. M. Dantsig and his associates established that profound physiological changes occur in human beings deprived of full-spectrum light for long periods. The same authors also found ultraviolet radiation to be of marked benefit to agricultural animals, with the ideal doses of radiation varying according to the species and the age of the animals. The action of ultraviolet radiation stimulates enzyme reactions and metabolism, increases the activity of the entire endocrine system, and increases immunological responses.

This last benefit is probably largely responsible for the overall improved health of creatures exposed to ultraviolet radiation. They are less likely to fall victim to disease, and are less prone to suffer from allergies. Of course, the heightened, immunological response is not the whole answer, the endocrine system also affects both susceptibility to infection and to allergic reactions.

But isn't Ultraviolet Light Dangerous?

I know, I know. Too much ultraviolet can be harmful. It's like water: too little and you die, too much and you die. In our world of biology, to thrive we need things more or less just so.

You have surely heard that too much ultraviolet light can cause premature aging of the skin and skin cancer, which is true, especially in fair-skinned individuals.

If I had any of the following disorders, I would consult my dermatologist before installing full-spectrum lights:

1. Keratoses (dry, precancerous lesions on the skin, which should be removed).

2. Leukoplakia (precancerous lesions on the lip or other mucous membrane, which should also be removed).

3. Porphyria (a rare biochemical disorder characterized by abdominal pain and mental symptoms).

4. On medications (like the major tranquilizer, Thorazine).

It is my personal opinion that skin cancer would be greatly reduced, or perhaps nearly eliminated, if they ate a proper diet and took the correct nutritional supplement, especially vitamins A and C, plus beta-carotene, calcium, magnesium, zinc, selenium, and vitamin E, as well as unsaturated fats.

INTERESTING FACTS

Apparently quite unrelated facts add further weight to the increasing evidence about the importance of light stimulation:
- Eskimo women during the long Arctic night do not menstruate and are infertile.
- Children in tropical zones mature earlier sexually than do those in more northern latitudes.
- Apples grown under glass, which cuts out ultraviolet radiation, never ripen.
- Chinchillas raised under blue colored light produce 85% female offspring.
- Under artificial light, many tropical fish die; others produce offspring with a 20% rate of birth defects.
- Mice kept under pink light stimulation for up to twelve hours a day eventually lose their tails.

   (I once mentioned this last bit of information during an address before the Society of Clinical Ecology in Albuquerque, New Mexico. At the time of my lecture, the participants at the meeting had been indoors for approximately three days, receiving only the usual inadequate light stimulation. I suggested that the assembled physicians might want to check their posterior anatomy upon returning to their rooms. The next day I found an impressive array of my colleagues sunbathing during the lunch recess. I've always wondered what their mirrors revealed.)
- Employees of the Well of the Sea, a well-known Chicago restaurant located in the Sherman Hotel, were found to have significantly lower rates of illness and absenteeism than people working in other parts of the hotel. Ultraviolet lights, "black lights" are used to activate fluorescent decorations.

The Light of My Life

Since learning about the importance of full-spectrum light, I've put it to good use. This newly acquired knowledge has not magically healed all the emotionally ill people who consult me, but using full-spectrum light along with vitamins and minerals and diet has helped many of my patients reach a higher level of improvement.

I practice what I preach. I've installed Vita-Lites in my office and home. I started out gingerly with only one or two such lights in the rooms where I spent most of my time. Soon I became quite fond of this type of illumination, and began to find other types of light annoying. I ended by installing Vita-Lites everywhere. I simply no longer wished to be exposed to ordinary lights.

I've had my glasses changed to an optical glass that transmits the full-spectrum light, including ultraviolet light.

The reflected light from the written page is a major source of stimulation to the retina of the eye. Since full-spectrum light stimulation is so important, it is mandatory to wear reading glasses made of full-spectrum (ultraviolet-transmitting) material.

If you wear glasses at all times you should be especially interested in obtaining these full-spectrum lenses. They are also available in dark shades (gray), which reduce the total amount of light stimulation but do not distort the spectrum. The net effect is that you still receive full-spectrum light stimulation, even though the light passes through a dark lens. Nowadays, I wince when I walk down the street and see people wearing ordinary dark glasses, knowing to what an extent they are distorting the amount of light stimulation they receive, thereby almost certainly impairing their health.

My apartment has been equipped with ultraviolet-transmitting plastic windows (quarter-inch) so I get the full-spectrum light blocked out by ordinary window glass. An added benefit is the great reduction of noise entering the office from outside.

Has full-spectrum light improved my life?

With full-spectrum light I feel better and get more work done. I forget how fond I've grown of full-spectrum light until I go to a medical meeting and spend a morning in ordinary indoor light. I can hardly wait for the noon break so I can get outside and enjoy some full-spectrum light.

CHAPTER TWENTY-ONE

GOOD FOOD,
GOOD SEX

At the turn of the century, Sigmund Freud concluded that good sexual adjustment was important for mental health. In fact, he went further and hypothesized that emotional illnesses were essentially sexual in origin. For nearly half a century this idea seized and held the imagination of the western world, including the psychiatric profession. It's surprising that Freud should attach such importance to sex. He was a virgin until thirty and became impotent in his early forties, which must have greatly contributed to his intellectual preoccupation with sex.

I often find that seriously disturbed patients report that their sex lives are unsatisfactory. But it is a great mistake, in my opinion, to attribute their emotional illnesses to poor sexual adjustment. I find they usually have unsatisfactory sex lives for the same reason they are emotionally disturbed. When we correct the biological defects that are causing their emotional problems, their emotional condition improves and their sex lives usually become satisfactory. In my view, you improve your sex life by improving your emotional health; not the other way around. Had Freud adjusted his vitamins and diet properly, very likely he would have eliminated his depression, his phobias, his hypochondriacal complaints—and his sexual disorder.

269

IS MORE SEX BETTER SEX?

Many people equate more sex with better sex. That is like saying that a five-pound steak is better than a one-pound steak, that a Pontiac is better than a Porsche. A patient who saw me the other day is a prostitute and has intercourse more than a hundred times a week, yet she's completely frigid and does not enjoy sex at all.

Another of my patients, a vigorous seventy-eight-year-old man, jets to Chicago once a month to visit his girlfriend. When he returns to New York and tells me of the sexual encounters there, his face dissolves into a saintly expression of glory as if speaking of a miracle. Sex may not come to him as frequently as in the old days, but it is beautiful and endearing when it does.

When we are happy and secure, we may not feel as much need for sex as when we are tense and frightened. It may be the same way with money. The insecure man may be forever trying to make another dollar to put with all his other dollars in the hope he will somehow find security through wealth. He desperately runs from business deal to business deal and stores away his money, but no amount of savings will produce the inner peace he seeks.

Thus a restless man may have a great need for sex and may indulge in it frequently, but it may not give him satisfaction. Indeed, each encounter may leave him less satisfied than the one before. This man frequently uses sex in an attempt to relax. We all know that orgasms tend to be followed by a period of relaxation. He, or a woman like him, may use sex the last thing at night in an attempt to fall asleep.

Sex may have nothing to do with love for a person, and may not even have anything to do with sex itself. Rather, it becomes a mechanism by which he tries to reduce tensions. Such a person does not derive great satisfaction and pleasure from the act.

So before you answer the question, "How good is my sex life," be sure to ask yourself what you mean by good sex. Do you mean a wonderful experience that leaves you feeling fulfilled? Or are you talking about relieving a nervous itch?

Poorly nourished people tend to go through periods of tension when they have more sex than well-nourished people—but don't have more enjoyment.

To carry this observation to its logical conclusion, let me point out that populations explode in parts of the world where malnutrition and starvation are chronic problems. Examine the birth statistics of the poorer South American countries and you will discover that their populations are rising at a staggering rate. Study the population figures for a country such as India, where semi-starvation stalks the whole nation, and you will discover the birth rate to be enormous when compared with that of such stable and relatively well-fed countries as Denmark and Sweden.

Mother Nature Tells Us Why

Apparently the increased sex drive among the semi-starved and poorly nourished is an attempt on nature's part to preserve the species. Nature seems to know when a person weakens. When premature death stalks the land, sex flourishes. Nature wants an individual to reproduce before fading away, and it encourages a frenzy of sexual activities, never mind whether there will be enough food to feed the offspring. Some of them will probably live to carry on; certainly none will live if there is no sex, no new life.

DEATH STIMULATES SEX

Men and women have increased sexual drives in their forties. Again, we see nature pushing them for sexual activity and reproduction before sexual death overtakes them. By "sexual death" I refer to the inability of women to have children after the menopause and to the waning sexual performances of many (though by no means all) men in their fifties and in later life.

We all know that wartime stirs up sexual activities. Soldiers ready to go overseas or into battle experience a strong need for sexual relations and women tend to be particularly receptive to men in uniform. Again, this is sex being prodded to the foreground by death.

One of the most interesting stories I heard from physicians who served overseas during World War II was told to me by a surgeon who was operating in a tent not far from the front lines. Returning casualties were divided into two groups. The first group consisted of soldiers with not very serious wounds. It was possible to save them. The second group were so badly injured that it was unlikely that surgery would save their lives. The largest number of patients could be saved by first treating those who had a good possibility of living.

The surgeon who told me this story was walking past the second group, the men so badly injured that there was little hope of saving them. As the surgeon walked by, accompanied by his operating room nurse, one of these nearly-dead men reached out, grabbed the nurse's leg, and ran his hand up toward a part of her anatomy that interested him very much.

"Let's take that soldier next," the surgeon said. If there was that much will to live, then he wanted to give the man every chance. In fact, what the surgeon saw was a dying man's natural reaction to sexual stimulation.

Physicians who have spent years of apprenticeship as interns and residents in hospitals know that it is the rule for people to die with their hands clutching their genitalia, a last desperate expression of their sexual drive as they fade away.

Such activation of sex by the threat of extinction happens throughout the animal and even in the plant kingdom. For example, we know that when grass is poorly nourished it goes to seed, puts its last strength into the formation of seeds that can produce new life and thence preserve the species.

It's hardly necessary to add that if malnutrition goes beyond a certain point, sexual activity ceases. Sex increases only through the gray band that extends from good nutrition to true starvation. After true starvation begins, all sexual interest quickly wanes. By starvation, I mean a total lack not only of calorie intake but a prolonged lack of adequate vitamins and minerals.

If frequency of sexual activity is your goal, and each one of us must decide for ourselves exactly what our goals are, then the remainder of this chapter should give you some new ideas for increasing the frequency of your sexual encounters.

The first obvious conclusion from these remarks is that, to have frequent sex, it is best to be malnourished. I don't advocate that road since being malnourished is not desirable for your general health. If you are malnourished you will be more susceptible to infections such as the common cold, pneumonia and tuberculosis. It is quite possible that malnutrition will increase your chances of getting other diseases such as AIDS.

To be obsessed with sex is not a sign of good health, physical or mental. Quite the contrary. This is true for societies as well as individuals. Some people have decried the similarity between the decadence of ancient Rome and the peep shows and porno movies in Times Square, and in one way, they are correct. A society responds to the threat of disintegration, just as an individual does. Never have the American people been under more biochemical stress from inadequate diets, air and noise pollution, and toxic and allergenic substances in their food and water—and never have Americans been so obsessed with sex.

YOUR PRESCRIPTION FOR THE GOOD LIFE

Many people who feel less than their best, hope to find some magic way to improve their sex lives, going along with the old Freudian belief that their other problems will fade away if they can only achieve good sex. You should know by now that such is not true. There is no magic cure for an ailing sex life, and if there were, it would not cure all your misery. To have a truly fulfilling sex life, it is necessary to be healthy.

The most responsible advice I can give you: Apply what you have already learned in this book about achieving your own best nutritional program. Once you have eliminated depression, fatigue, anxiety and other emotional symptoms caused by deficiencies, allergies and poor diet, your energy and zest for living will increase—and so will your sex life.

If you are chronically toxic from eating the wrong foods and not having proper vitamins and minerals, eventually your sex life will suffer.

Many people have experienced a hangover from drinking too much alcohol. A hangover is nothing but a toxic state. Did you ever see anyone with a hangover who had great sex while in that state?

Many people are toxic from the foods they eat and from lack of proper supplements. It's as if their lives were spent struggling through one long hangover.

NUTRITION AND POTENCY

You hear talk about vitamin E as a cure for impotence. It has come to be known as the sex vitamin, probably because it was found to prevent spontaneous abortions in many animals. While the claims are almost surely exaggerated, I think it important that anyone with an impotence problem pay attention to vitamin E. It often helps to increase energy levels, and thus is a boon whether or not you are impotent or frigid.

Vitamin E probably produces this effect because it helps to detoxify environmental pollutions that slow us down. It also supplies more oxygen to each cell, so that they burn their metabolic fuels more efficiently.

Some patients swear by vitamin E—1,500 to 3,000 units taken on an empty stomach one hour before having sex. I remember a traveling salesman who was a patient of mine. This man was something of an authority on sex. He seemed to have a woman waiting for him in every small town he visited. As he made his rounds and did his thing, he popped vitamin E capsules.

Remember that a rare person has an elevated blood pressure from this vitamin.

I have had a number of patients tell me that they felt stimulated when taking 200 mcg selenium tablets once a day. The effect was felt only after they had been taking selenium for a week or more. As a test they tried leaving off selenium for a week or more, then going back to it, then stopping and starting it again. The sexual stimulation they felt from it was quite definite. Certainly suggestion had nothing to do with it because I had given each of them other supplements before and I personally had no knowledge that selenium might improve their sex lives.

I especially remember one man in his mid-seventies. When I started him on selenium—as a preventative against cancer—he shyly asked me if selenium might be changing his sexual habits. It seemed that he had come to desire intercourse three or four times a day. A single man, he remarked that it was ironic that a man started and ended his sex life with masturbation.

I told him that I was sure there was a rich widow in Palm Beach who would be delighted to meet him and support him in a princely fashion.

Fatigue and depression are the great enemies of sexual desire and performance. Therefore, the nutritional factors that most often counteract depression are the ones most likely to help a sexual problem. These are thiamine and niacin, which often give people a lift, and vitamin C, which is also a detoxifying agent and will help you to deal with pollutants and allergens. For a lift you might also include a trial on glutamine.

How Sexual Wishes Come True

I should point out that while none of these substances alone can cure impotence, your confidence in their value could have a positive effect.

Let me tell you an anecdote about the effect of belief on sexual performance. I once had a patient, a college student who was quite religious but was able to reconcile sex with his girlfriend with his fundamentalist religion. Once when her period was late, he was certain that she was pregnant. But he was not able to marry her. His father had told him that he would cut off the allowance if he married while in college.

When the young man learned that his girlfriend's period was late, he knelt down and prayed to God for the young lady not to be pregnant. If God would only not let the woman be pregnant, he would never have intercourse again. He pointed out to God that he was aware that he had offended Him with his sexual behavior, but that he was now a new person and had seen the light. He requested that God reciprocate by having his girlfriend menstruate.

A week later, the girlfriend did get her period. As you might guess, the boy began to have second thoughts about his vow of chastity. Unhappily, the next time he visited his girlfriend and wanted to have intercourse, he discovered that he was completely impotent—and remained so for over a year!

Sex is between the ears as well as between the legs.

What About Aphrodisiacs?

In ancient Egypt radishes were touted as a sexually stimulating food. The Romans sang the praises of onions. The French believe that eating frog's legs makes them passionate. Catherine de' Medici swore by artichokes. Others praise mushrooms, carrots, spinach, turnips, celery, and even asparagus. Caviar and oysters have their advocates, and a great authority on love, Casanova, and the ribald physician Rabelias both reported good results from truffles.

I cannot attribute aphrodisiacal qualities to any of these foods, but it might be a pleasant pastime for you to try them. Conceivably, your findings just possibly might agree with those of Casanova and Catherine de' Medici.

Here are my personal experiences.

Once Susan Hecht, my office assistant, was testing a woman for an allergy to tomatoes. During the test, the patient came over and whispered in her ear.

"What are you testing me for?" she asked.

Susan explained that she could not tell her until after the test was ended. When the testing session ended, the patient asked the same question.

"Do tomatoes ever make people passionate?" the patient asked after learning what she was being tested for.

"Why do you ask?" Susan wanted to know.

"I feel like I could make love for six hours straight," the woman said and added, "Now I know why I always let men go home with me after they take me to an Italian restaurant!"

We've had other patients report the same feeling from tomatoes, diet cola, celery, and other foods.

It's my personal impression that in some people sexual stimulation can be one manifestation of an allergic reaction. I suspect that's why so many different foods are reported to be aphrodisiacs. Different people are allergic to different foods.

Perfumes are often used as sexual stimulants. I suspect scientific studies would show that they are effective. People are frequently allergic to perfumes.

If the allergic reaction to perfume happened to be depression, then certainly perfume would be counterproductive. But if a perfume-sensitive individual happened to feel slightly confused or excited by an odor, or happened to have sexual excitement as an allergic reaction, then it's quite possible that sexual appetites would be increased.

In any case, most people get the cue that perfume means that the wearer is trying to appear sexually attractive. Effort and enthusiasm alone are certainly turn-ons. The ugly man who courts energetically often wins over the handsome man who pouts in the corner.

Words and stories whispered during the sex act can be an aphrodisiac.

Let me reemphasize: Whatever anyone believes will increase sexual appetites is likely to do so. If a woman wears a perfume in which she has absolute faith, she will certainly be more bewitching and she herself will be turned on from her efforts and her faith in the new product.

If a man swallows 1200 units of vitamin E before undressing and believes with all his heart and soul that the vitamin E is going to make him more potent, then it almost surely will.

CHAPTER TWENTY-TWO

DON'T LET AGE DESTROY YOUR MIND

Although aging is an invariably fatal condition that pursues us all, its complications—the mental disorders of senility—can be dealt with far more readily than most people realize.

So far, medicine's frequently applauded success in prolonging man's average lifespan is largely an illusion. We have greatly reduced the rate of infant mortality, which makes the statistics for average life expectancy look good. We have also decreased early deaths from infectious diseases so that the second largest killer of young adults, after accidents, is suicide.

That suicide should be a major cause of death poignantly illustrates that, while medical science has improved our chances of living, it has—by feeding every generation more and more junk food—done little to improve the quality of those extra years.

In 1850, the average lifespan was 38.7 years. In 1900 it was 49.2 and now that figure has been extended by twenty-plus additional years. Unfortunately, the lifespan past the age of 40 is almost what it was 300 years ago. Indeed, as our civilization continues to mechanize the food industry, resulting in the removal of more and more essential elements from the diet and the addition of chemicals, the sum total of man's modern ecology may already have caused a shortening of our potential life span all over again.

Even if our leading killers—cancer, heart and circulatory disease, kidney and respiratory disease—were all eliminated, we wouldn't

278

live much longer unless we discovered some way to hold back aging.

THE PRICE FOR SEX IS HIGHER THAN YOU REALIZE

In nature, death is not necessarily an inevitable part of life. A single-celled creature, like an amoeba, reproduces by subdividing. One cell simply splits into two halves, creating two living creatures where there had been one. Such cells have no particular prepro-grammed lifespan and can theoretically subdivide indefinitely, except when environmental circumstances cause their demise.

Only when such cells gather together, each specializing in a particular function, and form a more complex animal, does the prospect of death enter into the process of life.

Man, of course, is a collection of cells living together in an enormously complex symbiosis which arrived at the present advanced state through a series of adaptive evolutionary modifications that were a technical marvel.

This extraordinary creature, however, is in some ways not as successful as the amoeba. Unlike the amoeba, man hasn't learned how not to die.

SEXUAL AND ASEXUAL REPRODUCTION

The one-celled animal's splitting in two is known as asexual reproduction.

Sexual reproduction through mating is reserved for complex animals. Only when we have sexual reproduction do we have death. Death is the price we pay for sex. I leave it to you to decide whether the trade was worthwhile. In any case, I'm afraid you and I have little say about the matter.

Young people have only a vague conception of death, which is one reason why they are so often quick to rush into dangerous, even life-threatening situations. Once in our twenties, we tend to take the world about us a bit more seriously and look at it more realistically. Still, thoughts of death are far away. Not until the thirties do we begin to lose our omnipotent delusions of youth.

The thirties is the decade that brings the knowledge that few will become Nobel prize-winners, movie stars, or president. Vague notions of physical decay and death begin to stir in us occasionally when we look in the mirror and view our midriffs and thinning hair.

In the forties, many people experience a relative lessening of zest for life. Sexual interest may wane, stairs may become a bit more difficult. Reflections concerning old age, the loss of mental faculties, and the reality of ultimate death come to occupy a more prominent place in our thinking. These reflections proliferate with increasing momentum during our fifties, sixties, and seventies.

Age Thirty: The Turning Point

Archaeologists tell us that 50,000 years ago man was a short-lived mammal. Only five percent of primitive men lived past the age of 30, and only one percent past 45.

Was man designed to die at about age 30? Quite possibly. Old age even for us begins at that time. That may seem like a very startling statement today, but if you will contemplate it for a moment, perhaps you will agree. We know, for example, that the most taxing sports are dominated by young people. Teenage girls are often at the peak of their achievement in speed swimming contests. Boxers are at their best during their twenties, as are long distance runners. This is why, at about age 30, the hope that helped carry us forward during difficult times in our teens and twenties often begins to fade. Experience, as well as the subconscious knowledge of our waning powers, cause an onset of half-cynical, half-wistful resignation.

If you contemplate your life, chances are that you can detect a sort of natural turning point around the age of 30. Carl Gustav Jung, the noted Swiss psychiatrist, wrote about the "two halves" of life, and believed firmly that the problems of the first part (ending at about 35) of life and those of the latter part were totally different, and had to be approached psychotherapeutically in entirely different ways.

WHY CHEMISTRY IS CRUCIAL

I agree with the end result of Jung's findings, though not with his theoretical underpinnings. Jung was, of course, a psychoanalyst, and remained one even after his break with Freud. His explanations of the emotional turmoil of the second half of life were therefore strictly psychoanalytic. Once I might have shared that view, but today I feel very differently. During the decades I have spent trying to help emotionally ill people, I have come to a belief that psychological problems are largely chemical problems.

I have—and sometimes still do—use psychological as well as chemical and nutritional techniques to treat emotionally disturbed people. The fact is, however, that I have been able to help people achieve much higher levels of performance and happiness by using nutritional approaches. Once we normalize the chemistry of the central nervous system, problems that appeared to be psychological have a habit of melting away. Patients become emotionally stronger once we correct their chemistry. Then they gain the strength needed to deal with the slings and arrows of outrageous fortune that come to all of us.

Gradually the chemical approach to emotional illness is taking over the field of psychiatry. Even conventional psychiatrists are moving away from psychoanalysis. The analysts—like the dinosaurs—have had their day. Time was when psychoanalysts had waiting lists of people anxious to be seen five times a week for five years or more. Today these analysts spend a great percentage of their time doing practical, supportive—"eclectic"—psychotherapy. Often they come down from their ivory towers and bow to biology by prescribing tranquilizers and antidepressants. Freud himself anticipated this state of affairs when he wrote: "We must recollect that all our provisional ideas in psychology will some day be based on organic structure. This makes it probable that special substances and special chemical processes control the operation.

Since the advent of the major antipsychotic medications of the mid-1950's, we have been rapidly approaching the era of psychochemistry predicted by Freud. And since chemistry for all living creatures involves nutrition, it is particularly appropriate to pay more attention to nourishment in all its forms. Unless the cells of the body are properly nourished, they cannot achieve or maintain their full efficiency.

As I discussed earlier, all chemical reactions in the body depend on enzyme systems to carry out their work. These enzyme systems are very efficient in youth, but gradually, as part of the aging process, lose their efficiency. The girl swimmer who broke records at 16 achieved championship status partly because she had the good luck to be born with efficient enzyme systems. They allowed her muscles to work effectively and her nervous system to coordinate her muscular activity with great precision. The longer she is properly nourished, the longer her enzymes will work effectively. Up to a point, that is.

Gradually, no matter how well nourished she may be, her enzyme systems will begin to deteriorate and at some point she will lose her championship status.

The purpose of proper nutrition is to furnish ideal amounts and forms of proteins, minerals and vitamins for our enzyme systems so that they can reach whatever inborn potentials they possess, and remain at their ideal level for as long as possible. It goes without saying that, no matter how well nourished a person may be, he will eventually reach a period of senility and old age. The question is: When?

Also, let me add: If you eat foods which your enzyme systems cannot metabolize, then you will be toxic (in an allergic state, if you will) and your body chemistry will not be able to work up to the level of its true potential.

The point of this chapter is to discuss how you can avoid the foregetfulness and emotional illness that too often beset the later years, or at least postpone them as long as possible.

To Postpone Aging—Start Now

It's never too early to begin a program of good nutrition. Now is the time to stop drinking soda pop, eating hot dogs and french fries, and going on ice-cream sprees. If you are a mother-to-be, let me remind you also that the food you eat and the nutritional supplements you take affect not only you, but to an equal extent, the child you carry. And remember that what your baby eats even during the very first months after birth will influence him until the day he dies.

Although periodic depressions frequently occur during the first half of life, these are usually short-lived and relatively mild.

A profound, long-term depression in a young person is relatively rare, and often indicates severe trouble.

In the second half of life, depressions are so frequent some people consider them almost the norm. Together with receding energy levels, feelings of depression are perhaps the most important difficulties associated with the aging process. In fact, since loss of energy and a feeling of depression are so very common in middle-aged and elderly people, we must consider that these are themselves symptoms of the condition we call aging—that is, of the growing inefficiency of our enzyme systems. Uncorrected, these enzyme systems deteriorate at an ever-increasing pace, and the symptoms escalate until they reach the dreaded end point of senility, with its loss of memory, disorientation, misperceptions, and degeneration of all intellectual life. To treat the disease we must find out how to delay or prevent the breakdown of enzyme systems that cause it!

How Your Body Can Attack Itself

Roy L. Walford, a professor of pathology at the University of California School of Medicine, has spent much of his life investigating the immunological aspects of aging. He presents a convincing argument for the theory that in part, old age is caused by failures in people's immunological system. The immunological system produces antibodies to fight infections, and to control substances to which one is allergic; it is also the system that forms autoimmune antibodies. Forming autoimmune or self-immune antibodies is what the German bacteriologist Paul Ehrlich called "the horror reaction"—the immunological reaction in which the body puts out antibodies against its own tissues and thereby destroys itself.

Hashimoto's disease is the classic "horror reaction" and the one most studied. In this disease, the body forms antibodies against its own thyroid tissue and eventually destroys it as if it were a foreign invader like a germ. We now know that such autoimmune reactions are quite common and that they increase with advancing age. There is a growing medical belief, for example, that the inflammatory, crippling type of arthritis is in fact an autoimmune reaction. Also, when a person has a heart attack and part of the heart muscle is destroyed, the body often forms antibodies against the heart muscle, and may go on to destroy more of the heart muscle than was originally damaged.

The work of L. Robert suggests that arteriosclerosis (hardening of the arteries) is in part an autoimmune phenomenon. It is most likely that immunological failure explains why people get cancer. More and more it looks as if all of us get cancer from time to time, but, if our immunological system is strong enough, it kills off the cancer cells and we hear no more from them.

Just as proper intake of vitamins, minerals, and proteins greatly improves your ability to fight disease such as flu and pneumonia, immunological response is probably much better in persons who eat foods that their enzyme systems can readily metabolize. In all probability, full-spectrum light stimulation is important for maintaining a sound immunological system.

Everything suggests that nutrition is vital to the maintenance of normal immunological functions, thereby providing one possible way of delaying the onset of old age.

How I See Autoimmune Diseases

As you might guess, my views about autoimmune diseases is quite different from the profession's conventional wisdom.

In my view, all "autoimmune" diseases result from allergies and should be treated as such. Usually the allergic reaction is triggered by foods and environmental substances, common "new foods" like grains, milk products, table sugar, and environmental hazards such as fire retardants in mattresses, household cleaning products, laundry detergents, etc.

In regard to arthritis, I feel that an allergic reaction causes destruction of the joint. As the joint tissue breaks down, particles of it enter the blood stream. The immune system reacts to the particles in the blood stream and forms antibodies against them.

The horror reaction is not a matter of the body mindlessly attacking itself, but allergic reaction destroying tissue.

ALZHEIMER'S DISEASE

In my view Alzheimer's disease is the end result of many small tissue-destroying allergic reactions. I suspect grains, table sugar, and milk and milk products are the most common offenders.

As I have mentioned before, my brain is made disorganized by eating wheat, and I become tired and depressed after eating most cheeses. I suspect each time I eat such foods and experience cerebral symptoms, a small part of my brain is destroyed. If I continued eating those foods, I suspect I would end up with Alzheimer's.

I don't eat those foods.

Preventing Alzheimer's Disease

Simple: stay away from foods and chemicals that give you cerebral symptoms. Usually these are grains, table sugar, milk and milk products, and chemicals such as gas from the kitchen stove, sterilizing cleaners used in the home, formaldehyde from wall-to-wall carpeting, pets, etc.

Alzheimer's disease is becoming more common. I suspect it will continue to increase until people start eating more red meat and animal fat, and fewer simple and complex carbohydrates. From a food standpoint, our society is headed in the wrong direction. Fears about cholesterol have reached the state of group madness.

Also, prevention of Alzheimer's is helped by taking proper nutritional supplements.

Poor memory is the first symptom of approaching Alzheimer's disease. Take it seriously. At first it's reversible. The longer you wait, the more difficult it is to reverse.

Treatment of Alzheimer's Disease

It's no different from treating any other allergy: spot the allergens and remove them. See above for the foods and chemicals most often at fault.

No alcoholic beverages—not even wine.

Take adequate nutritional supplements. Often a vitamin dependency disorder is present and must be treated. Pay special attention to vitamin B_{12}.

If the disease is not too far advanced, one can expect excellent results.

Biggest problem: people with Alzheimer's will not follow a proper diet. Someone must force them to eat foods to which they do not react.

The other day I saw a wealthy older man with moderate Alzheimer's. His young wife did nothing to make him follow my program. She wanted him to hurry and take his trip and leave her a wealthy widow.

Wealthy old men take note!

It is dangerous to offer "just a little" wine, a little pizza, a little ice cream. Kindness kills.

They must clean up their environments and get outside and walk.

My biggest problem: people don't believe what I tell them!

Why don't they believe me? Mostly because they don't want to. It's easier to take a pill than change their habits. No change, no gain.

ANTIOXIDANTS

Another theory of aging holds that its primary cause is the cross-linking between certain large molecules in the body, such as proteins and nucleic acid. "Cross-linking" refers to the abnormal joining of proteins, and could involve genetic materials such as DNA, thus interfering with the cells' metabolism and their ability to divide. Or the cross-linked connective tissue might be less permeable to the body chemicals. In that case, aging would cause a choking of the cells, rendering them unable to receive essential nutrients.

For that reason, antioxidants are in all probability very important to our bodies. They help prevent cross-linking of molecules, and thus help prevent the choking of the tissue cells. Selenium, vitamin E, and vitamin C are effective antioxidants. In all likelihood they delay the aging process, and therewith the onset of the emotional illnesses associated with age.

CAN VITAMIN E SLOW DOWN AGING?

Vitamin E, like all vitamins, is still a controversial issue despite years of reliably reported therapeutic successes in many areas. The very experienced Drs. Shute in Canada used it over several decades. They were particularly impressed by vitamin E's ability to spare and even repair blood vessel damage.

Drs. Lester Packer and James R. Smith of the University of California extended the growth limit of artificially grown human lung cells by adding vitamin E to the media in which they were living. The "hayflick limit"—the end of their normal reproductive life— of 50 reproductions passed the 120th reproduction and at the time of the report was still going strong.

The verbal gyrations of some people who are supposed to be authorities on vitamins never cease to amaze me: A few years ago, the New York Academy of Science held a symposium on vitamin E. At its end, spokesmen for the attending members told newspapers that the scientists had no concrete evidence that vitamin E plays an important role in human disease. A year later the academy published the results of that symposium in book form. Entitled *Vitamin E and Its Role in Cellular Metabolism*, the volume is composed of papers presented at the symposium, and is full of information on the vital importance of vitamin E and its use by every cell in the body. Some of the papers even discussed its specific therapeutic uses favorably!

The book repeatedly refers to vitamin E as an antioxidant, and speaks of its role as a hydrogen ion transporter. The fact that it is an antioxidant means that, in all probability, it does slow down the aging process. The fact that it is active in the transfer of the hydrogen ions means that a high level of vitamin E might well enable the cells which are partly choked off by a cross-molecule to function better than they would without this vitamin.

These Are the Most Important Vitamins to Slow Aging

Let me remind you once again that the intake of any single vitamin is of limited usefulness. To get the maximum possible benefit from vitamins you must maintain a proper diet, and take all the vitamins and minerals you need, since they work together like the members of an orchestra.

To prevent aging, however, several nutrients are of extra importance: magnesium, zinc, selenium, vitamin E, vitamin C, and vitamin B_{12}.

VITAMIN B_{12} IN THE AGING PROCESS

The autoimmune reactions discussed earlier are often found in people with low serum vitamin B_{12} levels. The body cannot absorb vitamin B_{12} unless a special factor with enzyme-like properties is present in the stomach.

Autoimmune reactions may block or bind the intrinsic factor in the stomach, preventing vitamin B_{12} from being absorbed. Also, autoimmune reactions may be directed against the parietal cells in the stomach, and thus destroy the cell's ability to produce the vital intrinsic factor. As we grow older, we may develop stronger and stronger autoimmune reactions, so that less and less of the intrinsic factor is produced by the stomach, until we reach the point of not absorbing sufficient vitamin B_{12} to satisfy the body's needs. Furthermore, proper blood levels of B_{12} also require an extrinsic factor, which is found largely in meat. Vegetarians therefore run a special risk of receiving too little of that factor, and therefore too little vitamin B_{12}. If you eat little meat, watch B_{12} closely.

I saw a patient this afternoon who suffered from bulimia and had eaten no meats for four years. Her B_{12} level was a dangerous 77. With that level, she could be getting not only brain damage but also spinal cord damage that could result in paralysis. In the end she could die of pernicious anemia.

The Patient Who Wept for Six Months

Several years ago a 76-year-old woman was brought to my office by her daughter, who stated that the mother had been weeping uncontrollably for the past six months and had recently become so incapacitated that she was unable to do her housework. She had been to see five physicians who had treated her in five different ways, mostly with antidepressants and tranquilizers. One doctor had given her injections of multiple vitamins, which had not helped.

In spite of her normal B_{12} level, I gave her a trial injection of 1000 mcg of vitamin B_{12b}. I told myself that unless she quickly improved, she could need antidepressants. If the antidepressants didn't help her a great deal within a month, she would need electro-convulsive therapy.

When she returned to my office three days later, she was considerably improved. She was no longer crying, and reported that she felt much stronger and had slept throughout the night for the first time in many months.

At the time of her next visit three days later, she looked happy and told me she could do her housekeeping again.

During subsequent visits the daughter was taught to administer the injections to her mother twice a week, or more frequently if she seemed in greater need of the vitamin. When she returned several weeks later, the elderly lady told me that she could feel herself becoming depleted of the vitamin every three or four days, and always felt completely restored after receiving another injection. At the time of that visit she was feeling the way she had felt ten years earlier, and was busy with all the household chores which she, like so many good German housewives of her generation, immensely enjoyed.

She was instructed to take the injections more often. If the injection gave her a lift, then she had waited too long.

This woman is a good example of a vitamin-dependent individual. I am sure we had elevated her serum vitamin B_{12} level to enormous heights. It would have been a waste of money to retest her.

Perhaps she was one of those people whose enzyme functions gradually fade with age. But this patient was restored to normal by giving her massive amounts of vitamins. It is even possible that certain metabolic pathways, not normally employing vitamin B_{12}, switched pathways, and made use of this invigorated set of enzymes. At any rate, a few injections of B_{12b} turned a crying, shuffling old woman into a bright-eyed, merry, elderly housewife who could once more take an active role in life and enjoy her remaining years.

Such transformations are what chemistry and nutrition are all about.

The Special Nutrition Needs of Older People

One of the reasons the old have more emotional disorders than the young is that they tend to skimp on their diets. They often have no family to cook for, and don't consider it worthwhile to prepare good food just for themselves. Their reduced energy encourages them to take shortcuts in food preparation. They stop shopping for fresh vegetables, fruits and meats. Too often they subsist on processed foods like TV dinners. Financial problems also play a part. Since more retired people must live on curtailed incomes and value some of the diversions of life more than sound food, they tend to save money by living on cheap, nonnutritious foods.

Yesterday, while lunching in a restaurant, I observed an elderly lady sitting at a nearby table. Her lunch consisted of a tiny hamburger lost in a large bun, an anemic slice of tomato atop a dollar-size lettuce leaf, and a generous helping of mashed potatoes with gravy. For dessert she had a vanilla ice cream sundae. From her tired movements and the sad look on her face I suspected that this was a rather typical meal for her. When I see people eating such food, especially when they also appear depressed or otherwise emotionally disturbed, it always makes me feel depressed, too. I have a great urge to talk to them about good food. I hope this book will reach such people.

SPECIAL HELP FROM NIACIN

Many elderly people feel better on extra doses of niacin, a form of vitamin B_3. Aside from its other benefits, discussed in an earlier chapter, this fascinating vitamin has an additional effect that has nothing directly to do with its action as a vitamin.

Niacin counteracts blood clotting tendencies and is therefore of special interest for the older age group that is more prone to blood clots in the brain (stroke). In some circles, niacin is also thought to give protection against blood clots in the blood vessels of the heart—the condition known as coronary thrombosis (or heart attack).

One theory says that some heart attacks are caused by blood platelets that stick to the blood vessel walls. A clot then forms around the platelets.

Niacin often makes the anti-clotting drug work more effectively. Thus the dosage must be carefully adjusted.

As early as 1938, T. D. Spies found that the abnormal electrocardiograms of cardiac patients reverted to normal after patients were given niacin.

Luigi Condorelli, writing in a book entitled *Niacin in Vascular Disorders and Hyperlipemia,* states that he considers niacin a "most efficacious drug for the treatment of cerebral thrombosis."

In another chapter of that volume, Elaine Bossak Feldman describes her use of niacin in the management of severe disorders of fat metabolism, in which large fatty deposits were visible in the skin. The photographs of the lesions taken before and after treatment with niacin are spectacular. They make it easy to imagine the cholesterol deposits in one's own arteries disappearing in a like manner.

The same volume also has an article by Drs. Ernst Ost Stenson and Svend Stenson, entitled "Regression of Atherosclerosis During Nicotinic Acid Therapy: A Study in Man by Means of Repeated Arteriographies." They present graphs of pulsations in the arteries of the leg which clearly demonstrate that circulation is vastly improved by treatment with niacin.

CAUTION: Anyone taking niacin must be under the close supervision of a physician experienced in its use. Many people do not tolerate large amounts of niacin. Also, niacin can cause serious liver damage. Liver tests must be done at frequent intervals. See chapter 16 on vitamins.

Niacin, when taken in adequate doses, puts a negative electrical charge on the red blood cells which affects their oxygen-carrying ability. As we grow older, our red blood cells develop a tendency toward "slugging": the red blood cells stick together and go through the blood vessels in clumps like grapes. This has been observed by studying the small blood vessels in the eye through a microscope.

These slugged red blood cells obviously cannot travel through the finer arteries of the body, and thus do not deliver adequate blood supplies to their ultimate destination, the tissues of the body.

Also, since these blood cells touch each other, the surfaces of the red blood cells exposed to oxygen are reduced. Gas exchange is no longer rapid and efficient. Once the slugging is broken up with niacin, the red blood cells' full surface area is again exposed to the oxygen in the lungs, so that it can quickly and efficiently receive their full saturation of oxygen. Not only does such breaking up of the slugged red blood cells help the circulation in the brain and therefore forestall senility in its early stages, it also is of obvious aid to people suffering from narrowing of the heart arteries, and in disorders where the blood vessels of the legs are narrowed and insufficient blood supply is the result.

Linus Pauling has reportedly said that if one could only get enough oxygen to the brain cells, depression could be altogether avoided. It is easy to see how niacin would enter into the picture of supplying more oxygen to the brain cells.

If you take niacin, I would suggest that you take capsules, not tablets.

How Overfeeding Hastens Death

More than a generation ago, C. M. McCay and his associates described an experiment in which they prolonged the life of laboratory animals by about a third merely by underfeeding them from birth. Only the total calorie intake was reduced. In all other respects, the animals' diet was kept entirely normal.

I can imagine how mothers will react to the suggestion that they underfeed their babies!

Pediatricians know that it's best for babies to be underweight, but they're under so much pressure from mothers that often the pediatricians don't pay enough attention to obesity.

To mothers the advice to cut down on their baby's food sounds antimotherhood, un-American, and almost godless.

Because mankind has lived with hunger throughout the ages, mothers have a strong instinct to overfeed their babies. Keeping babies fat is a holdover from the time when a well-fed baby meant that he had a better chance of surviving.

Today, overfeeding is not only useless, it's dangerous. Babies are fed formulas made with sugar. Canned baby foods commonly contain sugar. The more sugar the foods have in them, the better the mothers like them.

Given the composition of present-day babies' food, if you cater to Junior's appetite, you'll shorten his life. If you want your children to live longer, to ward off for as long as possible the senility that may come with old age, underfeed babies from birth, and keep on underfeeding them for as long as their food is under your control.

A baby should be slightly below the weight that is "normal" for his age. Pinch (gently!) to test for fat. You know fat when you feel it.

Although each of us has an inherited preprogrammed time to die, our lifespan probably can be influenced for the better by correct nutrition. McCay's laboratory animals, like us, also had a preprogrammed life span, and yet their lives were increased by a third through low-calorie diets. Translated into human terms, such an increase would mean that a person biologically programmed to die at 66, and underfed from birth, could increase his lifespan to 99.

HOW PANTOTHENIC ACID HELPS LONGEVITY

Some years ago, Roger Williams, Ph.D., of the University of Texas, grew interested in royal bee jelly because of its extraordinary effect on longevity. If female larva of a bee is fed in the usual way, the result is a drone, an infertile worker bee, whose life as a rule lasts only for a few short weeks in the summer. But if the same larva is fed royal jelly, the result is a fertile queen bee with a lifespan of 6 to 8 years. Williams traced this effect to the royal jelly's high pantothenic acid content.

He took two groups of laboratory mice and fed them the standard laboratory diet (which, I might add, is far superior to the diets of humans. We're the only civilization in which mice and dogs eat better than man). The diet contained all essential nutritive elements, including some pantothenic acid. But one group of mice had additional pantothenic acid added to their drinking water, so that they averaged 0.3 mg of extra pantothenic acid daily. The mice in both groups were then observed over their entire lifespan.

The 41 mice on the standard laboratory diet lived for an average of 550 days; the 33 mice that were fed the standard chow *plus* the pantothenic acid in the drinking water lived for an average of 635 days.

Translated into human terms, the first group would have died at age 75; the second group would have lived to be 89. This makes me think it's worthwhile to add a few pennies' worth of pantothenic acid to our diets. It seems a relatively cheap way of buying a possible postponement of the old age and senility that haunts us all.

Liver Spots and Aging

A hallmark of aging is the appearance of brown spots (as mentioned in the chapter on beauty) not only on the skin but also in the internal organs. They're most visible on the backs of the hands.

Before I became interested in nutritional supplements, these brown spots were regularly appearing on my own hands. After I began taking vitamins, minerals, and unsaturated oils and following a good diet, I saw a marked regression in brown spots. Today, a number of years later, I can only find two small ones.

In London to deliver a scientific paper on vitamin B_{12}, I had an opportunity to discuss this with Mark Altschul, M.D. of the Harvard University School of Medicine. He expressed the opinion that this disappearance of pigmentation was probably due to my large intake of vitamin C. Apparently, in at least one individual, this particular aspect of aging was reversed by megadose of this vitamin. While full substantiation of such a statement would require control studies, there is little doubt in my mind that my observations would be proved accurate because I have often seen the same thing happen in my patients.

PABA and Aging

In 1931, S. Ansbacher produced achromotrichia (gray hair) in rats on a diet deficient in PABA. He restored the hair color by giving them PABA. Since graying of the hair is one of the most common signs of aging in humans, Ansbacher's work deserves attention.

Ana Aslan, M.D., for many years advocated injections and tablets that contain a special type of procaine (H-3 or Gerovital, an acidified form of procaine buffered with magnesium and potassium) to retard aging. She even claimed to reverse some of the effects of aging.

Procaine is the local anesthetic known in this country as novocaine. You may well ask what a local anesthetic could possibly have to do with aging. The answer is quite simple. PABA makes up part of the molecule of procaine. The procaine, or novocaine, molecule is broken down in the body to release PABA, a fact that seems to have escaped some observers.

For years a dispute has been going on in the international medical community regarding Dr. Aslan's findings. Her work has been rejected by the American medical establishment.

Nutritionist Herman Goldman, M.D., visited Dr. Aslan's clinic in Romania on several widely-spaced occasions and reported that some of the patients who appeared to be vegetating when they went into treatment in their sixties became actively engaged in useful pursuits, and were full of life and vigor, ten years later. Perhaps this isn't very conclusive proof of the efficacy of procaine injections, but certainly it is enough to make procaine deserve some attention.

Three Patients Try H-3

I have, however, three patients who on their own have become involved with H-3. One of them jetted to Romania and spent a couple of weeks at Aslan's clinic. The only thing that impressed him was the poverty of the country. He felt no better after the treatments.

Two of my women patients, on the other hand, take H-3 and swear by it. They say that they simply feel better when taking H-3. both of these patients are rather sophisticated in the ways of nutrition as well as food and environmental allergies. They would probably know if they were getting nothing more than a placebo effect.

One thing I can say for certain about H-3: if patients took H-3 and ignored their diets and nutritional regime, they would not feel significantly better.

Even Aslan put patients on vitamins and minerals and reduced the sugar and white flour in their diet. She took them off of alcohol and tobacco. If nothing else were done for patients, this program alone would make a high percentage of patients feel better and look younger.

Are patients helped by H-3 tablets and/or injections? I'm not certain. If it were harmful, I think we would know about it by now.

CELL THERAPY AND AGING

No discussion of the aging process and its retardation would be complete without mentioning cell therapy. Although this form of therapy does not involve a nutritional supplement taken by mouth, in a sense it's a form of nutrition.

Cell therapy, rests on the scientifically shaky medical myth that "like cures like." Patients are given injections of cells from various organs of animal fetuses. The cells are supposed to rejuvenate the corresponding organ in the human patient.

Paul Niehans, a Swiss physician, brought cell therapy into prominence in Europe. Although Niehans himself died some years ago at the age of 88, his method continues to be used by thousands of physicians all over Europe. Some of the injections still consist of fresh animal fetus cells; the majority of the injections now come from freeze-dried organs, organs preserved by a cell-preserving process known as lyophilization.

In Germany, for example, the preparation of the cell therapy substance is in the hands of the Hygiene Institute of the University of Heidelberg, and is controlled by the German Ministry of Health.

The treatment, which consists of a series of injections, also involves the avoidance of all alcohol and tobacco. A high percentage of people are going to feel better and look younger if they do nothing more than leave off alcohol and tobacco.

I am not convinced about the benefits of the Niehans cell therapy, but I am keeping an open mind on the subject. Not so the FDA, which has prohibited the use of cell therapy, and the import of lyophilized cell-therapy material into this country.

People who are interested in such treatment must travel to Europe, where their purses are considerably lightened by many practitioners of the technique.

No one was reassured about cell therapy after it was involved in a disaster in Florida a few years ago. A physician—he was not an M.D.—was going out to the local slaughterhouse, getting fetal material, making a suspension of it and injecting it into patients. All this is standard practice for cell therapy.

Unfortunately, some of his material was contaminated. One or more of his injected patients developed gas gangrene. As I recall there were several deaths.

One of the worse aspects of the case was that the physician apparently did not make the diagnosis of gas gangrene and hence did not seek prompt authoritative help for the patient.

Prior to this disaster, out of curiosity I once attended a lay meeting where this physician spoke to a group of interested people—potential patients. During his speech he kept mispronouncing common medical terms such as "diabetes mellitus."

In order to feel out his medical knowledge, I asked him (he didn't know I was an M.D.) several somewhat technical questions.

He evaded the problems my questions gave him by giving folksy, nonsensical answers such as "I'm not a professor. I'm just a practical, practicing doctor."

Transferring Genetic Material

In the prestigious scientific journal *Nature*, Drs. Kari R. Merril and Mark I. Greier reported that genetic material had been successfully transferred from bacteria to human cells, and that this genetic material was capable of activating enzymes that could be used by cells grown under artificial conditions, cells that could not metabolize milk sugars properly.

This successful transfer of genetic material from one cell to another suggests that cell therapy deserves more scrutiny by serious scientists, who can now use the more sophisticated apparatus and techniques available for research in cellular enzyme chemistry.

We might write an entire volume on the aging process, its possible causes, and its mental disorders. We might investigate, for example, the reason for the "pockets of longevity" such as exist in remote rural areas of Russia, Tibet, and South America, where people are said to live active lives to age 150, 160, and even beyond. We might look at the intriguing phenomena presented by many schizophrenic patients who often appear much younger than their chronological age (and, incidentally, have an exceedingly low rate of cancer). But such discussions would exceed the practical limits of this book.

Final Advice About How to Slow Aging

With your physician's approval:

1. Take the unsaturated oils, the minerals and vitamins as outlined in chapter 18.

2. Follow the diet as put forth in chapter 15.

3. Walk outdoors at a fast pace for one hour and five minutes *every* day. If you can't walk, crawl.

Walking is the easiest and cheapest, but it's the hardest thing for me to get patients to do.

CHAPTER TWENTY-THREE

SAVING MONEY ON YOUR NUTRITIONAL NEEDS

Sadly, people try to save money on basic foods so they'll have more to spend on fun items. I know a high school principal whose wife feeds their children a diet that contains much cheap food such as peanut butter, bread, hot dogs, and drinks laden with sugar.

This same family will send their children to the orthodontist to have their teeth straightened (made necessary by poor diet), to a psychologist to straighten out their minds (also mixed up because of their poor diet), and to summer camp. They will house their children in a fine home in an expensive suburb, and will later send their children to college.

They've completely missed the essentials.

Given a good diet, most other things would fall into place.

Don't quote me as saying I'm against higher education, but it's ten thousand times more important for a child to have a good diet than to have a "good education."

EXAMPLES OF MONEY SAVING—OR MONEY EARNING

Here's what's happened to some of my patients. Several years ago a 24-year-old woman (call her Joan) visited my office for the first time. She had been holding an important behind-the-scenes job in television until three months previously when she was demoted to routine office duties with a 60 percent cut in salary. The manager called her to his office and as kindly as possible told her that her work was no longer adequate. She had missed one or two days of work every few weeks and seemed to have lost her intelligence and her enthusiasm. The company vice president hoped that the reduction in salary and job responsibility would "shake you up enough to bring you back to your former good senses."

The young woman sitting across the desk from me wept as she told her embarrassing story. Her face was puffy. Her skin was so pale she looked as if she had spent six months chained in a dungeon.

A year and a half before she had had hepatitis and had never recovered her energy. She was so weak that she drank a pot of coffee a day and still could barely drag herself to the office. Saturdays and Sundays she spent in bed, partly because she was too weak to do anything else and partly because she was trying in the only way she knew to regain enough strength to go to work on Monday morning.

During the four years before her slump, Joan had a good marriage. Finally, her husband had decided she was lazy, inadequate, and anything but the energetic, interesting girl he had married. After she had been exhausted for a year, he insisted that her doctor consult with another internist for a complete workup. Both physicians agreed she was in good health, but depressed and should see a psychiatrist.

Joan visited several times a psychiatrist who also thought she was depressed and began probing into her marriage and past life to explain her lack of enthusiasm. When this tactic did not produce results, she stopped "therapy."

At that point her husband became thoroughly disgusted and left her.

When she saw me, 18 months had passed since the beginning of her hepatitis. She still complained of all the difficulties I mentioned earlier, plus weak legs, eyes that burned, and a puffiness and swelling of her face, hands and ankles. Her hair was dry and she said that she was excessively sensitive to cold. The history revealed that she was taking vitamin tablets, lecithin, and vitamin E.

I require all my new patients to have a physical examination. In the case of Joan, because of her history of hepatitis, I felt that a workup for possible chronic liver disease was indicated. I sent her to a liver specialist at Mount Sinai Hospital in New York. He hospitalized her for a thorough examination, including a liver biopsy. He concluded that she had no liver disease and felt her symptoms were due to a psychoneurosis.

Here is what I found on a routine clinical work-up: Her six-hour glucose tolerance test was abnormal; a sharp drop (87 mg/dl) in her blood sugar level during a one-hour period indicated hypoglycemia. At the time of the drop, she became nauseated, weak, and sweaty. Her estrogen and serum folic acid levels were also abnormally low.

Blood tests showed that she was also low in Vitamin B_1 and B_6. Challenge tests revealed that she was allergic to 21 out of 24 substances for which she was tested. She became very tired when tested for fish. When tested for cats she became flushed in the face, began sweating and fell asleep for about fifteen minutes. She felt excessively tired after being tested for corn, and developed a headache and pains in both knees after being tested for milk.

I put Joan on a diet that eliminated the foods to which she was most sensitive. Others foods to which she was only mildly allergic were rotated so that she ate them only every four or five days, a technique that helps reduce all-over sensitivity. I gave her a vitamin-mineral regimen to correct her deficiencies, and, because of her history of sensitivity to cold, her dry skin and hair, and her low morning temperatures, I prescribed thyroid tablets even though her thyroid tests were normal.

In spite of her normal serum vitamin B_{12} level, to learn whether she might have a vitamin B_{12} dependency disorder, I gave her a trial injection of vitamin B_{12b}. She felt a great deal more energy after having B_{12b}. (She now gets an injection every week from a neighborhood nurse.)

During the first two months of therapy, this patient made slow but quite definite progress. Her energy increased and her taste for life began to return. But we noticed that sometimes she became depressed and tired after visiting a cottage on Long Island in which she owned a share. Then we discovered that she had trouble only on rainy weekends. We concluded this was due to her mold allergies. After we eliminated her visits on rainy weekends, her bouts of fatigue and depression lessened. (Incidentally, when Joan went into her mold allergy slump, her face, ankles and hands became swollen. This swelling—edema—is a typical allergic reaction. A traditional physician would prescribe a diuretic to promote water loss—exactly the wrong treatment for a person like Joan: It does nothing to treat the allergy that causes the problem, and it drains the system of sodium and other minerals, leaving the patient even more allergic.)

After three months Joan was greatly improved. She had a sparkle to her personality again. Her face had lost its sallow puffiness. She was able to think clearly and her memory had returned. She had regained her old efficiency at work—and with it her old job. Her lost interest in sex returned and she began dating. I did not retest her estrogen level and did not give her estrogens because I felt that her hormone levels would return to normal after her biochemistry was corrected. Her periods, which had stopped altogether, returned. At first they were painful and unpleasant but soon they became quite normal.

Soon Joan reported that she got a $3,000 raise in salary. She now earns more money because she has the energy, the will to work. Once more she had her old intelligence and enthusiasm.

Like this patient, in plain dollars and cents, many people who follow the directions in this book will earn more money. Who can say what it's worth to also feel energetic and happy? As I so frequently tell patients, an investment in good health is a capital investment that will pay off. It is not money down the drain like spending money for a night on the town. The catch is that the money must be spent for good medical care, not the inadequate care that most people get when they fail to have a good nutritional workup.

The Honor Student Who Clerked

Let me tell you next about Ann, an honors college graduate who came to me while barely holding on to a three-day-a-week clerical job because she was almost incapacitated by schizophrenia. She had not been helped by the treatment she received at a famous private clinic, nor had she made any progress with the three private psychiatrists who had treated her.

After six months of nutritional therapy she took a full-time job and now has moved up to a very gratifying position in one of New York's major industries. Now that she is healthy again, she not only earns more money but has gotten back her self-respect and is alive once more.

The Depressed Patient from Philadelphia

A few years ago I saw a patient from Philadelphia who had been in a severe depression for more than a year. He had made two serious suicide attempts. He had been admitted to a famous psychiatric hospital in Maryland on two occasions and was receiving psychotherapy when he first came to my office.

He was borderline low in testosterone (male sex hormone). I put him on injections of testosterone, and on mineral and vitamin supplements. If he felt too ill to test for food allergies, we guessed at the correct diet for him and put him on it.

After about two weeks his depression began to lift; eight weeks later, he returned to work. When he first visited me he was about to lose a very responsible position because he simply had not been able to function. He will probably be a more effective executive than in the past.

The economic advantages gained by these three patients are obvious. Because they feel better, they can earn more money. Before they corrected their nutritional and hormonal deficiencies they were disorganized and depressed. They used up most of their energy merely holding themselves together. They had little left to give to an employer.

PENNY WISE, POUND FOOLISH

In the long run, remember that rib steaks are cheaper than peanut butter and hot dogs.

Buying vitamins is less expensive than skipping them.

My advice: Give nutrition a trial. Experience has taught me that preventive medicine pays for itself many times over, not only with improved income, but with better health, more happiness, and a longer life. Only you can be the judge, but you can't judge nutrition until you try it.

What to Buy at the Health Food Store

1. Vitamins.
2. Minerals
3. Unsaturated oils.
4. My books.
(Not necessarily in that order!)

ORGANIC FOODS?

Frankly, I've been disappointed in the benefits to be had from "organically" grown foods. I have personally used them and have had patients use them, but have seldom found them worthwhile.

"Organically" grown meats are particularly poorly tolerated, possibly because they're aged to make them more tender and often have no fat on them.

INEXPENSIVE MEAT

Most towns and cities have a source of wholesale meat. Search these out and hang around them enough to find out what goes on. Most of them will sell you a rib of beef. Many will even cut it up for you.

Consider cheap cuts of meat: heart, kidney, chuck. Hamburger is often not tolerated.

IF PRESSED TO THE WALL

If my budget were strained to the limit, there are certain basic items of nutrition I would buy even if it meant limiting my diet to beef hearts, beef kidneys, and vegetables.

The first of these is vitamin B-complex. I would pray that I wasn't allergic to it. If allergic, I would try a smaller amount. If that didn't work, I would try spacing what I took, even if it meant going as low as half a teaspoon every three days.

GETTING VITAMIN C (ASCORBIC ACID) THE LOW-BUDGET WAY

The next essential basic is vitamin C. Ascorbic acid powder is much less expensive than buying vitamin C tablets or capsules. It is also better tolerated, provided you take it well diluted. Remember to *buy fine powder, not crystals.*

Some crystals, are mistakenly labeled "powder." The powders look like baby powder, the crystals like sugar. The crystals are often poorly tolerated. Be sure the powder contains no filler. You may be offered a powdered form of vitamin C that costs less per bottle than pure ascorbic acid. If the strength is not close to 4000 mg per teaspoon, then the powder has been cut and is no bargain.

(Some hot-shot vitamin pushers have begun to copy heroin pushers and cut their vitamin C.)

GETTING VITAMINS A AND D THE LOW-BUDGET WAY

The third essential is a teaspoon every day of cod liver oil.

VITAMIN E AND CALCIUM ON A TIGHT BUDGET

Vitamin E is expensive. Nevertheless, I consider it an essential to counteract the effects of stress and pollution and to combat aging. If you can possibly afford it, take a 200 IU capsule a day; if not, cut down to 100 IU daily.

Those are the vitamins I consider most basic. In an emergency, I would cut down on solid food before cutting these out.

MINERALS

Only slightly lower on the priority list stands dolomite powder, ½ teaspoon in water three times a day. If I could beg, borrow—or, perhaps, steal—one or two 60 mg zinc gluconate capsules a day.

PRISON

A few years ago one of my most food-sensitive patients was sent to prison. I wrote to the doctors there and told them about his allergies, but I felt certain they would ignore my letters. (It turned out that they did.)

Five years later the patient returned to see me. I told him I'd been worrying about him and asked him how he had made a go of it.

"I traded," he said. "Other men wanted my apple pie. I would swap it to them for their hamburgers, and on and on."

With my allergies, I hope to miss the opportunity of checking out this means of survival, but it might give you some ideas if you ever get in a tight spot.

CHAPTER TWENTY-FOUR

WALKING'S
WHERE IT'S AT

Life on planet Earth has developed biochemistries that depend on what surrounds them. For example, most life forms have encountered things like oxygen, light, and water and cannot live without them.

Movement has been a part of animal life for one and a half billion years, so it's not surprising that our biochemistries have come to depend on movement almost as much as air and water. Our immediate ancestors have been walking upright on two feet for four million years. To function properly, it's hardly surprising that our biochemistries have come to depend on walking.

To give a simple example: if a person goes to bed and stays in bed, no matter how good his diet, his bones will lose calcium. The chemistry of bone—as well as muscle and every other organ—has come to depend on the jarring motion of walking to produce minute electrical currents that our chemistry requires to function properly.

GOOD NUTRITION IS NOT ENOUGH

No matter how perfectly you adjust your diet and your vitamin-mineral program, your chemistry will not function at its best unless you exercise.

307

I advise all my patients to walk for an hour and five minutes each day. Understand that I said walk, not stroll. You should walk at your best pace, not wander around shopping malls pausing here and there to buy items you suddenly realize you can't live without. It's far more beneficial if you walk the straight hour and five minutes without stopping.

"What about going to the gym or riding a bicycle for an hour and five minutes every day?" patients frequently ask me.

"Fine," I tell them, "Go to the gym if you like or ride a bicycle, but don't let it interfere with your walking. Nothing takes the place of walking.

"If it's raining, walk anyway; if necessary, get wet. Your body can take an hour and five minutes of being wet better than an hour and five minutes of not walking.

"If it's cold, wear more clothes. Eskimos walk in the wintertime; so can you. Put a thin cotton terrycloth towel over your mouth to breathe through if it's really cold.

"If you absolutely can't walk, crawl!"

CHAPTER TWENTY-FIVE

YEAST AND YOU

MRS. MAYES

Mrs. Mayes was a middle-aged society woman, a neighbor of Richard Nixon in an exclusive section of New Jersey. She consulted me because she suffered from tiredness, depression, and recurrent yeast vaginitis. Two psychiatrists and four gynecologists had been unable to cure her. She had decided that the vaginal yeast infection caused all of her trouble. She wanted me to give her something that would kill the yeast once and for all so she would permanently recover.

To help her understand what had happened to her, I started off by giving her a speech. I said, "Yeast, Candida, is a 'disease' of civilization. For more than 2 million years our ancestors lived on a diet of mostly meat and animal fat, with small amounts of vegetables and sometimes a little fruit.

"From 5 to 10 thousand years ago our ancestors settled down and changed to a mostly agricultural diet, a diet that got many of its calories not from animal fat but from grains (such as wheat) and tubers (like potatoes). About 150 years ago they added table sugar in significant amounts.

"Evolution hasn't had enough time to adjust our biochemistry to handle efficiently 'new foods' such as grains, tubers, and sugar.

"When we examine the fossil feces (coprolites) of primitive man, we see no evidence of yeast. When we examine the feces of modern man, we find yeast a universal inhabitant.

"Like many other ills that plague mankind, yeast infections are a disease of civilization. If you eat mostly red meat and animal fat, small amounts of non-root vegetables, and very small amounts of non-sweet fruits, the yeast in your vagina—and everywhere else—will starve to death and disappear."

Mrs. Mayes asked, "Can't you give me something that will kill off the yeast?"

"Yes, but the yeast infection will come back when you stop the medication."

Mrs. Mayes Wants What She Wants

Like many wealthy people, Mrs. Mayes was accustomed to having life go her way. She wanted to have her cake and eat it too.

"You're in a battle with Mother Nature," I told her. "Mother Nature has no interest in you. Mother Nature doesn't make an exception for you because you're pleasant, generous, and kind. You can only win in a battle with Mother Nature by learning her laws and obeying them.

"For example, if your house is in the path of an earthquake, you are in a battle with Mother Nature. You must get out of the house or have it fall on top of you. You can't save your house by standing on the front porch and saying to the earthquake, 'I am Mrs. Mayes. This is my house. Last year I gave two thousand dollars to the United Save The Children Fund and did 150 hours volunteer work at the local hospital.'

"Battling the earthquake, one of Mother Nature's forces, will get you nowhere. You can't have it both ways. You get out or you die."

Mrs. Mayes didn't like my answer. She expected me to kill the yeast so she could be done with it forever.

Books on Yeast Infections (Candidiasis)

People who read books telling how to cure yeast get much misinformation.

True, if people will follow the directions in the books on yeast (Candida) infections, many will improve. They improve because all of the books advocate reducing the carbohydrates in the diet, which means reducing the amounts of "new foods" eaten: grains, root vegetables, and table sugar—foods to which people are commonly allergic.

Many people will not recover until they cut out almost all carbohydrates. Most people don't want to do that. They are addicted to carbohydrates. They look upon carbohydrates as fun foods. They want to go to parties and eat "normal foods." They want to continue drinking alcoholic beverages, a no-no for most people with yeast infections.

Eat a "Normal Diet," Suffer from a "Normal Infection"

At parties Mrs. Mayes eats finger foods and sips champagne, "normal foods" for our society, but not "normal" for her particular biochemistry. Most of the women at the party are also suffering from fatigue, depression and vaginitis. It's a "normal" part of our civilization.

Having Your Cake and Eating It Too

Like many wealthy people, Mrs. Mayes felt she knew more than most people. She might not admit it, but she thought she knew more about curing yeast infections than I did. She insisted that I give her medication to kill the yeast.

I didn't tell her that people who tell the doctor how to treat them are not getting their money's worth.

Because it wouldn't injure her, I gave her a prescription for the powdered form (the only effective form) of Nystatin. To suppress her yeast vaginitis, she had to take large doses, one teaspoon 6 times a day.

As I told her it would, every time she reduced the dose of Nystatin or stopped it, her vaginitis returned. Only by changing her diet could she kill off the yeast and keep it killed off.

She felt a slight lessening of her fatigue and depression.

She was satisfied to take the Nystatin and continue following her "normal diet."

THE DARK CONTINENT

Then she went to Africa on a safari. She forgot her Nystatin and left it on the plane. In the middle of the wilds of nowhere, her vaginitis returned full force, more than full force. The weather was hotter than the Devil's furnace. The bathing facilities were primitive.

Mrs. Mayes became more depressed and so tired she could hardly get up in the morning. It wasn't her greatest vacation. Even though Mrs. Mayes was wealthy, Mother Nature stuck her tongue out at Mrs. Mayes and laughed at her.

END OF STORY

Mrs. Mayes continued her "normal" diet and her Nystatin. She has now gone through menopause. The yeast infection has cleared, as it often does at menopause. Her depression and fatigue, however, grew worse, as they often do at menopause. Clearly, the yeast infection had only been a minor cause of the fatigue and depression she had felt earlier.

"You're allergic to some of the carbohydrates you eat," I said. "Why don't you give me a chance to cure you?"

She visited a psychiatrist for antidepressants. They didn't do the job. She came back to see me. Finally, she decided that she couldn't win a head-on fight with Mother Nature. She allowed me to test her. We eliminated several classes of foods to which she was allergic. She replaced her gas stove with an electric stove and made some changes in her bedroom.

She now does very well.

Here's What a Book on Yeast Promises to Cure

Acne, allergies, anxiety, asthma, constipation, depression, diarrhea, earaches, fatigue, headaches, infertility, lost sex drive, poor memory, muscles weakness, persistent coughs, premenstrual syndrome, recurrent vaginitis, skin irritations.

The above list of symptoms, disorders and diseases are claimed to be caused by yeast (Candida) infections. Much to the distress of traditional physicians, the diagnosis and treatment of yeast infections has become a major medical industry. My view is that if you work out your food and environmental allergies, the troubles listed above—along with many others—will disappear.

Yeast Infections (Candida Albicans)

The last few years have brought a growing interest in the diagnosis and treatment of *Monilia albicans* or *Candida albicans* infections. (Also called "fungus infection," "yeast infection," or "candidiasis.") This interest was spurred by books written by C. Orian Truss, M.D. and William G. Crook, M.D.

Apparently almost everyone has *Monilia albicans* (a form of yeast) growing in the gastrointestinal tract. The yeast is a more or less permanent guest. Since monilia is almost always present in everyone, looking for the yeast in stool specimens is not the way to diagnose the disorder. Also, almost everyone is allergic to *Monilia albicans,* so it's a waste of time to skin test patients for sensitivity to monilia.

A careful history is the best way to diagnose this disorder. A therapeutic trial on medication that kills the yeast is also helpful in diagnosing the condition.

Candidiasis is more common in women than in men. If a woman has a vaginal discharge that keeps recurring, it's very likely she has a chronic yeast infection. If a man or woman has an itching, burning, redness, or irritation around the anus, again a monilial infection is likely. Anyone who eats a diet high in junk food, has recently been pregnant, or uses adrenal cortical hormones ("steroids"), estrogens, birth control pills, or antibiotics is a prime suspect. Many people with hypoglycemia have monilial infections. Everyone with diabetes has a monilial infection until proven otherwise.

People with chronic yeast infections are often very sensitive to molds and will not feel well in damp weather. They are especially likely to have trouble in summer cottages that have been closed up for long periods of the year. They display symptoms when they are in low, damp, shaded areas or damp basements. They may react poorly to foods that contain yeast, such as brewers' yeast or bread; eating sweets may cause a flare-up as well.

TREATMENT

The first and most important step in the treatment of candidiasis is to change from a high-carbohydrate to a high-fat diet. Yeast thrives on carbohydrates and dies on fats. In all probability the yeast has moved into our bodies because many people in our culture eat a diet very high in carbohydrates—such foods as pasta, bread, cereals, corn, etc., and sweets such as cake, cookies, pie, ice cream, and candy. Sweet fruits and high carbohydrate vegetables like potatoes and carrots also favor the growth of monilia.

When you come off carbohydrates, what do you eat? The answer seems to be a mystery to most people, both patients and doctors.

One fact must be borne in mind: the human body can function by using either carbohydrates or fats as fuel. People cannot survive on protein alone. Most people with food allergies and/or monilial infections do poorly both on carbohydrates and foods that contain mold, such as cheese.

Fresh (unaged) beef rib steak is usually the best tolerated form of fat. The deckle of beef must not be eaten. Most people are allergic to it. Only the inner white fat should be eaten—along with the lean. Do not eat the browned or burned fat and do not cook the meat with gas.

Other good sources of fat: olive oil, safflower oil, linseed oil, cod liver oil, butter, porterhouse beef steaks, pork, fatty fish (such as blue fish, black fish, sword fish, mackerel, salmon), and chicken or duck (if tolerated). Because much of the fat in fowl is the skin, eat it as well.

I have had an opportunity to use Nystatin and/or Nizoral (as Truss and Crook do) to treat several hundred patients and have had a chance to evaluate its effectiveness first hand. Although these drugs are often helpful, I feel that much of the improvement reported is brought about by the reduced-carbohydrate diets Drs. Truss and Crook give their patients when administering these drugs.

There is little doubt that monilial infections produce a general toxicity in many patients which can stimulate any emotional or mental symptom you can name—anxiety, depression, generalized tiredness, confusion or psychotic delusions.

Too many symptoms blamed on monilial infections, however, are often caused by allergies. In my opinion, monilial infections usually start in tissue that has been either damaged by allergic reactions or has poor immunity because of vitamin and mineral deficiencies. For example, it is well known that thrush, a monilial infection of the mouth, appears in children who are poorly nourished. I have a woman patient who develops burning in her vagina after she eats oranges. Of course she's allergic to oranges. The day after eating oranges—her favorite food which she keeps trying "only one more time"—she develops a vaginal yeast infection. Her vaginal tissue is injured by the allergic reaction. The injury weakens the tissue and monilia is able to take over and start growing.

Because oral yeast infections may be a first sign of AIDS, it must not be ruled out whenever yeast infections are found—particularly in the mouth.

FURTHER TREATMENT

As indicated, to control monilial infections, a change in diet from carbohydrates to fats is essential. Foods to which a patient is allergic must be avoided. Most patients benefit from taking more than minimum amounts of vitamins, minerals and unsaturated oils. An exercise program that involves walking is also beneficial. Only white, all-cotton clothes should be worn next to the skin, especially if the monilial infection involves the anus or the vagina. (This clothing should be soaked first in white vinegar, then washed with baking soda. After the first washing, use only baking soda. Hang— rather than machine—dry. Women with vaginal infections should *never* wear panty hose or slacks; whenever possible, wear a skirt without panties.)

Avoid antibiotics if at all possible. If antibiotics absolutely must be taken, ask your doctor if Mysteclin-F is appropriate. This antibiotic includes a drug that kills both monilia and bacteria.

Acidophilus is helpful but most people are allergic to it. I find the best tolerated product to be Vital-Dophilus powder made by Klaire Laboratories. Widely available in health food stores, acidophilus promotes the growth of "good" bacteria that tend to keep monilia in check. The usual yogurt is worthless in this regard, and most people are allergic to it.

The LaPacho herbal tea—from the bark of a South American

tree—has been touted as an effective treatment for monilial infections. I understand, however, that Dr. Truss has actually grown monilia in LaPacho tea. (I have some of the ground up LaPacho bark in my kitchen cabinet, but to be quite honest, I'm afraid to try it. So far as I know, no scientific studies have been done on possible side effects or long term damage. In my own radical way, I'm very conservative!)

Nizoral

Nizoral is a widely available medication that effectively kills monilia. Don't forget, however, if your diet and nutritional supplements are not correct, the infection will only return again after discontinuing this or any other medication. I have seen brilliant results from the use of Nizoral; however, in my experience it's a dangerous drug and should only be taken under the close supervision of a physician experienced in its use. Liver function tests should be closely monitored; if they become abnormal, the drug should be discontinued. I check such tests carefully because almost every patient I've had on Nizoral had to be taken off the drug because of positive liver function tests.

Nystatin

Nystatin powder, oral, is usually the drug of choice. Your local doctor may not be familiar with the use of the oral powder, which is the only worthwhile form. Most pharmacies do not carry Nystatin powder for oral use. They will have the tablets (not very effective) or the powder for use on the skin (do *not* take that type by mouth). If your druggist wishes to stock Nystatin for you, he may order it in billion-unit batches from Lederle Laboratories: (800) 533-3753. The volume and weight of a unit vary from batch to batch. Your druggist may not want to order it because he has relatively few calls for it.

DIRECTIONS FOR TAKING NYSTATIN POWDER

Always take Nystatin in an inch or so of room-temperature water. Using a spoon, swish it back and forth to dissolve it. Then put the solution in the mouth and swish it around for two minutes before swallowing it. Take it first thing in the morning, last thing at night, and four times in between. Usually I start patients on ⅛ of a teaspoon, then gradually increase the amount to ½ to 1 teaspoon as I seek the best level.

Many doctors interested in Nystatin will tell you that no one is allergic to it. Not so. *Allergy to Nystatin is common;* reactions are generally dose-related and often it can be tolerated at a lower dosage.

During the first four days of taking Nystatin, patients may feel markedly worse. Reactions include nausea, dizziness, tiredness, headache—and almost any other symptom you can name. If the symptoms last more than four days, allergy must be considered and the dose adjusted accordingly.

I seldom find medication needed for the treatment of yeast infections. Diet plus vitamins and minerals will almost always take care of the problem.

The treatment of monilial infections, as you have gathered by now, is definitely not a do-it-yourself project.

CHAPTER TWENTY-SIX

FOOD, BRAIN CHEMISTRY AND "SOCIAL PROBLEMS"

It is the superb paradox of our time that in a single century we have proceeded from the first iron-clad warship to the first hydrogen bomb, and from the first telegraphic communication to the beginning of the conquest of space; yet in the understanding of our own nature, we have proceeded almost nowhere.

ROBERT ARDREY

WHY DID ARTHUR BREMER SHOOT GOVERNOR GEORGE WALLACE?

On May 15, 1972 Arthur H. Bremer shot George C. Wallace. Wallace, governor of Alabama, was campaigning in the democratic primaries to run for the presidency of the United States. The bullet left Governor Wallace paralyzed from the waist down.

On the day after the shooting, I read a newspaper article based on an interview with Arthur Bremer's mother.

The mother told the reporter, "He [her son] must have eaten something that disagreed with him."

The tone of the article sounded as if the reporter thought that Arthur Bremer's mother lacked human feelings, that she understood nothing about child-rearing or human relationships. The reporter left the impression that a mother with such a distorted view of life would naturally raise a son who would grow up to become a killer.

The mother's statement—"He must have eaten something that disagreed with him"—is one of the saddest quotes in all of history. Why?

Not for the reasons you think.

It's sad because what the mother said was undoubtedly true, yet because her statement—"He must have eaten something that disagreed with him"—did not fit within the framework of our society's general knowledge, she was totally rejected. Because of the reporter's and society's lack of information about food and brain chemistry, the mother's statement was taken as a sign of ignorance.

MOTHERS' SPECIALTY

I suppose it's not currently fashionable to say so, but mothers—whether college professors, housewives, or illiterate mountaineers smoking a corncob pipe—are specialists in the care and feeding of children. Mothers know when children want to eat, what they want to eat, and which foods agree with them and which do not.

Mothers, with their talent for making detailed observations about their children, know more about food incompatibilities than all the allergists put together. A mother knows that cabbage gives her child gas, or that her child becomes groggy and falls asleep after eating sweets, or that her child has diarrhea after drinking cow's milk.

Not rarely children become irritable and negativistic after eating wheat or other grain products.

Many children—and grownups—are constantly toxic from foods that they are unable to metabolize properly and hence do not notice a dramatic change after eating a toxic food. What we eat remains in our bodies from four days to a week. Hence if you are toxic from eating wheat in the form of cereal for breakfast and have wheat in the form of a doughnut for lunch and wheat in the form of a roll for dinner, you are always reacting from wheat.

If you load up on wheat by eating too much of your birthday cake, you may pass your body's capacity to handle wheat and develop symptoms. The next day you might feel irritable and depressed, for example. (Probably you will, however, incorrectly attribute your bad mood to being a year older.)

To test for wheat sensitivity, leave absolutely all grains out of your diet for 1 week, then eat a meal made up only of wheat. Have no more grains, and then another all-wheat meal the next day. For the ultimate wheat test, you might have an all-wheat meal for three days running.

(As always, check with your physician before carrying out any test or taking any supplement.)

Arthur H. Bremer's Mother

The reporter who interviewed Arthur Bremer's mother failed to consider that Mrs. Bremer might have special knowledge about her son's reaction to certain foods.

Many of my patients become angry and paranoid after eating certain foods, especially is that true of wheat. It's quite possible that Bremer's mother knew that he became angry and aggressive when he ate wheat (or some other food.) Perhaps Bremer ate wheat (or some other food that made him aggressive) in excessive amounts for day after day prior to the shooting. Possibly he ate a breakfast of wheat cakes on the morning of the shooting.

DR. KIM

The other day I saw a patient in my office, a psychiatrist I've been seeing on and off for years. He's quite sensitive to most foods and to many common environmental chemicals. As a result he must eat little else other than beef rib steaks.

He went to a medical meeting one night last week. He became hungry. During a break between speakers he left the building, went to a nearby fruit and vegetable stand, bought and ate a carrot. He knew he shouldn't have a carrot, but he thought he would just try one.

After eating the carrot and returning to the meeting, he found himself becoming more and more angry with the other psychiatrists at the meeting. During a question and answer session, he stood up and made some blazing remarks to one of the speakers on the hospital staff.

"My God, the carrot made me paranoid!" Dr. Kim realized when he sat down. Wisely, he left the meeting and went home, suspicious all the way.

Because you are probably eating other foods that give you toxic symptoms, you may not react in such a clear way to eating a food incompatible with your chemistry. As you become less toxic, your reactions will be more clearly highlighted.

TWENTY-THREE KILLED: GEORGE HENNARD BREAKS THE RECORD!

In Killeen, Texas George Hennard broke the mass murder record on October 16, 1991.

Sad-faced TV news announcers tell about the tragedy: twenty-three people murdered.

Then the next flash on the screen we see amusing plays featuring make-believe loving mothers feeding their children breakfast cereals: feeding them wheat products so they too can get their names in the headlines by breaking George Hennard's record!

Then come the TV "wise men" speculations: Hennard wasn't able to form stable relationships, Hennard had an unfulfilled childhood, Hennard was unemployed.

Nonsense. Hennard's brain—like the brains of Sir Robert McCarrison's mice, soon to be discussed—had been made toxic by the food he ate and he turned into a cannibal.

Take away the guns?

Not the solution. The Hennards of the world will simply blow up airplanes or start wars or derail a train as it crosses a canyon— or find how to trigger an atomic bomb.

ONLY TWO POSSIBLE SOLUTIONS

One:

Let Evolution continue her merry way and gradually kill off those people who cannot thrive on grains, milk, and sugar, and remove their genes from the human gene pool. (At the very least, come

Saturday night Hennard won't be having sex and passing along his genes.)

Two:

Remove grains, milk, and sugar from the human diet: let them eat vegetables, fruits, and mostly meats and animal fats.

We must make our choice: it's one or the other.

Don't blame me for setting mankind up that way: I didn't do it: speak to God about it: I only make observations.

DOHAN

Dohan at the University of Pennsylvania—you'll find some of his references in the bibliography at the end of the book—has been writing about the association between wheat and paranoid schizophrenia since the early 1960's. (Anger and paranoid schizophrenia are kissing cousins.)

I had a paper published on the subject in 1973.

No one's paid much attention to Dohan. Why should they? The pop crackle and snap breakfast cereal people have all the money, sponsor all of the "research," imprison all the minds with their clever ads.

The cereal people learned from Hitler: keep telling the common man a lie enough times long enough and a lie becomes the 14-carat truth.

I used to think Robert Atkins was a little paranoid when he spoke that way about the food processors. He was right. I was young and naive.

EXAMPLES AMONG MY PATIENTS

Last evening I talked with the father of one of my patients. We'll call his daughter Barbara. This usually attractive 19-year-old college student lives at home with her father. Several months ago he brought her to see me because of her outbreaks of anger, troubled social relationships, and difficulty concentrating on her school work.

Her moods rotated between depression, hell-raising, and anger.

By maneuvering her diet—by taking out first one group of foods and then another and later reintroducing them to her diet—I have other several months' time learned that her main incompatibilities are grains, milk and milk products, and table sugar: the usual story.

We also found that she had a vitamin B_6 and vitamin B_{12} dependency disorder. Giving these vitamins in large amounts considerably reduced her food sensitivities.

A short time ago this patient went to St. Louis to spend the weekend with a girlfriend. Barbara's girlfriend thinks her diet is silly. Barbara went wildly off her diet and ate ice cream, cake, hot cakes, Coca-Cola, and cheese.

When she returned home on Sunday evening, she physically attacked her father. (Her father told me he visits the gym regularly to keep in good shape so he can keep winning when Barbara attacks him!)

When Barbara visited me on the Monday following her holiday, nothing I could say pleased her. She argued about every point I tried to make. Usually we have a good relationship, but this time she became angry and accused me of having her visit my office too often.

You've seen people like her: hard exterior shell that you can't penetrate. Everything you say is wrong. You feel like telling them to go to hell and not to come back.

They are like Charlie when he's hungry at five in the afternoon.

In both cases they simply have disturbed brain chemistries that must be corrected before you can deal with them.

Barbara is by no means rare. I see patients like her all the time. The other day after cheating on her diet, one of the patients said, "To hell with your diet!" and walked out of my office as I reminded her, "It's not my diet. It's your diet."

Another multimillionaire who has an enormous apartment on the best part of Park Avenue went on a trip, cheated on his diet, got angry with me and walked out without paying his bill.

You don't need to visit Harlem or an Indian reservation to find poor relationships. Toxicity is everywhere.

Breakfast cereals should show news clips of people attacking and killing each other, not smiling actresses acting like loving mothers.

SIR ROBERT'S WORLD

In England, Sir Robert McCarrison and H. M. Sinclair used a large cage to build a world they could control. They populated their experimental world with twenty laboratory mice. When the mice were fed rough, straight-from-the-farm-food, they had slick, smooth hair. They remained free of disease.

Not only did the mice thrive physically, but they were happy and lived together peacefully without complications.

McCarrison and Sinclair then changed the diet from straight-from-the-farm foods to processed foods: white bread, jam, sugar-laden products and canned meats.

The mice stopped living in harmony. They turned restless and tense. They tried to bite their attendants; they fought with each other and killed each other; three of the animals not only killed their companions but cannibalized them.

Why did "social problems" develop?

What we see as "social problems" are only reflections of disrupted brain chemistry caused by deficiencies of victims, minerals, and fats, and by eating foods incompatible with the biochemistry of individuals.

"Social problems" are symptoms, not causes.

THE WORLD OF THE SALVATION ARMY

In London, the Salvation Army studied seventeen delinquent girls, ages 11 to 15 living in their world. While eating a diet in which most of their calories came from processed foods—white bread, margarine, jam, sweetened tea, and canned meats—the girls had become a problem both to themselves and to society.

After they stopped eating processed foods and ate whole foods, their complexions improved, they developed a feeling of well-being. Although formerly bored, they began taking an interest in life. They quickly became less aggressive, less angry, less quarrelsome. Their antisocial behavior disappeared.

Dozens of studies have revealed similar correlations between foods eaten and behavior. (If you're interested in more details, the bibliography at the end of this book lists articles by Swanson, Prinz, King, Rapp, O'Banion, Schoenthaler, Politt, Newbold, and others.)

Again, what we see as "social problems" are only reflections of disrupted brain chemistry caused by deficiencies of vitamins, minerals, and unsaturated fats, and by eating foods (incompatible with the biochemistry of the individual's brain hemistry.

"Social problems" are symptoms, not causes.

WE LIVE IN SIR ROBERT'S WORLD

Like the laboratory mice living in Sir Robert's miniature world, we too live in a miniature world floating through the infinity of space.

Most people—even scientists, and especially politicians—do not accept that all of us—including Popes, presidents, dictators, kings, and senators—are, like the white mice in Sir Robert's world, a collection of chemical reactions.

Because we are a collection of busily bubbling chemical reactions does not mean that we cannot fashion a Pietà from raw stone or string words together to construct a sonnet. Without his bubbling chemistry, however, Michelangelo would have fashioned no Pietà. When Shakespeare's chemistry sputtered to an end, so did his clever pen.

THE RETURN OF CHARLIE

Do you remember Charlie, the 5-year-old who became combative at 5 o'clock and struck his mother because he was hungry? Do you remember how he calmed down and lost his "social problem" and became lovable after his mother fed him?

Had your son Charlie been an African-American and had you given him a glass of milk to solve his biochemical problem (hunger), you might have solved one problem only to cause a second problem: *Charlie might have stopped his combative behavior only to become sleepy, sullen, and depressed.*

Harrison's textbook of medicine says, "Five to fifteen percent of the adult white population shows intestinal lactase deficiency, but in black Americans, Bantus, and orientals, the incidence has been reported as high as eighty to ninety percent."

Similar figures are widely quoted. (Blacks from the Masai tribe in Africa and a few other milk-consuming tribes are exceptions. Evolution adapted their biochemistry to effectively metabolize milk.)

The widespread belief that lactase intolerance (a lack of an enzyme needed to metabolize milk sugar) only causes stomach or intestinal upsets is false. Both cerebral and generalized manifestations of toxicity—such as mental dullness, depression and physical tiredness—are the rule. For example, in his 1621 treatise entitled *The Anatomy of Melancholy,* Robert Burton stated, "Milk and all that comes from milk increase melancholy."

Dr. Joe Edozien, professor of nutrition at the University of North Carolina and an authority on the biochemistry of blacks, tells me that blacks utilize calcium more efficiently than whites. Blacks lay down more calcium in their bones at an earlier age and have fewer problems with osteoporosis.

Possibly an intolerance to cow's milk was designed by evolution to protect blacks from excessive calcium.

African-American Principal

I once had an African-American patient who was the principal of a grammer school attended mostly by African-American children. She knew that studies showed that a high percentage of African-Americans and African-Africans suffer from milk intolerance. She and the teachers had observed that after the students drank milk they became withdrawn, sullen, and sleepy: entirely unreceptive to learning.

In spite of strong efforts, she found herself unable to keep milk out of the school. When she explained the problem to her superior, he stated that the Federal government required all schools to serve milk. When she approached her congressman, he referred her to a committee chairman in Washington. When she contacted the chairman, he suggested that she speak with the FDA. Around and around my patient traveled on a bureaucratic road to nowhere.

Several years later I had a patient who was high in the politics of the milk industry. When I told him about the African-American principal's attempt to keep milk out of her school, the patient chuckled and said that the milk industry spent millions of dollars every year to make milk mandatory for schools. Millions were contributed to the champagne funds of congressmen and senators in an attempt to equate cow's milk with good health, motherhood and the American flag.

When I mentioned that blacks often suffer from milk intolerance, his comment was, "They got their problems, we got ours."

(Compare a photograph of your mother's face with a photograph of a cow's face. Not very similar, are they? Still, their faces are more alike than their milk.)

It would seem that most blacks exposed to milk would not only be poorer students, but later would perform less well and thus take home less money when they sell their services in the marketplace. Indeed, the depression brought on in part by the use of milk would make street drugs more attractive to African-Americans than to Euro-Americans.

What a pity that African-American leaders do not use their resources in more positive ways, such as removing cow's milk and milk products from African-Americans' diet!

THE FOLLOWING WORDS ARE THE MOST IMPORTANT YOU WILL EVER READ

In our original discussion of the 5-year-old Charlie at 5 o'clock in the afternoon, after correcting Charlie's biochemical problem by feeding him, Charlie's aggressive behavior disappeared. Once again he smiled and welcomed hugs of affection. He could happily play with his toy space ship or concentrate and sit still while listening to a fairy tale.

If fed milk, the African-American Charlie turned sleepy, sullen, and depressed.

The simple act of feeding both Charlies completely changed the biochemistry of their brains and thus changed their behavior.

If you can fully understand and appreciate the three paragraphs above, you will understand not only why Bremer shot Governor Wallace, but much more about our world.

Now you know why our prisons grow every year, why our medical bills soar, why insane people camp on our streets, why families live on welfare generation after generation.

Incidentally, you also know why Johnny can't read.

FACTS AND SPECULATIONS

Hitler would not have started World War II if he had not disrupted his brain chemistry by being a sweet- and junk-eating vegetarian.

In the Middle East they have been eating wheat longer than any other place on earth. What has it done to the people's brain chemistries?

My prediction is that we will never see the end of the conflicts in the Middle East until all people made aggressive by wheat incompatibilities kill off each other and their genes are removed from the genetic pool in the Middle East. They have a chemical problem, not a social problem.

What would happen if we put an embargo on the entire Middle East to keep all grains, milk and milk products, and table sugar out of the area and let them eat meat, vegetables, and fruits?

Probably they would stop fighting. Probably their "social problems" would fade away like the morning dew.

Such a course would be far less expensive than building bombers, missile launchers, and atom bombs.

We've tried bombers, missile launchers, and atom bombs and learned they have not settled the problems.

Why not try my way? Why not be scientific and experiment with new approaches? Will the minds of mankind stay locked into the rigid patterns of the authoritative Middle Ages forever?

> *History is little more than the register of the crimes, follies, and misfortunes of mankind.*
> —GIBBON

> *We're two-footed animals gobbling wheat and chocolate bars, killing, dancing, and copulating to a tune played by Evolution.*
> —NEWBOLD

Here's how prison riots and hijackings should be handled:

Send in water, fresh red meats and fish, fresh raw vegetables, and fresh raw fruits. Send in no tobacco, grains, table sugar, milk or milk products. No processed foods.

Within five days the rioters and hijackers would lose interest in disruptive behavior.

Johnny can't read (or do much of anything else except watch TV and shoot at arcade figures) because his brain is carbohydrate junk-food shot. That's why the people in the world get angrier and crazier every year and will keep on getting angrier and crazier as long as we follow the Pied Pipers pushing grains, table sugar, milk and milk products, and processed foods.

Why will people follow a leader to war and death, but won't follow a leader into a junk-food-free land and life?

As Charles Darwin said:
With me the horrid doubt always arises as to whether the convictions of man's mind, which has been developed from the lower animals, are of any value or are at all trustworthy.

As Robert Adrey said:
We are creatures of reason only in our own eyes.
We are a mathematical improbability.

We are an evolutionary failure, trapped between earth and a glimpse of heaven, prevented by our sure capacity for self-delusion from achieving any triumph more noteworthy than our own self-destruction.

A FEW LAST WORDS

Don't bother visiting an allergist for diagnosis and treatment. Allergists don't understand food and environment incompatibilities. Allergists say that only 1% of the population has food allergies. That's absolutely not true. The figure is closer to 99%.

The average allergists spends fifteen to thirty minutes with new patients. He then orders various allergy tests, usually skin tests and/or blood tests. The tests, especially for food and environmental substances, are close to meaningless.

For example, the skin may react to a skin test for apple. That doesn't mean that the brain also reacts to apple. And what kind of apple is he testing you for: Granny Smith, Yellow Delicious, Red Delicious? He doesn't know.

Also, usually he doesn't know that people react differently to different types of apples. People may even react differently to Granny Smith apples grown in France and Granny Smith apples grown in Washington state. The soils are different, therefore the chemical composition of the apples is different.

People react differently when the apple is not quite ripe and when the apple is fully ripe and juicy.

I can eat Yellow Delicious apples without reacting at certain times of the year. If they've been stored too long, I react unfavorably to them.

Also, the volume of the food eaten is important. Some people can eat one apple every third day without reacting, but react if they eat an apple every day.

Allergies are too complicated to handle in the superficial, mechanistic ways they are handled by most allergists. Most allergists practice good show business, but they do little or nothing to cure patients.

I spend 15 to 30 minutes every week or two with every patient, usually for week after week until I carefully go over exactly what they eat and how they react to it. I have them eat one food at a time and write down their reactions, sometimes 3 or 4 times with each food.

I get to know the patient and the patient's biochemical requirements.

What allergists have patients keep food diaries to correlate their symptoms (including mental symptoms) with what they eat and to what environmental toxins they are exposed?

None do. If they did, they would be poor like me.

The other day an allergist told me he would never recommend my books for his patients as long as I advocated no in-office testing!

If allergists did that they would cut their incomes by half, as I did when I stopped in-office testing. Understandably, they fight my approach.

To tell you the truth, allergists don't even understand inhalant allergic reaction to things like ragweed.

If you remove things in the environment and food to which people react, ragweed allergies disappear on their own.

I ought to know. I've had an allergy to ragweed since 1924 and have had a good chance to observe it first hand.

Example of what I mean: if I cheat and eat something that I'm allergic to in February, I may become tired, or grouchy, or develop dandruff.

If I eat that same cheat during the ragweed season, I get the above symptoms *plus sneezing and itching eyes.*

If I don't cheat and eat foods to which I'm sensitive during the ragweed season, I have no symptoms from high ragweed pollen counts.

Unlike the public beliefs, people are not allergic to one thing. It's one thing on top of another that pushes them into a reaction.

And so it goes. . . .

VITAMINS, MINERALS, AND UNSATURATED FATS

One of the most important facts about the brain is its enormous biochemical activity. The brain is a seething cauldron of chemical activity. The human brain makes up only 2% of the body's weight yet uses 25% of the body's energy. Because of the brain's extraordinary biochemical activity, any defects in its chemistry will be magnified. A small change in the brain's nutrients will make enormous differences in how it performs.

In my view everyone should take nutritional supplements. The truth is that no one knows just how much. We know how much vitamin C will keep you from developing scurvy, which is only the last desperate stage of a vitamin C deficiency. The question is, how much vitamin C do you need to keep from getting pneumonia? How much vitamin C do you need to become mayor of your town instead of dog catcher? How much vitamin C does a baseball player need to take to hit 302 instead of 232?

Those not knowledgeable about nutrition (and those simply hostile toward everything having to do with nutrition) will tell you that you will simply lose excess vitamins in your urine.

True, but your brain and the rest of your body will be able to use them while they're still in your body.

Ask them: Why drink excess water? You will only excrete it as urine. Yet few people advocate drinking less water.

Those opposing good nutrition simply don't know. Most of them don't spend their days and months and years in an office with sick people they cure by using purely nutritional techniques.

It's nice to stay out of the poorhouse, the crazy house, and the jailhouse. It's even better to feel great and to be able to develop your full potential as a human being.

If we are on the wrong food and drink and do not have proper supplements, we are not likely to reach our potential.

If I eat wheat, it shoots down my brain's ability to correlate information. When I come to write in the morning, some facts I need are over here and some over there. I can't properly integrate them into the needed whole.

That's one reason I don't eat wheat.

It's not that I'm following a banner. It's not that I'm a great and noble person. It's that eating wheat paralyzes a part of me that I don't want paralyzed. For purely selfish reasons, I don't eat wheat.

You say wheat doesn't do that to you.

You never know until you leave out all grains, then test them one by one.

(But only with your physician's approval and supervision.)

If you have any "mental," "emotional," or physical symptom, the chances are it's caused by a hypersensitivity.

No matter what the X-ray picture shows—whether spurs, arthritis, chips of bone floating in the joint—the ex-football player with a painful knee is probably having the pain because of a food or environmental incompatibility—no matter what his orthopedist has told him.

The same is true of your emotions—no matter what your psychiatrist has said about your sad childhood and the boss that doesn't understand you, your real troubles and the answer to those troubles almost surely lie in the field of food and environmental sensitivities, and nutritional supplements.

THE CRAZIES

> *If we all worked on the assumption that what is accepted as true is true, there would be little hope of advance.*
>
> ORVILLE WRIGHT

My Grandfather Newbold owned a moving company (moving company!—one T-model Ford and one dear old African-American semi-alcoholic employee named Garland who would buy me delicious vanilla ice cream cones and help my grandfather lift the furniture) in Elizabeth City, North Carolina.

One December day in 1903, my grandfather returned home for supper and told my grandmother, "I moved a flying machine off a railroad car and loaded it onto the Fulton. A couple of crazy fool Yankee brothers named Wright are going down to Nag's Head to try to fly. They'll get their necks broke for sure. Pretty soon I'll be loading them back on the train in pine boxes."

(The Fulton was a coastal freighter that plied the Pasquotank River, the Albemarle Sound, and neighboring waters.)

PEOPLE THINK THEY PRETTY MUCH KNOW WHAT GOES ON IN THE WORLD

If a person doesn't believe what we believe and see the world as we see it, then there's something wrong with the other person. He's primitive, uneducated, stupid, or downright crazy.

Whether the explanations people cherish are scientifically true is of little importance as long as their beliefs are generally believed and accepted by their neighbors.

We humans hold "truths" dear. What we see as truth gives us security, peace of mind.

We have come to believe that all the people of the world need to be happy and cooperative and to live in harmony is good housing, adequate food, and more love: especially love.

Yet a moment's thought will tell you that such is not true.

We believe that people grow up to become criminals because they were treated cruelly by their parents, or because they didn't have enough love, or because they had poor housing or didn't finish school.

Like most things we believe, that's not true.

WHAT IS TRUE?

You and I are a skin full of bubbling chemical reactions.

If your chemistry doesn't go right, your world won't go right.

If you want a better life, you had jolly well better get your chemistry straight.

STRUCTURAL FATS

If you never read another word, read a book by Michael and Sheilagh Crawford entitled *What We Eat Today,* published in 1972 by Neville Spearman Limited, London.

At the time the Crawfords wrote the book, Michael Crawford headed the department of biochemistry at the Nuffield Institute of Comparative Medicine in London.

The main point made by the book: 60% of the human brain is made from what is called structural fat, a fat that cannot be made by the body, but must be eaten.

Structural fat occurs in fish and meats.

Because a large percentage of the human brain is formed during pregnancy, children can be born with normal brains only if their mothers eat structural fats, i.e., meats and/or fish, while carrying the baby.

By abnormal brains, I don't mean that the child will be mentally defective. I mean the child will grow up to be a killer, a pill taker, a member of society with difficulties relating with other people, a preacher or senator who can't stop fornicating, an alcoholic, an unhappy multimillionaire, a Hussein, a Hitler, or maybe your next-door neighbor who constantly fights with you about your leaves falling on his side of the fence.

You don't want to give birth to such a person. The world already has too many of them—and their numbers and percentage are growing every year.

Because it discourages the eating of fatty meats, the present insanity about cholesterol greatly helps in the destruction of the human brain. The crazies and ne'er-do-wells in our world are increasing. People are angry and looking for excuses to shout and curse and break windows and kill.

Browned, burned, and old meat and fish fats do not help the body in any way and indeed harm the body in many ways. Fats cooked with gas are carcinogenic and dangerous in other ways.

BREAST FEEDING

The developing fetus can have a normal brain only if the mother eats structural fats. The infant after birth can continue developing a normal brain only if it gets generous quantities of structural fats. The infant's structural fats can only come from good-quality human milk rich in structural fat.

Cow's milk, goat's milk and other milks of lower animals contain only trace amounts of structural fat. Unlike humans, cows and goats do not need to grow large brains in proportion to their body size; therefore, their young need less structural fats than do human infants. The relative brain size of humans is 50 times that of a cow!

Incidentally, the blood vessels of carnivorous mammals—like man, especially man—are also dependent upon a generous supply of structural fat. For that reason, most research done on cholesterol and hardening of the arteries has no bearing on the needs of man.

Mothers who do not nurse their babies for two full years are doing a great disservice to their young and to the human race. If they fail to nurse their infants for two years, mothers are robbing their babies of their most precious and human birthright: a normal brain.

The ability of humans to successfully reproduce seems also to be tied in with the amount of structural fat available to the developing brain.

While nursing, it's especially important for nursing mothers to eat a generous amount of structural fat. They must also have generous amounts of calcium and magnesium supplements, and vitamin D. That is their absolute minimum requirement.

Never take calcium without also taking magnesium, about 2 parts of calcium to one part of magnesium.

Other supplements are desirable. (Ask your physician for advice and guidance. Give him this book to read.)

After age two the infant's milk enzyme levels change, and with them the ability to use milk changes. No children, or anyone else, should have any milk or milk product after age two. This milk abstinence is important for whites but even more important for blacks and orientals.

(Two exceptions: I suspect many people can handle butter, especially clarified butter, without difficulty. As mentioned, some people, the Masai in Africa, for example, have been designed by evolution to handle milk products even as adults.)

Of course children should have generous amounts of structural fats, calcium, magnesium, vitamin D and other supplements. Seek your physician's advice.

It's easy to understand why evolution has given both men and women a compelling interest in the female breast. Within the womanly breast lies the future of mankind, both mankind's temperament and intelligence.

> *That the art of the physician is grounded on cooperation with nature is so well known, so intrinsically obvious, one would suppose that the point does not need repetition. Alas, I think it does. In this book I shall argue, among other things, that orthodox medical training has already drifted dangerously far from this fundamental perception of the physician's role.*
> —ROGER WILLIAMS

> *The doctor of the future will give no medicine but will interest his patients in the care of the human frame, in diet, and in the cause and prevention of disease.*
> —THOMAS A. EDISON

WHICH VITAMINS DO WHAT?

Here, for quick reference, are notes about the biochemistry of some of the more important vitamins.

I've included some information about which vitamins work together. This is to remind you that every cell in the body needs every vitamin and that every vitamin depends upon another to do its job.

I have also included a brief list of the chief dietary sources of each vitamin because natural crude sources of vitamins are always important. I have not attempted to report exactly how much of each vitamin is contained in each food, because, as you know, that fluctuates wildly according to where the food was produced, how long it has been stored, and how it is cooked. And I repeat, you should not rely on food sources alone to provide an adequate intake of vitamins.

While it's accepted medical practice to group vitamins according to whether they are fat- or water-soluble, I have chosen to list them here in alphabetical order for the sake of clarity.

Vitamin A. Fat-soluble.

Chief Functions: When adequately supplied, vitamin A helps maintain normal growth and bone development; it helps to provide protective sheathing around nerve fibers; and it helps to maintain healthy skin, hair and nails. It's especially crucial to healthy vision.

Vitamin A is present in the eyes themselves and is used up in the process of seeing; when it is deficient the eye has trouble processing light, particularly bright or artificial light. Vitamin A helps to maintain healthy mucus in the respiratory system, and thus helps to fight infection and allergic symptoms. There is mush evidence that vitamin A helps protect against some types of cancer.

Symptoms of Deficiency: Impaired vision, particularly "night blindness" and sensitivity to bright lights; poor growth and bone development, especially in children; impaired hormone production; dandruff, or other dryness or itching of skin and scalp; rough skin, especially over the back of the upper arms; dry brittle nails; susceptibility to colds and allergies; tooth decay.

Works With: Vitamins B_2, B_{12}, C, D, and especially E.

Factors Affecting Need: Exposure to bright or artificial lights, watching movies and television; exposure to environmental pollutants including air pollution, cigarette smoke, and toxic food additives such as sodium benzoate; insufficient proteins, fats, and liver bile (impairs absorption); liver damage.

Best Dietary Sources: Yellow fruits and vegetables such as carrots, yams, winter squash, peaches, and apricots; also spinach, parsley, turnip greens and other dark green leafy vegetables; liver, including fish liver and fish liver oils.

Minimum Daily Intake: 5,000 IU.

Overdose Symptoms: (Usually brought on by a daily intake of 50,000 to 100,000 IU over several months. A few people might be made toxic by doses as low as 25,000 IU per day over a period of time.) Headaches, nerve damage (with attendant nervous symptoms); fatigue, insomnia, loss of appetite, pain in bones and joints, jaundice, loss of hair.

Where Stored: Liver and kidneys. It is believed that vitamin A helps the liver to detoxify environmental poisons.

How Long Stored: Long term storage.

Vitamin B₁ (Thiamine). Water-soluble.

Chief functions: Helps in carbohydrate metabolism, growth, maintaining appetite and good digestion, and in nerve function.

Symptoms of Deficiency: Beri-beri; heart pain or failure; nerve death; depression, tension, insomnia, forgetfulness; weight loss; numbness in extremities; swelling in ankles and elsewhere.

Works With: Vitamins B_2, B_3, B_6, C, D, and pantothenic acid.

Factors Affecting Need: While it is present in many foods it is easily destroyed by soaking and cooking; older people may fail to absorb it adequately.

Best Dietary Sources: Wheat germ, yeast, rice bran, soy flour, ham, beans, eggs, beef, pork, lamb, turkey, mushrooms.

Minimum Daily Intake: 1.5 mg.

Overdose Symptoms: Edema, restlessness, sweating, rapid heart beat, cold sores; trembling, low blood pressure, liver disorders; vitamin B_6 deficiency.

Where Stored: Heart, liver, kidney, brain.

How Long Stored: Short term storage.

Vitamin B₂ (Riboflavin). Water-soluble.

Chief functions: Necessary in every cell in body; especially helps maintain respiratory system mucous membranes; necessary to healthy skin and eye tissue.

Symptoms of Deficiency: Dandruff; skin lesions, cracks in the corners of the mouth; inflamed tongue and mouth; nerve degeneration; hormonal defects; sensitivity to bright light, and other visual difficulty.

Works With: Vitamins A, B_1, B_3, B_6, B_{12}, folic acid, panthothenic acid, and biotin.

Factors Affecting Need: Riboflavin is easily lost in urine (i.e., your need may be increased if you drink and pass a lot of liquid); it is destroyed by light.

Best Dietary Sources: Yeast, kidney, liver, heart, avocados, beans, green vegetables, wheat germ.

Minimum Daily Intake: 1.7 mg.

Overdose Symptoms: Tingling in extremities; itching.
Where Stored: Heart, liver, kidney.
How Long Stored: Short term storage.

Vitamin B₃ (Niacin, Niacinamide, Nicotinic acid). Water-soluble.

Chief Functions: Co-enzyme in your fat metabolism (important in controlling blood fat levels); principally significant in complex chemical interactions affecting the working of the nervous system. For this reason, niacin has been critically important in the nutritional treatment of some forms of mental illness.

Symptoms of Deficiency: Pellegra (dementia, dermatitis, diarrhea); depression, nervousness, weakness, insomnia, headache; loss of appetite.

Works With: Vitamins B_1, B_2, B_6, B_{12}, D, panothenic acid.

Factors Affecting Need: While much may be lost in cooking, or through impaired absorption caused by illness, it is likely that one of the greatest thieves of niacin stores is emotional stress, which is also the most typical symptom of niacin deficiency.

Best Dietary Sources: Yeast, liver, heart, turkey, chicken, peanuts, tuna, halibut, swordfish.

Minimum Daily Intake: 20 mg.

Overdose symptoms: Nausea; vomiting; activation of peptic ulcer.

Where Stored: Liver, heart, muscle.

How Long Stored: Short term storage.

Vitamin B₆ (Pyridoxine). Water-soluble.

Chief Functions: Important in red blood cell formation and in production of hormones in the central nervous system. Used in metabolism of carbohydrates, fats, and all proteins.

Deficiency Symptoms: Nervous disorders, convulsions, tension, rashes; blood disorders; hardening of the arteries; edema.

Works With: Vitamins B_1, B_2, B_3, folic acid, biotin, C, E, and adrenalin.

Factors Affecting Need: Rapidly destroyed by heat (i.e., lost in cooking); also easily lost in water, through soaking food or frequent urination; B_6 is affected by estrogen levels. Nausea or morning sickness caused by pregnancy or the Pill is often helped by additional B_6. Since B_6 is used in protein metabolism, a high protein diet often causes a need for extra B_6.

Best Dietary Sources: Yeast, beef and pork liver, salmon, herring, brown rice, bananas, and pears.

Minimum Daily Intake: 2.5 mg.

Overdose symptoms: Nerve damage with numbness, tingling, loss of balance, etc., reported from doses of 2,000 mg or more daily.

Where Stored: Skeletal muscles.

How Long Stored: Short term storage.

Vitamin B_{12} (Cobalamin). Water-soluble

Chief Function: Used in production of nucleic acid (therefore important to the health of all body cells); affects protein and fat cells, including production of genetic material DNA and RNA; used to maintain sheaths on nerve tissue; important in blood formation.

Deficiency Symptoms: Poor growth, inflamed tongue; disturbed carbohydrate metabolism; fatigue; anemia, including pernicious anemia; spinal cord degeneration; brain degeneration; any emotional disorder up to and including insanity.

Works With: Vitamins A, C, E, B_1, folic acid, biotin, and pantothenic acid.

Factors Affecting Need: Vegetarian diet or any diet low in animal protein may cause B_{12} deficiency. Many people cannot absorb B_{12} when taken orally. In such people, B_{12} body levels can only be maintained by injections.

Best Dietary Sources: Lamb and beef kidney, lamb, beef and pork liver; beef brain; egg yolk; clams, sardines, oysters, crabs, salmon, herring.

Minimum Daily Intake: 6-8 mcg per day.

Overdose Symptoms: Generally unknown except for a possible high hemoglobin count.

Where Stored: Liver, lungs, kidney, spleen.

How Long Stored: Long term storage.

Folic Acid. Water-soluble.

Chief Functions: Many complex metabolic functions; important in production of nucleic acid, thus necessary to all body cells; important to maintaining healthy blood count.

Deficiency Symptoms: Intestinal disorders; fatigue; low white blood count; pernicious anemia; depression, nervousness; brain damage.

Works With: Biotin, pantothenic acid; B_1, B_2, B_3, B_6, B_{12}, C, E, and sex hormones in male and female.

Factors Affecting Need: Illness, intestinal disorders, genetic factors or aging may cause poor absorption; as much as 75% may be excreted in urine, and even greater urine loss may be caused by high vitamin C intake.

Best Dietary Sources: Yeast, dark green leafy vegetables such as spinach and beet greens; liver; asparagus; dried legumes such as lentils, navy beans; wheat.

Minimum Daily Intake: 4 mg.

Overdose Symptoms: None. However, the absence of either B_{12} or folic acid in the system can produce pernicious anemia, and if folic acid is taken while B_{12} is not, a patient can have irreversible nervous damage caused by a B_{12} deficiency without having the blood signs of the disease. For that reason, a prescription is required for 1 mg tablets.

Where Stored: Liver.

How Long Stored: Short term storage.

Vitamin D. Fat-soluble.

Chief Functions: Regulates calcium and phosphorous metabolism; necessary for bone growth; important in nerve excitation.

Deficiency Symptoms: Rickets; poor bone growth; increase in nervous system irritability caused by low blood calcium and phosphorous.

Works With: B_3, A, calcium, phosphorous; sunlight.

Factors Affecting Need: Growing children need more vitamin D; older people may need more to prevent loss of calcium from bones;

since vitamin D is made on the skin with sunlight, people whose clothing and lifestyle keep them out of the sun may need more; it is believed that dark-skinned people living in northern climates may not synthesize enough vitamin D; similarly for people who live where the sunlight is cut by smog.

Best Dietary Sources: Fish liver oils; egg yolks; fish.

Minimum Daily Intake: 400 IU.

Overdose Symptoms: loss of appetite; weakness; nausea; thirst; diarrhea joint pains; frequent urination; hardening of arteries; calcium deposits in tissues.

Where Stored: Liver, skin.

How Long Stored: Long term storage.

Vitamin E (Tocopherol). Fat-soluble.

Chief Functions: Promotes normal growth; aids normal functioning of muscle, vascular, and nerve cells; antioxidant (important for protecting essential fatty acids); aids absorption of unsaturated fats; acts as detoxifying agent; fights stress.

Deficiency Symptoms: Diarrhea; anemia; gall bladder disorders; liver diseases; fibrosis of pancreas; muscle weakness; nervous disorders; skin disorders, degeneration of reproductive tissue.

Works With: Vitamin A, B_6, B_{12}, C, K, folic acid; estrogen, testosterone.

Factors Affecting Need: Nervous or environmental stress increases your need for vitamin E; since it is used to protect unsaturated fats in the body, preventing them from turning rancid, a diet high in unsaturated fats will increase your need for vitamin E. Much is lost in heat from cooking and food processing; much is lost when foods are frozen.

Best Dietary Sources: Cold-pressed vegetable oils, especially safflower or sunflower oil; yeast; cabbage, spinach, asparagus.

Minimum Daily Intake: 30 IU.

Overdose Symptoms: Elevated blood pressure.

Where Stored: Muscle, fatty tissue.

How Long Stored: Short term storage.

APPENDIX TWO

REDUCING SERUM CHOLESTEROL BY FEEDING A HIGH ANIMAL FAT DIET

ABSTRACT

Multiple food allergies required a group of seven patients with higher than ideal serum cholesterol levels to follow a diet in which most of the calories came from beef fat. They were given nutritional supplements. Their diets contained no sucrose, milk, or grains. So far as the author has been able to learn, this is the only group of people in recent times to follow such a diet.

The triglyceride levels fell from an average of 113 mg/dl to 74 mg/dl in the study group patients.

At the same time, the patients in the group had a reduction of serum cholesterol from an average initial value of 263 mg/dl to an average of 189 mg/dl.

At the beginning of the study, patients had an average HDL% of 21. At the end of the study, the six patients retested had the HDL% rise to an average of 34.

The findings raise an interesting question: Are elevated serum cholesterol levels caused in part not by eating animal fat (an extremely "old food"), but by some factor in grains, sucrose or milk

345

("new foods") that interferes with cholesterol metabolism? Because the fat that accompanies red meats such as lamb, pork, and beef is high in cholesterol, it has been advised that such meats be eaten in limited quantities to help lower serum cholesterol levels and thus prevent coronary artery disease (CAD).

Nichols et al, however, reported that blood cholesterol studies on 4,057 people in Tecumseh, Michigan, showed no correlation between their diets and their serum cholesterol levels.

Others have found a relationship between serum cholesterol levels and types of carbohydrates eaten. For example, when sucrose replaced maize in a rat diet containing 0.5% cholesterol, serum cholesterol levels were raised.

Wiebe, Bruce, and McDonald discovered that a diet in which 55% of the protein came from beef raised serum HDL values, lowered serum triglycerides, and brought about no change in serum cholesterol levels.

It is generally agreed that raising serum HDL levels is especially important in the prevention of CAD.

Recently a national campaign has been mounted to make the general public aware of the importance of lowering serum cholesterol levels. The National Institutes of Health has advocated that serum cholesterol levels be maintained below 200 mg/cc.

PATIENTS AND METHODS

The author has treated a group of food-allergic patients who at the time of their initial visit were eating ordinary, varied American diets. They had higher than ideal cholesterol levels.

It was discovered that each of these patients could best tolerate beef rib steaks. For varying lengths of time these patients ate mostly unaged beef rib steaks. Some of the patients were able to tolerate lamb, pork, or chicken if eaten no more than once every three or four days. These patients occasionally ate pork, lamb, or chicken in place of the rib steak. They seldom ate other cuts of beef.

Because it has been observed that many patients have allergic reactions to meats cooked in gas-fired ovens, each patient cooked the meat with heat from electricity. Patients were instructed to ask their butchers to leave a large percentage of the fat on the steaks. After cooking, the burned or browned fat was thrown away. Only the white fat was eaten. (Browned or burned fat may be carcinogenic. Also, burned or browned fat is highly toxic. Patients may experience abdominal discomfort, tiredness and/or a number of other unpleasant symptoms if burned fat is eaten.) In order to satisfy caloric needs, patients were instructed to eat as much of the fat as they could comfortably tolerate.

The only other foods eaten were: zero to one cup of fresh raw vegetables one to three times a day, and zero to three cups of fresh raw fruit one to three times a day. No seasoning. Once or twice a week some of the patients had chicken, fish, pork, or a different cut of beef in place of the rib steak. They drank only bottled spring water (or self-distilled water), at least 1.5 liters daily.

The patients were given supplements of vitamins A, B complex, C, D, E, and polyunsaturated fat, 30 ml daily. They also took calcium, magnesium, selenium, and zinc.

Serum Cholesterol, Triglyceride, and HDL Levels on Patients Before and After High Animal Fat Diets

The blood for each laboratory test was drawn at 9 A.M. after the patient had fasted from 10 P.M. the night before. State-approved commercial laboratories performed the tests. Units for the figures given are mg/dl.

CASE 1. A 35-year-old white male.

First visit:		*Nine months later:*	
cholesterol	278	cholesterol	188
triglycerides	165	triglycerides	69
HDL	35	HDL	58
% HDL	13	% HDL	30
glucose	118	glucose	93

CASE 2. A 48-year-old white male.

First visit:		*Six months later:*	
cholesterol	298	cholesterol	191
triglycerides	149	triglycerides	87
HDL	57	HDL	65
% HDL	19	% HDL	34

CASE 3. A 56-year-old white male. At his first visit he was on oral medication in an attempt to reduce his blood sugar. The medication was discontinued after two weeks.

First visit:		After 12 weeks:	
cholesterol	234	cholesterol	166
triglycerides	102	triglycerides	75
HDL	40	HDL	32
% HDL	17	% HDL	19
blood sugar	216	blood sugar	98

CASE 4. A 58-year-old white female.

First visit:		One and a half years later:	
cholesterol	327	cholesterol	209
triglycerides	65	triglycerides	58
HDL	90	HDL	87
% HDL	28	% HDL	42

CASE 5. A 60-year-old white male.

First visit:		Four months later:	
cholesterol	224	cholesterol	168
triglycerides	128	triglycerides	84
HDL	47	HDL	42
% HDL	21	% HDL	25

CASE 6. A 63-year-old white male. At the time of his first visit he was eating a "low cholesterol diet" that included lean red meat only once a week.

First visit:		Three months later:	
cholesterol	252	cholesterol	220
triglycerides	92	triglycerides	75
HDL	74	HDL	92
% HDL	29	% HDL	42

CASE 7. A 72-year-old black male.

First visit:		*Five months later:*	
cholesterol	228	cholesterol	183
triglycerides	90	triglycerides	68
HDL	100	HDL not repeated	
% HDL	42		

RESULTS

Before starting a diet high in animal fat, a group of seven patients had an average serum cholesterol of 263. On a diet free of milk products, grains, and sucrose in which most of the calories came from beef fat, their average serum cholesterol levels fell to 189.

At the same time their triglycerides fell from an average of 113 to 74.

One of the patients failed to have a repeat HDL test.

In the 6 patients retested for HDL, the HDL percentages rose from 21 to 34.

COMMENT

Anthropologists generally agree that mankind ate a diet low in grains, sucrose, and milk products and high in meat and animal fat ("old foods") for 2.2 million years—more than 146,000 generations. This heavy intake of meat and animal fat was intensified in Europe during the last glaciation, the Würm glaciation, which lasted 65,000 years and ended about 11,000 B.C.

Mankind has gradually added milk products and grains ("new foods") to his diet for something like 7,000 to 9,000 years (350 generations). Sucrose, another "new food," has been eaten in significant amounts for about 150 years (25 generations).

In terms of evolutionary and biological time, the "new foods" have been eaten for a very short period compared to the time "old foods" were eaten.

It is only logical to postulate that certain members of our present society have inherited a biochemistry unsuitable for metabolizing the new agricultural diet. In the short time of 350 generations, evolution cannot completely change the biochemistry of an entire population that was fixed for 146,000 generations.

The ingestion of "new foods" along with "old foods" by certain people appears to bring about a defect in the metabolism of cholesterol from animal fat.

Given the "old foods" alone, i.e., animal meat and fat along with modest amounts of raw vegetables and fruits, the patients in the study metabolized animal fat very efficiently. On a high animal fat diet their cholesterol and triglyceride levels fell, and their HDL levels rose.

To my knowledge, no one since Stefansson in 1928 has fed a high animal fat diet to a group of people who have had milk products, grains, and sugar completely removed from their diets.

Until now, it has been the custom to blame high serum cholesterol levels in part on animal fat. Perhaps the real culprit lies with the grains, milk products, or sugar which, in some people, interfere with the metabolism of animal fats.

APPENDIX THREE

VITAMIN B$_{12}$
DEPENDENCY DISORDERS

H.L. Newbold, M.D., in the *Journal of the American Medical Association*, September 15, 1989. Reprinted by permission of the *Journal of the American Medical Association.*

The April 7 *JAMA* article by Drs. Lawthorne and Ringdahl ignores B$_{12}$ dependency disorders, and thus may leave readers with the false impression that only patients with low serum vitamin B$_{12}$ levels require the administration of vitamin B$_{12}$. Patients suffering from vitamin B$_{12}$ dependency disorders do not thrive without extra amounts of the vitamin.

The *Merck Manual* states: "Several specific disorders of cobalamin-dependent metabolism have been reported. In each there is some defect either in (1) cellular uptake of the vitamin precursor, (2) conversion of the vitamin to the coenzyme form, or (3) coenzyme-apoenzyme interaction. . . . These disorders usually respond to massive doses of vitamin B$_{12}$ (1000 mcg/day IM)."

Rosenberg reported on vitamin B$_{12}$ dependency disorders, and I have published a paper correlating psychological tests scores with serum B$_{12}$ levels in eight patients suffering from vitamin B$_{12}$ dependency disorders.

Patients with normal sreum B$_{12}$ levels who felt better on large amounts of hydroxocobalamin were given therapeutic tests to learn

351

the frequency and amount of hydroxocabalamin needed for the maximum feeling of well-being.

Serum B_{12} levels performed to record the levels at which the patients felt best. At this point each took a Minnesota Multiphasic Personality Inventory. Hydroxocobalamin injections were then discontinued for 5 to 7 days. The patients took another serum vitamin B_{12} test and another Minnesota Multiphasic Personality Inventory.

With the higher vitamin B_{12} levels (average 465,173 pg/ml), the Minnesota Multiphasic Personality Inventory patterns were more normal (Profile Elevation average 56.1).

With lower serum vitamin B_{12} levels (average 110,611 pg/ml), Minnesota Multiphasic Personality Inventory patterns showed much more emotional distress (Profile Elevation average 67.5).

The Michaelis-Menten equation helps us understand why large amounts of a vitamin are sometimes therapeutic.

$$ R = \frac{d\,[S]}{dt} = \frac{k\,E\,[S]}{[S] + (1/K)} $$

[S] is the concentrate of the substrate. E is the total concentration of the enzyme. K is the equilibrium constant for the formation of the enzyme complex ES. k is the reaction rate constant for the breakdown of the complex into the enzyme and the reaction products.

If $K = 2$ is the normal constant for the formation of an enzyme complex, then the enzyme complex will need only normal amounts of, say, a vitamin for the chemical reaction to proceed in a normal manner.

When defective, however, and $K = 0.01$, then the key substance, say a vitamin, must be increased by a factor of 200 for the chemical reaction to take place at a normal rate.

Thus a large increase in a vitamin level can sometimes help an abnormal biochemical reaction proceed in a normal manner.

I have found vitamin B_{12} dependency disorders associated with many different illnesses, from depressions to duodenal ulcers. I advocate that physicians test every patient for a serum vitamin B_{12} level and then test for a vitamin B_{12} dependency disorder.

I suspect that vitamin B$_{12}$ dependency disorders are common, are misdiagnosed (often as psychiatric disorders), and are poorly handled by the medical profession.

H. L. Newbold, MD
New York NY

APPENDIX FOUR

WHAT TO DO ABOUT PETS

IF YOU ABSOLUTELY CANNOT PART WITH FELIX, FIDO AND OTHER PETS

When the bond between a pet and an owner proves too strong to give up the pet, we can reduce the allergic exposure.

Reducing exposure, however, is definitely second best and is a great deal of trouble. No matter what you do, an incompatibility with your pet may well defeat you and condemn you to remaining ill.

HOW TO REDUCE AN IINCOMPATIBILITY WITH YOUR PET

1. The bedroom door must remain closed at all times and the pet must never be allowed in the bedroom.

2. Take a shower and have a shampoo each night before going to bed. Have no contact with your pet or with the contaminated part of your home after bathing.

3. Pets must be washed *all over* with warm water and a non-scented shampoo once a week.

Soak the animal with warm water. Work up heavy suds. Rinse with warm water. Repeat.

Sometimes cats are reluctant to allow bathing. It may be necessary to place a window screen in the tub to give them something to hold to. Sometimes owners must cross a cat's paws and tape them together with adhesive tape.

4. After washing your pet, Dust Seal your pet to hold down the shedding of dander.

Dust-Seal is the brand name of a product sold by Humphries Pharmacal, P.O.B. 256, Rutherford NJ 07070. Tel. 201-933-7744; or by Willner Chemists, 330 Lexington Avenue, New York NY 10016. Tel. 212-685-0448. (I have no financial interest in this or any other product or company mentioned in this book, unfortunately.)

Dust-Seal is an oily substance that is added to water before applying. Follow directions for diluting it. Apply with a sponge. *Do not spray.* (If you spray it, you might inhale some of it.

Before using Dust-Seal, you, and anyone who sleeps with you, must test it to make certain your body chemistry is compatible with it. I have only seen one patient who reacted unfavorably to Dust-Seal. Still we must be sure.

To test Dust Seal, dilute some of the Dust-Seal according to directions on the product label and use a sponge to apply it to a reasonably clean, old, all-cotton towel. Hang the towel up to dry in the air. After the towel's dry, drape it across your pillow and sleep on it. If you allergic to the Dust-Seal, you will know.

Always seek a physician's advice before performing any test. If you have asthma, it's especially important to get your physician's advice.

5. After washing and Dust-Sealing your pet for the first time, clean your home thoroughly, then go over everything with damp paper towels to remove all dust (and dander) from the floors, walls, ceilings, from above the door frames, picture frames, etc. Be sure to clean drawers and closets.

Air your home well and keep it aired out.

Before applying Dust-Seal to a fabric, test a small area in an out-of-the-way place to make certain the Dust-Seal will not harm the fabric.

Then Dust-Seal all the fabric in your home to reduce the dander in the air. It must be applied to *all* fabrics: mattresses (front, sides, and back, including the box springs), mattress covers, blankets (you may omit the sheets since, hopefully, you launder them frequently), draperies, rugs and carpets, upholstered furniture (top and bottom), pillows, stuffed toys—everything covered with fabric.

All of your clothes must be washed or cleaned to rid them of dander and vaporized oils from your pet.

Your pet needs to be bathed and Dust-Sealed weekly.

You will be pleased to learn that the fabrics in your home need to be Dust-Sealed only every five years, unless the fabric is washed or cleaned. If washed or cleaned, it must be Dust-Sealed again.

Your home must be kept spotless and well aired.

6. Dogs and cat can usually be made much less allergenic if their diets are changed so they will have a different composition to their saliva, urine, feces, and—especially—skin oils. Whether other pets can be made less incompatible by a change of diet, I cannot say from first hand experience.

Dogs and cat should *gradually* be changed to a mostly meat diet. Beef is usually best. *The meat must contain fat, otherwise your pet will starve.* Raw meat is usually best.

Some dogs and cats will enjoy a vegetable now and then: a small amount of fresh raw lettuce or carrot, for example.

Raw liver (but not raw pork liver) should be given once a week for vitamins. *Do not give your pet vitamins or minerals that have any yeast in them, or vitamins and minerals included in a yeast base.*

Kelp should be given once or twice a week for trace minerals. Dolomite powder and zinc gluconate powder must also be mixed in with the meat, along with cod liver oil and safflower and linseed oil. (You will, I'm sure, buy the linseed oil at a health food store, *not* at a hardware or paint store.)

The amounts of supplements will vary with the age and size of your pet. Seek your veterinarian's advice. Remember, however, that your veterinarian is not likely to know much about incompatibilities—especially is he unlikely to be familiar with the newer aspects of incompatibilities such as discussed in this book. Veterinarians might inappropriately try to discourage you from carrying out your project.

The biggest danger: people start by bathing and Dust-Sealing their pets regularly and put them on a proper diet, then gradually neglect to continue.

Do *not have a professional groomer care for your pet.* The groomer and his place of work will both be impossibly contaminated.

BIBLIOGRAPHY

NEWBOLD

1. Newbold, H. L. Relationship between spontaneous allergic conditions and ascorbic acid. *Journal of Allergy,* vol. 15, pp. 385–8, November 1944.
2. Newbold, H. L. Neurodermatitis. *Journal of the American Medical Association,* vol. 132, No. 11, p. 674, Nov. 16, 1946.
3. Newbold, H. L., et al. Aneurysm of the left ventricle secondary to myocardial infarction. *Southern Medical Journal,* April, 1949.
4. Newbold, H. L., et al. The use of chlorpromazine in psychotherapy. *Journal of Nervous and Mental Diseases,* March, 1956.
5. *Book:* Newbold, H. L., and Steed, W. D. The use of chlorpromazine in psychotherapy, p. 310. In *The New Chemotherapy in Mental Illness,* Ed. by H. L. Gordon, Philosophical Library, New York, 1958.
6. Newbold, H. L. Reduction of EST induced fractures by the use of sodium pentobarbital and succinylcholine. *Diseases of the Nervous System,* vol. 19, no. 9, pp. 385–387, Sept. 1958.
7. Newbold, H. L. How One Psychiatrist Began Using Niacin. *Schizophrenia,* vol. 2, no. 4, p. 150–160, 1970.
8. *Book:* Newbold, H. L. *The Psychiatric Programming of People.* Pergamon Press, New York, 1972.
9. Newbold, H. L. The Use of Vitamin B_{12b} in Psychiatric Practice. *Journal of Orthomolecular Psychiatry,* vol. 1, no. 1, 1972.
10. Newbold, H. L., et al. Psychiatric Syndromes Produced by Allergies: Ecologic Mental Illness. *Journal of Orthomolecular Psychiatry,* vol. 2, no. 3, 1973.
11. *Book:* Newbold, H. L. *Mega-Nutrients for Your Nerves.* Wyden Books, New York, 1975. (Pocket size: Berkley)
12. *Book:* Newbold, H. L. *Doctor Newbold's Revolutionary New Dis-*

coveries About Weight Loss, How to master the hidden allergies that make you fat. Rawson, New York, 1977. (Pocket size: NAL)

13. *Book:* Newbold, H. L. The use of B₁₂ in psychiatric practice. In *Physician's Handbook on Orthomolecular Medicine*, Ed. by Roger J. Williams, and Dwight K. Kalita, Pergamon Press, New York, 1977.

14. Newbold, H. L. *Vitamin C Against Cancer,* Stein and Day, New York, 1979. (Trade paperback and pocket size by Stein and Day)

15. Newbold, H. L. The reduction of serum cholesterol while feeding a high animal fat diet. *International Journal for Vitamin and Nutrition Research,* vol. 56, no. 2, p. 190, 1986.

16. *Book:* Newbold, H. L., *Mega-Nutrients,* The Body Press, (Price-Stern-Sloan, Inc.), Los Angeles, 1987.

17. Newbold, H. L. The Medical Origins of Duke University. *Southern Medical Journal,* vol. 80, p. 799, June 1987.

18. Newbold, H. L. Reducing Serum Cholesterol by Feeding a High Animal Fat Diet. *Southern Medical Journal,* pp. 61–63, Jan. 1988.

19. Newbold, H. L. Vitamin B₁₂, Megaloblastic Madness, and the Founding of Duke University. *Medical Hypotheses,* pp. 231–240, Nov. 1988.

20. Newbold, H. L. Vitamin B₁₂: Placebo or Neglected Therapeutic Tool? *Medical Hypotheses,* pp. 155–164, March 1989.

21. Newbold, H. L. Nystatin for Treatment of Acne Vulgaris, *Journal of American Academy of Dermatology,* p. 861, May 1989.

22. Newbold, H. L. Vitamin B₁₂ᵦ As An Antidote For Over-Sedation. *Medical Hypotheses,* vol. 30, no. 1, Sept. 1989.

23. Newbold, H. L. Dependence on Vitamin B₁₂ Injections. *Journal of the American Medical Association,* p. 1468, September 15, 1989.

24. *Book:* Newbold, H. L. *Dr. Newbold's Type-A/Type-B Weight Loss Book.* Keats, New Canaan Conn., 1991.

25. Newbold, H. L. Reducing the Blacks' Disadvantages in a White-Designed Ecosystem. Accepted *Medical Hypotheses.*

26. *Book:* Newbold, H. L. *Dr. Newbold's Nutrition for Your Nerves.* Keats, New Canaan, Conn., Spring 1993.

27. *Book:* Newbold, H. L. *The Newbold Syndrome: How to Cure the Incurable.* Completed.

28. *Book:* Newbold, H. L. *Dr. Newbold's How to Cure Diabetes Book.* Completed.

29. *Book:* Newbold, H. L. *Delusions We Live By.* In work.

BIBLIOGRAPHY

OTHER

Abrams, H. L., Jr. The Relevance of Paleolithic Diet in Determining Contempoary Nutritional Need. *Journal of Applied Nutrition,* vol. 31, pp. 43–59, 1979.

Ardrey, Robert. *The Hunting Hypothesis.* Atheneum Publishers, New York, 1976.

Ardrey R. *African Genesis.* Dell Publishing Company, Inc., New York, 1961.

Atkins, Robert C. *Dr. Atkins' Health Revolution.* Houghton Mifflin Company, Boston, 1988.

Baker, H., Frank, O., Khalil, F., DeAngelis, B., Hutner, S. H. Determination of metabolically active B_{12} and inactive B_{12} analog titers in human blood using several microbial reagents and a radiodilution assay. *Journal of the American College of Nutrition,* vol. 5, pp. 467–75, 1986.

Barnes, Brenda O. and Galton, L. *Hypothyroidism: The Unsuspected Illness.* Thomas Y. Crowell Co., New York, 1976.

Brothwell, D. and Brothwell, P. *Food in Antiquity.* Praeger Publishers, Inc., New York, 1969.

Bryant, V. M., Jr. and Williams-Dean, G. The coprolites of man. *Scientific American,* vol. 232, pp. 100–109, 1975.

Burton, Robert. *The Anatomy of Melancholy,* 1621. (Tudor, New York, 1955.)

Burton, B. T., ed. *The Heinz Handbook of Nutrition.* McGraw-Hill Book Company, New York, 1959.

Carlson, A. J. *The Control of Hunger in Health and Disease.* University of Chicago Press, Chicago, 1914.

Carney, M. W. P. and Barry, S. Clinical and subclinical thiamine deficiency

361

in clinical practice. *Clinical Neuropharmacology*, vol. 8, pp. 286–293, July–September 1985.

Coca, A. F. *The Pulse Test*. Arco Publishing Co., New York, 1972.

Cohen, M. N., *The Food Crisis in Prehistory*. Yale University Press, New Haven and London, 1977.

Congressional Record, United States of America. Proceedings and debates of the 94th Congress, second session, vol. 122, no. 125, August 24, 1976.

Crawford, M. A. and Crawford, S. *What We Eat Today*. Spearman, London, 1972.

Cunning, A. B. and Innes, F. R. *We Are What We Eat*. Salvationist Publishing and Supplies, Ltd., London, 1958.

Dohan, F. C., Grasberg, J., Lowell, F., Johnson, H. and Arbegast, A. W. Cereal-free diet in relapsed schizophrenics, Federation Proceedings, vol. 27, p. 2, 1968.

Dohan, F. C. Cereals and schizophrenia, data and hypothesis. *Acta Psychiatrica Scandinavica*, vol. 42, p. 125, 1966.

Eaton, S., Boyd, E., Shostak, M. and Konner, M. *The Paleolithic Prescription*. Harper & Row, New York, 1988.

Foran, J. A. et al. Increased fish consumption may be risky. *Journal of the American Medical Association*. vol. 262, no. 1, p. 28, July 7, 1989.

Foran, J. A., Cox, M. and Croxton D. Sport fish consumption advisories and projected cancer risk in the Great Lakes basin. *American Journal of Public Health*, vol. 79, pp. 322–325, 1989.

Friedman, M. A., et al. Subepidermal vesicular dermatosis and sensory peripheral neuropathy caused by pyridoxine abuse. *Journal of the American Academy of Dermatology*, vol. 14, pp. 915–917, May 1986.

Gaby, Alan, *Vitamin B₆. The Natural Healer*. Keats Publishing, New Canaan, Conn., 1987.

Gibbons, G. F., et al. *Biochemistry of Cholesterol*. Elsevier Biomedical Press, New York, 1982.

Gruberg, E. R., and Raymond, S. A. *Beyond Cholesterol*. St. Martin's Press, New York, 1981.

Grusky, F. L. et al. The gastrointestinal absorption of unaltered protein in normal infants and in infants recovering from diarrhea. *Pediatrics*, vol. 16, p. 763, 1955.

Hakami, H. et al. Neonatal megaloblastic anemia due to inherited transcobalamin 11 deficiency in two siblings. *New England Journal of Medicine*, vol. 285, no. 21, p. 1163, 1971.

Heyman, C. D. *Poor Little Rich Girl: The Life and Legend of Barbara Hutton*. Pocket Books, New York, 1986.

Horesh, A. J. Allergy to food odors. *Journal of Allergy*, vol. 14, p. 335, 1943.

Horrobin, D. F. (ed.) *Clinical Uses of Essential Fatty Acids.* Eden Press, Montreal, 1982.

Hsu, K. J. When the Mediterranean dried up. *Scientific American,* December 1972: also in *Nature,* March 23, 1973.

Isaac, G. The diet of early man. *World Archaeology,* February 1971.

Jolly, C. J. and Plog, F. *Physical Anthropology and Archeology.* Alfred A. Knopf, New York, 1982.

Lashley, K. S. Structural variations in the nervous system in relation to behavior. *Psychological Review,* vol. 54, p. 33, 1947.

Lessof, M. H. (ed.). *Allergy.* John Wiley & Sons, New York 1984.

Levine, M. New concepts in the biology of biochemistry of ascorbic acid. *New England Journal of Medicine,* vol. 314, pp. 892–902, April 3, 1986.

Lieb, C. W. The effects of an exclusive, long-continued meat diet. *Journal of the American Medical Association,* vol. 87, no. 1, pp. 25–26, July 3, 1926.

Linscheer, W. G., Vergroesen, A. J. Lipids (p. 103). In *Modern Nutrition in Health and Disease,* 7th ed. (Shils, M. E. and Young, V. R., eds.). Lea & Febiger, Philadelphia, 1988.

Lipkin, M. et al. The effect of added dietary calcium on colonic epithelial cell proliferation in subjects at high risk for familial colonic cancer. *New England Journal of Medicine,* vol. 313, no. 22, November 28, 1985.

Lippard, V. W. et al. Immune reactions induced in infants by intestinal absorption of incompletely digested cow's millk protein. *American Journal of the Diseases of Children,* vol. 51, p. 562, 1936.

London *Sunday Chronicle,* May 3, 1953. In Williams, R. J. *Nutrition Against Disease,* p. 43. Pittman Publishing Corporation, New York, 1971.

McCarrison, R. and Sinclair, H. M. *Nutrition and Health,* 3rd ed., p. 29. London, 1964.

McCay, C. M. et al. Growths, aging, chronic diseases, and life span in rats. *Archives of Biochemistry,* vol. 2, p. 469, 1943.

Michaelis, L. and Menton, M. L. Die kinetik de invertinwirkung. *Biochem, Zeitschrift,* vol. 49, pp. 333–369, 1913. From: Pauling, L. Orthomolecular psychiatry. Varying concentrations of substances normally present in the human body may control mental disease. *Science,* vol. 160, pp. 265–271, 1968.

Miller, D. R., and Hayes, K. C. Vitamin excess and toxicity. In: *Nutritional Toxicology,* Academic Press, Inc., New York, 1982.

Miller, N. E., Forde, O. H., Thelle, D. S. and Mijos, O. D. The Tromsö heart study. High density lipoproteins and coronary heart disease: a prospective case-controlled study. *Lancet,* vol. 1, p. 965, 1977.

Mintz, S. W. *Sweetness and Power, the Place of Sugar in Modern History.*
   Viking, New York, 1985.

Montagu, Ashley. *Man: His First Million Years.* 1957.

Montagu, Ashley. *Anthropology and Human Nature.* 1957.

Moore, T. J. *Heart Failure. A Critical Inquiry into American Medicine
   and the Revolution in Heart Care.* Random House, New York,
   1989.

Munro, H. N. and Crim, M. C. The proteins and amino acids (p. 34). In
   Modern Nutrition in Health and Disease, 7th ed. (Shils, M. E. and
   Young, V. R., eds.). Lea & Febiger, Philadelphia, 1988.

Nelson, J. Artificial sweeteners make you gain weight. *National Inquirer,*
   p. 63, January 20, 1987.

Nichols, A. B. et al: Independence of serum lipid levels and dietary habits:
   the Tecumseh study. *Journal of the American Medical Association,*
   vol. 17, p. 236, 1976.

Ott, J. N. *Light, Radiation, and You.* The Devin-Adair Company, Old
   Greenwich, Conn., 1982.

Packard, V. S., Jr., *Processed Foods and the Consumer.* University of
   Minnesota Press, Minneapolis, 1976.

Pauling, L. et al. *Orthomolecular Psychiatry.* Freeman Press, San Francisco, 1973.

Pauling, L., Orthomolecular psychiatry. Varying concentrations of substances normally present in the human body may control mental disease. *Science,* vol. 160, pp. 265–271, 1968.

Pfeiffer, J. E. *The Emergence of Man.* Harper & Row, New York, 1969.

Pinckney, E. R. The accuracy and significance of medical testing. *Archives
   of Internal Medicine,* March, 1983.

Politt, E. and Leibel, R. L. (eds.). *Iron Deficiency, Brain Biochemistry and
   Behavior.* Raven Press, New York, 1982.

Prange, A. J., Jr. et al. Enhancement of imipramine antidepressant activity
   by thyroid hormones. *American Journal of Psychiatry,* vol. 126, pp.
   457–469, 1969.

Price, Weston A. *Nutrition and Physical Degeneration.* Keats, New Caa-
   nan, Conn., 1989.

Prinz, R. J., Roberts, W. A. and Hartman, E. Dietary correlates of hyperactive children. *Journal of Consulting Clinical Psychology,* vol. 48,
   pp. 760–768, 1980.

Randolph. T. G. Descriptive features of food addiction, addictive eating
   and drinking. *Journal of Studies in Alcohol,* vol. 17, p. 198, 1956.

Randolph, Thomas G. Masked food allergy as a factor in the development
   and persistence of obesity. *Journal of Laboratory & Clinical Medicine,* vol. 32, p. 1547, 1947.

Rapp, Doris. *Allergies and the Hyperactive Child.* Cornerstone, New York, 1979.

Ratner, B. and Gruehl, H. L. Passage of native proteins through the gastrointestinal wall. *Journal of Clinical Investigation,* vol. 13, p. 517, 1934.

Raymond, C. A. Dietary cholesterol still a lively discussion topic. *Journal of the American Medical Association,* vol. 259, no. 11, pp. 1435–1436, March 11, 1988.

Reynolds, E. H. Neurological aspects of folate and vitamin B_{12} metabolism. *Clinical Haematology,* vol. 5, pp. 661–796, 1976.

Rinkel, H. J., Randolph, T. G. and Zeller, M. *Food Allergy.* Charles C. Thomas, Springfield, Ill., 1951.

Rosenberg, L. E. Inherited defects of B_{12} metabolism. *Science News of the Week,* vol. 98, pp. 157–158, 1970.

Rosenberg, E. Finding and treating genetic disease. *Science News of the Week,* vol. 98, p. 157, August 29, 1970.

Rosenthal, N. E. Antidepressant effects of light in seasonal affective disorders. *American Journal of Psychiatry,* vol. 142, p. 2, 1985.

Rowe, A. H. and Rowe, A., Jr. *Food Allergy.* Charles C. Thomas, Springfield, Ill., 1972.

Schoenthaler, S. J. The Northern California diet-behavior program: An empirical evaluation of 3,000 incarcerated juveniles in Stanislaus County Juvenile Hall. *International Journal of Biosocial Research,* vol. 5, no. 2, pp. 99–106, 1983.

Schwartz, R. M. 17% of doctors smoke. 87% nursing mothers in U.S. have traces of PCB in their milk. *National Inquirer,* January 6, 1987.

Seale, John, M.D., a member of the British Royal Society of Medicine, is quoted in *American Medical News,* Oct. 9, 1987. The AIDS virus is able to retain infectivity after seven days in water at room temperature and after being kept dry for a week. A virus with this degree of stability which persists in the blood and is shed in saliva cannot fail to be transmitted in many ways. People have been infected by blood touching chapped hands.

Shabecoff, P. 100 chemicals for apples add up to enigma on safety. *The New York Times,* p. 22, February 5, 1989.

Sheinkin, D., Schacter, M. and Hutton R. *Food, Mind, and Mood.* Warner Books, New York 1979.

Sherman, H. C., et al. Vitamin A in relation to aging and to length of life. *Proceedings of the National Academy of Science,* vol. 31, no. 4, pp. 107–109, April 15, 1945.

Smith, R. L. and Pinckney, E. R. *Diet, Blood Cholesterol, And Coronary Heart Disease: A Criticial Review of the Literature.* Vector Enterprises, Inc., 1930 14th Street, Santa Monica CA 90404 (213) 452-6134, July 1988 (Revision 1, January 1989).

Smith, A. D. M. and Duckett, S. Cyanide, vitamin B$_{12}$, experimental demyelinization and tobacco amblyopia. *British Journal of Experimental Pathology*, vol. 46, pp. 615–622, 1965.

Speer, F. (ed.). *Allergy of the Nervous System*. Charles C. Thomas, Springfield, Ill., 1970.

Stefansson, Vilhjalmur. *Not By Bread Alone*. The Macmillan Company, New York, 1946.

Swanson, J. M. and Kinsbourne, M. Food dyes impair performance of hyperactive children on a laboratory learning test. *Science*, vol. 207, pp. 1485–1487, 1980.

Taube, E. L. *Food Allergy and the Allergic Patient*. Charles C. Thomas, Springfield, Ill., 1973.

Thompson, P., Stern, M., Williams, P., Haskell, W. and Wood, P. Death during jogging or running: a study of 18 cases. *Journal of the American Medical Association*, vol. 242, pp. 1265–1267, 1979.

Time magazine. The murky time. pp. 57–58, January 1, 1973.

Torun, B. and Viteri, F. E. Protein-energy malnutrition. In *Modern Nutrition in Health and Disease*, 7th ed. (Shils, M. E. and Young, V. R., eds.). Lea & Febiger, Philadlephia, 1988.

Walford, Roy L. *The Immunologic Theory of Aging*. Williams & Wilkins Co., Baltimore, 1969.

Warin, J. J. Sensivitity to cyanocobalamin and hydroxocobalamin. *British Medical Journal*, vol. 2, p. 242, 1971.

West, J. B. *Best and Taylor's Physiological Basis of Medical Practice*. William & Wilkins Co., Baltimore, 1985, pp. 1227, 1235.

Williams, J. R. *Nutrition Against Disease*, Pitman Publishing Corp., New York, 1971.

Williams, R. J. *Biochemical Individuality: The Basis for the Genotrophic Concept*. Wiley, New York, 1956. (Available through the U. of Texas Press, Austin.)

Williams, R. J. *Physicians' Handbook of Nutritional Science*. Charles C. Thomas, Springfield, Ill., 1975.

Williams, R. J., Pelton, R. B. and Siegel, F. L. Individuality as exhibited by inbred animals: its implications for human behavior. *Proceedings of the National Academy of Science*, vol. 48, pp. 1461–1466, 1962.

Wurtman, Richard J. et al. Good light and bad. *New England Journal of Medicine*, vol. 282, pp. 394–395, 1970.

Yew, M. S. A plus for Pauling and vitmain C. *Science News*, May 5, 1973.

Yudkin, J. Dietary factors in arteriosclerosis: sucrose. *Lipids*, vol. 13, pp. 370–372, 1978.

Yudkin, J. et al. Sugar intake and myocardial infarction. *American Journal of Clinical Nutrition,* vol. 20, p. 503, 1967.

Yudkin, J. Dietary fat and dietary sugar in relation to ischemic heart disease and diabetes. *Lancet,* vol. 2, p. 4, 1964.

Yudkin, J., Diet and coronary thrombosis. *Lancet,* vol. 2, pp. 155, 1957 and 1964.

Yudkin, J. *Sweet and Dangerous.* Peter H. Wyden, Inc., New York, 1972.

Zamkova, M. A. and Krivitskaya, E. I. Effect of irradiation by ultraviolet erythema lamps on the working ability of school children. *Gigiena i Sanitariya,* vol. 31, pp. 41–44, April 1966.

Zamm, A. V. and Gannon, R. *Why Your House May Endanger Your Health.* Simon & Schuster, New York, 1980.

INDEX

369